SPEAKING OF SADNESS

SPEAKING OF SADNESS

Depression, Disconnection,
and the Meanings of Illness

Updated and Expanded Edition

David A. Karp

OXFORD
UNIVERSITY PRESS

OXFORD
UNIVERSITY PRESS

Oxford University Press is a department of the University of Oxford. It furthers the University's objective of excellence in research, scholarship, and education by publishing worldwide. Oxford is a registered trade mark of Oxford University Press in the UK and certain other countries.

Published in the United States of America by Oxford University Press
198 Madison Avenue, New York, NY 10016, United States of America.

© Oxford University Press 1996, 2017

First issued as an Oxford University Press paperback, 1997

Library of Congress Cataloging-in-Publication Data
Names: Karp, David Allen, 1944– author.
Title: Speaking of sadness : depression, disconnection, and the meanings
of illness / by David A. Karp.
Description: Updated and expanded edition. | Oxford;
New York : Oxford University Press, 2017.
Identifiers: LCCN 2016006605 | ISBN 9780190260965 (paperback) |
ISBN 9780190260989 (epub)
Subjects: LCSH: Depressed persons. | Depression, Mental. |
Depressed persons—Interviews. | Depression, Mental—Social aspects. |
Self-perception—Case studies. | BISAC: PSYCHOLOGY / Clinical Psychology. |
MEDICAL / Psychiatry / Child & Adolescent. | MEDICAL / Neuroscience.
Classification: LCC RC537 .K367 2017 | DDC 616.85/27—dc23
LC record available at https://lccn.loc.gov/2016006605

CONTENTS

Acknowledgments vii

Introduction: Voices and the Politics of Illness 1

1. Living with Depression 53

2. The Dialectics of Depression 83

3. Illness and Identity 125

4. The Meanings of Medication 167

5. Coping and Adapting 207

6. Family and Friends 253

7. Sickness, Self, and Society 301

Postscript: Sociology, Spirituality, and Suffering 337

CONTENTS

Appendix: Thinking about Sampling 349
Notes 355
References 383
Index 397

ACKNOWLEDGMENTS

Most authors find it difficult to distance themselves from their writing. Issues, worked on nearly daily for years, become so familiar that bringing them into clear focus sometimes seems impossible. Problems of perspective are further compounded when, as in this case, books are motivated by features of authors' lives that are at the core of their identities. Fortunate writers, therefore, have people around them who are willing to listen, to encourage, to suggest alternative views, and, above all, to provide honest, no-holds-barred criticism. By this standard, I am, indeed, a very fortunate writer. I am tremendously grateful for the emotional support and intellectual direction provided by my family, my friends, my colleagues, and my students. Their help has deepened my appreciation for the idea that all good writing is really a joint act.

Bill Yoels, a close friend and colleague, has influenced my thinking in too many ways to recount. Bill and I have collaborated on several books and articles beginning in the early 1970s. Since many of the chapters in this book pick up on themes in our earlier publications, it is truly difficult to gauge accurately his substantial impact on this project. Bill is among the most intellectually gifted persons I have ever met. He is insatiably curious and encyclopedic in his knowledge. He is an incredibly eclectic reader with an uncommon ability to synthesize ideas from a range of social science writing. The size of my telephone bills to Alabama is a good unobtrusive measure of how significantly I rely on him for friendship and sociological guidance.

Two colleagues at Boston College also deserve particular thanks. Charlie Derber and John Williamson have been ardent supporters of this project from its inception. Together, we form a small community in which the boundaries between personal friendship and academic work barely exist. Whether at lunch, watching Boston College play basketball, sweating together on StairMasters, or casually visiting in each other's offices, the talk invariably turns to our work. They have heard all my confusions along the way and always provided valuable advice as my arguments took form.

A great help in moving from the data collection to the writing phase of this project was a graduate course I directed in the spring and fall semesters of 1993. "The Sociological Craft" was a forum for advanced graduate students to talk about writing and offer mutual support for our work. As a member of that seminar I was, like everyone else, expected to present work in progress. My experience in the class reminded me how difficult it is to write with semester deadlines and to trust others enough to share very rough "working" drafts. I want to acknowledge Patty Bergin, Marlene Bryant, Platon Coutsoukis, Dan Egan, Cheryl Holmes, Vickie Levin, James Vela-McConnell, Michael Murphy, Ellen Robinson, Ruth Rosenbaum, Paul Stein, Jonathan White, Joanne Vasconcellos, and Youlie Venetis who helped me to refine the first two chapters of the book and a number of the theoretical ideas basic to the whole enterprise.

Others who read versions of chapters or provided important counsel at different stages of the writing are Robert Bogdan, Sev Bruyn, Donnah Canavan, Donna Darden, John Donovan, Carolyn Ellis, Melissa Kesler Gilbert, Lynda Holmstrom, Neil Katz, Sherryl Kleinman, Linda Marks, Stephen Pfohl, Morrie Schwartz, Bev Smith, and Diane Vaughan.

I also profited tremendously from the commentary of those who reviewed the manuscript prior to publication. There are several reviewers whose names I never learned, but whose responses to the writing helped to shape its evolution. However, I can explicitly thank Patty Adler, Peter Adler, Peter Conrad, Norm Denzin, and Jay Gubrium for their encouragement, knowledge, and insight. Early on, their expertise and enthusiasm supplied important motivation to push ahead.

The timely completion of this project is also significantly related to Boston College's support at critical moments. In 1991 I was awarded a research expense grant by the university in order to launch the study. By the end of 1993 I had completed and transcribed 30 of the interviews by myself. At a point of "transcription burnout," the university once again provided a grant to help with that task. It was the freedom to write rather than prepare the data for writing that significantly moved things along. In the fall of 1994 the university again helped with the cost of incidentals associated with the last stages of the work. During my nearly 24 years there, I have always admired Boston College's genuine commitment to all forms of scholarship. It has been a wonderful place to teach and to write.

Although I have relied on many people during the course of planning and writing this book, it absolutely could not have been completed without the support of my family. Writing a book requires that one have the freedom to spend an enormous amount of time alone. My kids, Peter and Alyssa, constantly chided me about how often I was hidden away in my study, laboring on the "interviews project," as they called it. When they wanted to know more about how I was spending my time, I discovered how delightful it is to reach a point where parents can talk seriously with their children about the work they do. My biggest debt of gratitude, though, is to my wife. Over the years, Darleen has unreservedly supported me in every way possible. Far more than anyone else, she understands just how important this research has been to me.

Chestnut Hill, Mass.   D.A.K.
April 1995

As indicated, the preceding acknowledgments were written in 1995. I remain thoroughly grateful to Boston College and all the persons named for their contributions to the original completion of this project. In preparing this updated and expanded edition of the book I yet again sought guidance as I first entertained the idea to refresh this volume and then completed the writing of the new introductory chapter. As previously, Charlie Derber, John Williamson, and Bill Yoels, friends and colleagues, provided gentle but insistent encouragement about the importance of completing this new edition. I am also grateful to Joan Bossert, my editor at Oxford University Press. Joan was enthusiastic about the project from the moment I first suggested it. She read early versions of the new introduction and offered valuable suggestions for its improvement. I also want to thank Anjalee Davis, Laura Delano, Darleen Karp, Steve Lappen, and Patricia Tueme who kindly read and helped me to refine the new material in this edition. Finally, I want to express appreciation for an organization called DBSA, The Depression and Bipolar Support Alliance. I attend the meetings of this vital support group nearly every Wednesday night. The DBSA has been critically important to me for both the personal nourishment it provides and its support of my writing efforts over many years.

Chestnut Hill, Mass. D.A.K.

June 2016

Introduction

Voices and the Politics of Illness

"It is more important to know what sort of person has a disease
than to know what sort of disease a person has."

                                                            Hippocrates

In this new introduction to the twentieth anniversary edition of
Speaking of Sadness, I welcome the unique opportunity to reflect
on the continuing validity of the book's approach and analyses,
my personal depression experiences over the last two decades,
and the strategic decisions that have reshaped psychiatry during
this same period. The research, the writing, and then the publication in 1996 of *Speaking of Sadness* was an exceptionally influential
time for me. My academic life to that point had been committed
to research on the ways that people interpret and give meaning to
their lives in such social domains as living in cities, aging, and leaving home for college.[1] Although I seemed to move easily along the
university career path, becoming an associate professor in 1977
and then a full professor in 1982, my life was dogged by sometimes
debilitating depression. By the late 1980s, it seemed perfectly
natural to begin a study based on conversations with fellow sufferers. The eventual completion of *Speaking of Sadness* became the

cornerstone for a series of books[2] on the complex experiences of mental illness, a subject that still absorbs me today.

The starting point for *Speaking of Sadness* was the urge to fulfill one of sociology's most enduring mandates—to give voice to the experiences of those whose accounts are typically marginalized, shunted off to the side, or discounted altogether. In particular, early American sociologists, part of the celebrated "Chicago School of Sociology,"[3] were committed to extensive, in-depth descriptions of such normally invisible worlds as those of hoboes, professional thieves, gang members, immigrants, and slum dwellers.[4] These sociological ancestors were ideologically prone to taking the side of society's underdogs,[5] believing that their stories were perhaps even more conceptually important for understanding the functioning of society than the lives of those comfortably ensconced in society's mainstream cultural worlds. I should add that I also embarked on my new book project with the hope that listening to the experiences of others would give me greater insight into my own depression predicament.

Among those who have written extensively about the significance and power of telling and listening to stories, Arthur Frank has eloquently shown how stories bind us together, construct our identities through both telling and listening, and have the potential to heal. Our lives are shaped by the stories we tell and hear. Indeed, Frank suggests that there is no such thing as a simple "self" story. All stories are "self–other" stories because they are told to others, and in that sharing the stories we listen to become part of our own biographies. With a focus on illness accounts in particular, Frank suggests that "The voices of the ill are easy to ignore because these voices are often faltering in tone and mixed in message. . . . These voices bespeak conditions that most of us would rather forget our vulnerability to. Listening is hard but it is also a fundamentally moral act. . . . In listening for the other, we listen for ourselves. The moment of witness in the story crystallizes a mutuality of need, when each is for the other."[6] In short, our lives and supportive communities are shaped and enriched by each other's narratives.

During the years leading up to this first depression project, I had been attending a support group nearly every Wednesday evening at McLean's Hospital in Belmont, Massachusetts. The stories that I heard at MDDA (The Manic Depression and Depression Association)[7] meetings staggered me. They were unfathomably complex, revealed the nearly unimaginable pain of depression, illustrated the sheer confusion generated by mental illness, and spoke to the extraordinary heroism of those living with affective disorders.[8] Shortly after the tragedy of 9/11, the organization's president wrote the following in his yearly address entitled "A Time of Sorrow, Reflection and Renewed Connection":[9]

MDDA has been for me, and I dare say for many, a most welcome antidote to the yawning silence of an illness that aches to be heard, understood, and soothed. Membership in MDDA is a return to a fellowship and community that strengthens our resolve to be authentic beings who share our tragedies and triumphs alike. We are emboldened by our reliance on and being relied upon in this community. Our nature has been restored; we are, after all, not alone. Our sufferings and our strengths will no longer "echo in the wells of silence."

Once I became serious about offering a sociologically informed analysis of the depression experience, my role in the group shifted. As previously, I sought solace each week in the company of fellow travelers. Equally, though, I now arrived as an ethnographer listening carefully for themes in the words of my comrades. My first published article on depression based on my MDDA observations, entitled "Illness Ambiguity and the Search for Meaning,"[10] helped to solidify both my thinking on depression and my commitment to a more extended project. To this day, I still regularly attend the weekly support group meetings because I feel a connection and commitment to other members, because I continue to be informed by the accounts I hear, and because I value the opportunity to be with those who viscerally understand depression.

Despite the seemingly obvious value of collecting and analyzing stories, those who do qualitative research these days are distinctly a minority. Collecting and recounting stories is typically seen as an interesting exercise that yields a measure of insight. However, for those committed to a scientific vision of sociology, the primary goal of research is to gather statistical data from large samples of individuals to establish fundamental causal connections among variables. Although the tendency to slight the narratives of individuals is clear in the study of all aspects of social life, such an omission is perhaps most awkwardly and inappropriately evident in the efforts to learn about the experience of mental illness. To preview a later argument in this chapter, I maintain that, since 1980, the push toward scientific legitimacy within psychiatry has had the effect of muting patients' stories. The relative disinterest in hearing about the social contexts surrounding their struggles diminishes patients' trust in their healers. More troublesome still, the failure to respect and rely on the perspectives of patients may foster medical treatments that many are now claiming to be ultimately more hurtful than helpful.

Although interested readers can find a substantial number of memoirs describing lives bounded by mental illnesses,[11] I find it striking that twenty years after its publication, *Speaking of Sadness* remains among the few sociological treatments of depression rooted in careful analysis of firsthand accounts. After years of listening to stories in the MDDA/DBSA support group, the completion of well more than one hundred additional interviews for more recent books, and reading the relevant literature on the subject of depression, I feel confident that the analyses offered in *Speaking of Sadness* remain relevant. This large universe of additional data is consistent with my original description of the sequence of identity changes constituting a distinctive "depression career." Thus, I have chosen to leave the original chapters intact.

The aim of this new introductory chapter is to help readers frame critical questions about the importance of listening well to the kinds of depression stories they will encounter in the book. I especially want to sensitize readers to the political significance of honoring the stories of those who are typically dismissed and thus personally diminished. Long ago, Karl Marx taught us that all productive social change arises from collective storytelling.[12] Immediately, as a continuing step in describing how *Speaking of Sadness* has continued to influence my thinking about the political and therapeutic importance of personal narratives, I want to share a few of the many responses to *Speaking of Sadness* that readers have sent along to me.

READERS SPEAK THEIR MINDS

Among the most exhilarating rewards from my writing on mental illness have been the many emails, letters, and phone calls from people who want me to know that they feel less alone after reading my work and understand their own situations more deeply as a result of my analyses. I have been greatly privileged to write about things that I find deeply meaningful, are profoundly important to readers, and can make a difference in people's lives. I treated the responses of readers as I would any other set of collected data. I carefully re-read what they expressed and looked for patterns in their comments. An immediate observation was the number of communications that contained fairly detailed descriptions of readers' own stories. Beyond thanking me for the book, it was plain that these folks desperately wanted to share their stories, even with a relatively anonymous professor, but someone they believed would understand their plight. Although it was not a central theme of their commentaries, several individuals mentioned how important it was that I am a depression veteran. I believe that my own depression experiences were indispensable in establishing my credibility with those I interviewed and thereby fostered the kind of rapport and genuine trust necessary for open discussion of emotionally difficult questions.

The most consistent reaction to the book has been that hearing the stories of others is personally liberating. Over and again letter writers expressed the feeling that the book diminished their isolation by allowing them to see themselves in the experiences of others. They often said that those who tell their stories in the book were speaking for them. They felt represented and personally validated through the words of my respondents. Such personal validation, rooted in common experiences, affirms the power of stories to diminish the marginalization and discrimination typically associated with mental illness. In the latter part of this chapter, I elaborate on the intimate connection between shared stories and social movements meant to "emancipate" those labeled mentally ill.

You will read in Chapter 3 just how significantly depression isolates sufferers. Indeed, I describe depression as an "illness of isolation." In the middle of a depressive episode, persons withdraw from others, believing that no one could possibly understand their feelings. They believe themselves trapped by and utterly alone in their unfathomable pain. Such a belief, moreover, makes those ill with depression feel individually responsible for their presumably unique, personal, and idiosyncratic circumstance. It is no wonder, then, that those who speak in the book help readers to feel far less alone and less responsible for their suffering. Here, then, is a small sampling of the gratitude expressed for a book that gives voice to common experiences.

> Hello, my name is Lauren and I'm a sophomore at Boston University. I'm emailing you because I just read your book *Speaking of Sadness.* . . . I don't think I've ever read anything else that quite encapsulates depression the way this book does. . . . Your book beautifully illustrates the trials and tribulations of depression. I now realize that I am not alone in this and that others actually *do* (her emphasis) understand this illness.

> Thank you, thank you, thank you for writing *Speaking of Sadness.* . . . As I read in their own words, [the] tortuous and bumbling lives . . . of those interviewed, my own suffering from depression was validated in a profound way. I know now that it hasn't all been in my head.

> I just finished your book *Speaking of Sadness* and am so full of thoughts and feelings that I decided to write to you. . . . I want to . . . applaud your grass roots approach and honest personal sharing which made your study worthwhile, not just for fellow colleagues, but for us all. I come from a social science

background myself and am interested in what [that] community has to say. But far more valuable to me are the firsthand testimonies of those actually afflicted with depression, to help me deal with my own [depression] and feel less alone as I struggle with it.

I have just finished reading your book *Speaking of Sadness.* . . . I find it heartening to read a rigorous but human account of depression from a non-medical perspective, and I admire your courage in writing about your own experiences. As a sufferer from depression I constantly found myself saying, "Yes, that's what it's like" as I read the accounts by you and your interviewees.

I just wanted to thank you for putting to words the turmoil of emotions I have been going through for some time now. I am twenty-three years old and I thought I was just going crazy. It's very comforting to know that I am not alone.

The following comment is particularly revealing because it suggests that even among those hospitalized for depression, it is sometimes taboo to talk at length about personal experiences:

It was such a relief to hear what others have been through and what they have to say about depression. Even when I was hospitalized depression wasn't a thing to be spoken of, only by the staff who basically told us what it was, what it wasn't, and what we should do about it. Those "inmates" who tried to express their thoughts were silenced and threatened to be removed from the "group" because negative talk wasn't good for the "therapeutic" process. Wish I could get the [money] back from the hospital and send it to you because your book was much more therapeutic and helpful than anything they did for me.

In a way it made me feel more "normal," and for people like us that's nothing to sneeze at.

The fact that even persons hospitalized for depression may not share detailed accounts of their illness experiences connects with additional letters I received from mental health practitioners. These folks felt out of step with their profession because they still value listening to their patients' travails. As earlier promised, I will shortly comment on the direction that psychiatry has taken in recent years, a therapeutic orientation in which symptoms trump stories. Some of those responding to *Speaking of Sadness* identify with a sociological approach to therapy that tries to understand the plight of patients within the contexts of their lives. These persons preview my later comments by bemoaning an approach to healing that discounts patients' experiences and expertise. For example, several letters echoed the sentiments of a clinician who told me, "I would heartily recommend your volume to any of my practicing colleagues . . . interested in how the medical culture shapes our understanding of ourselves at this time in our nation's history."

I have been greatly pleased by another repeated theme in the way *Speaking of Sadness* has influenced readers' perspectives and insights about depression. Since I am, after all, a sociologist, it was not enough for me to simply relate stories. My job was equally to become deeply intimate with those "data" to discover repeating, underlying conceptual themes in the depression experience. As I scoured my data, I increasingly thought of my respondents as following a distinctive illness "career." Although we normally associate careers with such professionals as lawyers, businesspeople, doctors, and teachers, the sociological turn of mind equally appreciates that criminals, lovers, prisoners, and patients follow predictable career paths.[13] Moreover, just as each stage in a "conventional" career generates new identities, so also should we expect that a predictable depression career will spawn a succession of new identities. You will see that all the data-based chapters in the book pursue the idea that depressed persons typically move through a predictable sequence of "identity turning points."[14] My analytical approach, discovered in the stories I heard, provided many readers a kind of vocabulary for re-visioning their depression experience:

> I had thought that it would be highly improbable that anyone could write so accurately and incisively of "the career of depression" in all its horrific manifestations for the victim and its almost equally devastating role on the lives of others. *Speaking of Sadness* proved me wrong and I am glad for common humanity.
>
> A few months ago I had the good fortune of finding your book *Speaking of Sadness* while browsing in the new book section of . . . the public library. . . . Joining head with heart, you succeed admirably in relating personal experience and interview material to various sociological perspectives. . . . I found much in your book to identify with and to reflect on. It was both validating and stimulating.
>
> I was diagnosed with clinical depression about a year ago and since then have been reading much about the topic. Your book addressed issues related to many of my experiences, which for the most part I have been unable to adequately articulate. . . . To read about the experiences of the interviewees in your study and to see similarities in their accounts [through] your discussion . . . has really blown me away.
>
> It is a privilege to be writing this letter to you. I am very nearly finished with your new book *Speaking of Sadness*. . . .

I wonder if you know what a significant contribution you have made! My undergraduate degree is in sociology . . . and it was delightful (not to mention thought-provoking) to read a sociological perspective on depression. . . . Your analysis of the individual's process of becoming aware of his or her depression was right on target in my experience.

I have just finished reading your new book, *Speaking of Sadness*, and I want to tell you that it has had a transformative effect on me. Your book helped me [to] much more clearly identify some longstanding patterns of depression that have profoundly affected my ability to work, possibly destroyed my marriage, and led me into some self-destructive patterns of substance abuse. . . . Although there are many parts of the book that have been powerful reading, I think the most significant thing I take away is the extent to which depression has a career and is something to live with, learn from, and use as a grounding for a form of community.

In these last few pages, I have touched on the central responses readers have had to *Speaking of Sadness*. I might briefly add that several were glad that I had not written just another self-help book with greatly oversimplified agendas for defeating depression. They were appreciative that I did not hold out false promises of easy cures. Others, tired of the advice to simply pull themselves up by their bootstraps, were glad to have a book that could inform family members and friends about the nature of profound depression. A few took a more political stance suggesting that stories like those told in the book are necessary to dismantle the stigma and incomprehension attached to depression. Equally political, many readers expressed chagrin about the inadequacy and alienating aspects of medical treatments that discounted their personal experience.

Consider how one person expressed concerns about the unyielding "medicalization"[15] of depression.

> Like you, I wrestle with the whole "disease" model and heavy reliance on drugs to avoid deeper lying problems or emotional issues too painful to confront. Part of me welcomes the pill revolution and [I] will do whatever it takes to stop hurting. But another part just wants to be heard on a feeling level. . . . That part feels ignored by all the helping professionals who try to heal by just turning pain off. [I feel] invalidated when I am not allowed to speak for myself in their efforts to treat me.

The general tone of the readers' comments offered in the last few pages speak to the way that the accounts in *Speaking of Sadness* provoked changes in the ways they think about themselves, their illness, and the character of psychiatric treatment. In a similar fashion, my own consciousness about the meanings of depression and role of psychiatry has evolved since 1996. I was in my late forties when I first began to research the depression experience, and I am now seventy-two years old. My own depression career keeps advancing, and I continue to listen to others' stories. I have, of course, also witnessed dramatic changes in the way that psychiatry views depression. You should not be surprised that these experiences keep reshaping my own personal and political understanding of the meanings given to profound sadness. You will see that the original first chapter in the book recounts my depression journey through the early 1990s. Allow me, then, to bring my story up to date in the following section. I want my personal account to preface a fuller analysis of the state of psychiatry today. In particular, I want to reflect on the downside of professional claims to "expertise."

RESPONDING TO TREATMENT

I rarely remember jokes. So when one occasionally sticks with me, it carries some kind of special emotional or ideological significance. Among these few select stories is one about a middle-aged, highly successful businessman. Despite his economic triumphs, our entrepreneur feels a profound void in his life. Success has not brought the meaning and personal fulfillment he imagined it would. So, having plenty of money, he decides to go on a spiritual quest. He learns that a famous guru can be found in a remote area of Asia. At great expense, he sets out to find the wise man. After several weeks of travel and arduous trekking, he arrives on the mountaintop inhabited by the sage. Even then he must wait days for an audience. Finally, the long anticipated moment arrives and the excited pilgrim poses his burning question. "Sir, please tell me, based on your lifelong spiritual journey, 'What exactly is the meaning of life?'" After a few moments, the prophet replies with great solemnity, "Life is a river." Thoroughly dismayed, the businessman replies, "You mean, I've come all this way at great personal, physical, and financial cost and all you have to tell me is that 'life is a river?'" With a deeply perplexed look, the wise man finally responds: "You mean it isn't?"

I suppose that when I repeat the guru joke I am thinking about all the alleged experts who presume to know with absolute clarity what troubled people should do with their lives. An occupational lifetime of trying to understand human behavior persuades me that social life is a very messy affair and that efforts to document absolute, invariable truths about any human experience are doomed to failure. There simply are no social laws that are independent of human communication. Human beings in collaboration with each other are constantly reconstructing the meanings attached to their behaviors and experiences. The large majority of social scientists seek to document "truths" about society. In contrast, my research begins with the alternative presumption that the most realistic goal for sociologists is to write trenchant contemporary history—to provide novel and engaging analyses about critically important social phenomena.[16] In short, when it comes to human affairs, I believe we should listen well to those who have systematically studied certain issues. At the same time I reject the notion that we should unthinkingly hand decision-making powers to practitioners who claim to have the "right" answers about profoundly complex human problems.

Despite my general sociological skepticism, I have not always been quite so suspect of therapeutic expertise. When I was first diagnosed with "clinical" depression in my early thirties, I certainly had misgivings about handing myself over to psychiatrists. But I was relatively young, had little knowledge of depression, was strongly urged by my family to get help, and had grown up in an era when the advice of physicians was rarely questioned. The doctor I finally saw also seemed so certain in his assessment. After only twenty minutes or so, he told me that I absolutely needed to begin a course of treatment with the latest generation of antidepressants. He was so utterly persuasive in claiming that psychiatrists now understood that illnesses like mine were the result of chemical imbalances in the brain. Although years of thinking about how culture shapes emotions gave me pause, I was desperate. He offered a solution, and I bought the idea that I had a broken brain. At the beginning, I was like a religious convert, filled with hopes and expectations of a happier future.

Like most initiates into new belief systems, early failures did not dim my enthusiasm. I was confidently told that depressed people often must try a number of different medications before finding the "right one." So I dutifully spent six weeks or so working up to a therapeutic dose of each new pill, suffering a range of distressing side effects, and then remaining on the drug for several months before concluding that it had transient, minimal, or no positive effect. Then, I had to spend several weeks weaning myself from the current drug before beginning the next. Each new failure eroded my enthusiasm and confidence, but by now I was firmly ensconced in a cultural world dominated by talk of disease, neurotransmitters gone awry, and the drug miracle that patience and proper experimentation would eventually bring. Instead, I have unsuccessfully tried more than twenty different medications since the mid-1970s. This repetitive and unsuccessful process continued for years before I began to seriously question the expertise of those who never expressed much concern about past failures or doubts about the next treatment.

Every now and then my doctor would change because of retirements or bureaucratic needs. Early in my illness journey, because of the misguided idea that I would have been a "deserter," I never left a psychiatrist or therapist. Still, with each change I hoped to discover someone who would have a better handle on my depression dilemma and the clinical knowledge to come up with the right combination of drugs. To be sure, I had graduated from serial pill taking to swallowing multiple pills simultaneously, a practice that bears the nearly lyrical scientific label "poly-pharmacy." I accepted the idea that this new approach was necessary to tame my especially stubborn depression and anxiety. Despite my continued participation in a treatment that was growing more confusing, I was becoming increasingly dubious about the knowledge base of my doctors. I especially remember my association with a "healer" who put me on pills that, I believe, have seriously undermined my well-being. Of course, I did not realize this until years after we "stopped seeing each other."

Doctor D. was a slight, forty-something woman who spoke with a distinctively foreign accent. Each time we met, I might spend ten minutes describing my symptoms. Sometimes new options were then discussed, but normally the conversation quickly turned to matters that seemed far afield from my "medical condition." Doctor D. seemed to like hearing about my work, my family, a recent vacation, or a new writing project. The deal seemed to be that after a bit of inconsequential chatter about my life, she had earned the right to talk about the accomplishments of her two daughters. I often left these sessions thinking that they had been an utter waste of time, unless, of course, there was some therapeutic agenda to the talk that I did not properly appreciate.

Had Dr. D. done nothing but talk about her kids, I would have been better served. At one point, though, she wanted me to try something new for my insomnia. She suggested that I take a drug called Klonopin. Like the properly compliant patient that doctors most cherish, I asked few questions. In turn, Dr. D. never mentioned anything about the habituating potential of a class of drugs called benzodiazepines (drugs like Klonopin, Xanax, Valium, and Ativan). To give her the benefit of the doubt, Dr. D. might have been equally ignorant at the time about the difficulties of stopping this drug after long-term use. As documented in a 2006 book,[17] I made a failed attempt to get off Klonopin about fifteen years ago. Tonight, I'll take the same pills that I have been taking for years, not because they work, but because I am "hooked." The suspicion that my chronic anxiety might be partly the result of daily withdrawal from Klonopin makes me angry. Although I certainly do not think it was her intention, Dr. D. unwittingly violated the Hippocratic oath to "do no harm."

My decades-long dependence on benzodiazepines has sensitized me to another aspect of the quest for mental and physical health. Visits to doctors specializing in addiction have called attention to the way that a patient's age can affect treatment options. After the horrible distress caused by earlier efforts to stop taking Klonopin, I began to read up on the matter. My discomfort and anger were certainly deepened when I learned that long-term users of "benzos" might suffer from cognitive impairment and brain damage. The drug, moreover, can lead to a "far worse addiction than to heroin."[18] In the words of one addiction specialist I visited, "There will be hell to pay if you try to stop taking Klonopin." A second agreed that after decades of use, the withdrawal effects could persist for years, and the choice to stop the drug was "not a good idea for someone your age." Quality of life considerations for a man in his seventies suggested that it was better to remain on the drug and to deal as gracefully as possible with the anxiety resulting from the drug's daily "rebound effect."

The more dubious I became of psychiatric healers, the more I started trusting my own experientially based knowledge. Once I realized that psychiatrists were often making recommendations about pills based on arbitrary experimentation—what I now think of as "black box medicine"—the more recalcitrant a patient I became. I fooled around with my medication doses. I stopped taking certain pills without reporting it to my psychiatrist. I often simply lied about how I felt because I knew the truth would only provoke another unwanted experiment. I stopped making regular appointments and now see a psychiatrist primarily to get the prescriptions I need to avoid drug withdrawal. I also have tried other therapeutic avenues over the years such as cognitive behavioral therapy, conventional talk therapy with a social worker and then a clinical psychologist, meditation and relaxation exercises, programs such as co-counseling, yoga, acupuncture, and herbal remedies for sleep.

I have also become bolder in cutting ties with practitioners who seem too narrow in their approaches or dismissive of ideas that do not conform to their favored treatment notions. In one case, I tried to engage a doctor in conversation about the contributions of anthropology and sociology to a culturally relativist view of mental illness. Nearly immediately this psychiatrist was dismissive of such ideas, suggesting that if fuzzyheaded academics shared his direct clinical experience they would recognize how their views were largely theoretical abstractions and of little practical use. Disenchanted with his lack of curiosity, I switched psychiatrists yet again. In another case, a therapist devoted to cognitive behavioral therapy gave me a book to read on the subject. When I returned for a second visit and raised a few critical questions about the approach, he told me that he did not think we could work together because the treatment would succeed only if I fully "believed" in it. Not wishing to convert to his religion, we parted ways.

My writing over the years, based on long conversations with depressed people, has sensitized me to the ways that many patients come to wonder about psychiatric expertise. It is hardly surprising that in all the stories I have heard during the last two decades, the role of healers has been central—psychiatrists, psychologists, psychotherapists, psychiatric social workers, psychiatric nurses, and counselors of various sorts. As well, people regularly turn to such "alternative" or "complementary" healers as massage therapists and spiritual guides.[19] I have heard how patients begin their pilgrimages to obtain professional help, how they choose healers, how they evaluate their knowledge, how they combine the efforts of several clinicians, and why they frequently "divorce" mental health practitioners. To be perfectly fair, I have also heard several stories of gratitude about having found a psychiatrist or therapist who "saved my life."

I now believe that there are two fundamental domains of expertise. There is the professional knowledge that comes primarily from academic training and clinical experience. Then there is the experiential knowledge of patients that comes from years of suffering. Moreover, these two distinct knowledge bases are often at odds with each other. Over time, I suggest, there is typically a shift in patients' cognition about the treatment they are receiving. As in my own case, there is often a gradual erosion of faith in the once-trusted knowledge of healers who typically grant scant legitimacy to the theories, perspectives, and voices of those "under" their care. Rather like the gradual shifting of tectonic plates that eventuate in severe geological ruptures, the disjunctions between domains of experience regularly lead to powerful healer–patient collisions.

As you read the later chapters of the book, you should think about how the accounts of my interviewees suggest tentative answers to these questions: How do those suffering from depression initially decide to seek out therapeutic professionals? How do they evaluate healers at the outset of their troubles? How do their own theories about their difficulties comport with the explanations of psychiatric professionals? What reservations do patients have about their treatment? If they seek change, how do patients decide that they need to see a different doctor or therapist? How does a person's feelings about various forms of therapy shift over time? How does a patient's own sense of expertise about his or her life circumstance emerge over time? How do patients differentiate the place of trained therapists from the concern and responses of friends and family members? At what point do some patients begin to treat themselves, sometimes in opposition to "doctors' orders?" Why and at what point in their illness careers do individuals seek out complementary or alternative healers? Which patients lose faith altogether in professional healers and, consequently, stop all treatments?

You will see in the last chapter of the book, entitled "Sickness, Self, and Society," that I quote one of my graduate student mentors, a medical sociologist named Eliot Freidson. I believe his words are powerful enough to repeat here. In his book, *Profession of Medicine*, written more than 45 years ago, Freidson (1970: 336) maintained that "The relationship of the expert to modern society seems in fact to be one of the central problems of our time, for at its heart lie the issues of democracy and freedom and the degree to which [people] can shape the character of their own lives."[20] These words have a prophetic character. After all, experts dominate contemporary American life. They are ubiquitous, advising us on virtually all aspects of our lives.

I might well say that experts have successfully "colonized" the life course. There are prenatal experts, birthing experts, early childhood experts, experts on adolescence, professionals to help upper-middle class kids find the right colleges, life coaches to guide people negotiating career options, retirement advisers, and gerontologists who specialize in the circumstances of the "young–old" and the "old–old." The mass media highlights the advice of such healers as Dr. Drew, Dr. Phil, and Dr. Oz. These well-known public figures are there to guide us through the complexities of maintaining physical and emotional health. Their daily prescriptions strengthen a powerful cultural mandate to seek expert intervention should we feel anything less than full happiness and personal fulfillment.

Before readers conclude that I am advocating greater patient autonomy as an unequivocally positive event, I should say that disregarding or abandoning professional advice sometimes has catastrophic consequences. Patients, for example, who unilaterally stop their medications without proper guidance may suffer agonizing withdrawal. Failed drug experiments may lead to hospitalization. The unwillingness to follow doctors' orders frequently generates conflicts between patients and family members. In effect, patients reclaiming personal responsibility for their well-being often find themselves between the proverbial rock and a hard place. After a time, they may realize that their own efforts to deal with their mood disorder only creates additional "causal confusion" about the nature of their illness and helpful responses to it. For most consumers, then, coping strategies become an uneasy balancing act between clinicians' recommendations and their own judgments.

Let me offer still a bit more clarification about my intentions here and in the other chapters of *Speaking of Sadness*. Despite my personal frustrations and critical questioning, I believe that the vast majority of psychiatrists are honestly committed to the well-being of their patients. I also believe that the major mental illnesses (in particular, clinical depression, bipolar disorder, and schizophrenia) cannot be fully understood apart from the workings of biology. Certainly, continuing research efforts to understand the neurobiology of these illnesses are necessary. Finally, I appreciate that the use of medications is absolutely critical when persons are in the throes of dangerous episodes of illness. At the same time, I would be remiss in this new introduction to *Speaking of Sadness* if I did not attend to the historical, political, economic, and scientific factors that have shaped contemporary psychiatry in ways that may not always be in the best interests of patients. In the next section, I will broadly consider how and why psychiatry has become so committed to exclusively biological explanations of emotional pain and the efficacy of its current "pill paradigm."

A QUESTIONABLE REVOLUTION

Speaking of Sadness was published at a very propitious moment in the history of psychiatry. In 1986, Prozac ushered in a virtual revolution in our thinking about mood disorders. An influential moment in that revolution was the publication of Peter Kramer's book *Listening to Prozac*.[21] The book told remarkable stories about people whose lives had been utterly rejuvenated by this new "wonder" drug. Equally important, the appearance of Prozac, the first in a new category of drugs called SSRIs (selective serotonin reuptake inhibitors), clearly moved psychiatry away from an older psychological paradigm of the causes of psychiatric disorders. Now, we were told via endless public communications that problems like depression are clearly the product of neurotransmitter dysfunctions in the brain.

Depression, the mantra repeated, was unquestionably the result of a brain deficit of a neurotransmitter called serotonin. It appeared from the pervasive and coordinated messages that psychiatry had actually now found the elusive cure for depression: the promised cure that had for so long been "just around the corner." While some critical voices were raised, the joint public relations campaigns of psychiatry and the pharmaceutical companies largely overwhelmed dissent. Most Americans became believers. Drug company representatives pushing pills and patients eager to eradicate the slightest feeling of unhappiness flooded doctors' offices. Indeed, it became virtually a cultural mandate to swallow "meds" for nearly every emotional discomfort.[22] The relentless touting of Prozac, and then a whole new generation of SSRIs (e.g., Celexa, Lexapro, Paxil, Zoloft), coincided with the reconstruction of the *Diagnostic and Statistical Manual of Mental Disorders* (the DSM), often called the bible of psychiatry. To understand the emergence of psychiatric experts and their accelerating hegemony in determining which human behaviors are abnormal, pathological, and require "treatment," we need to briefly put things into a larger historical perspective.

In his brilliant and sweeping "archeological analysis," Michel Foucault traces the changing meanings attached to "madness" from the Middle Ages to the modern era.[23] During the Renaissance, the mad were largely thought to be harmless. Indeed, theirs was the frenzy produced by rare wisdom about the cosmic mysteries of life and death. Beginning in the seventeenth century, those considered "lunatics" were separated from the society and placed in brutal "houses of confinement." The birth of the asylum toward the end of the eighteenth century coincided with the emergence of the "medical model" of disease and the power accorded to physicians as the recognized experts on the definition of and proper responses to mental illness. The idea of mental illnesses as medical conditions requiring humane treatment took root in cultural consciousness. The shift to "hospital" asylums clearly began with noble intentions. However, as the often-cited proverb has it, "The road to hell is paved with good intentions." Perhaps nowhere has the truth of this observation been more evident than in the discovery of new treatments, offered in the name of science, to "cure" the hospitalized mentally ill.

Too often, what seems like progress at a given moment is later understood as laughable and inhumane. Many of the nightmarish therapies used in early psychiatric hospitals were considered, at the time, cutting-edge techniques.[24] Those with depression were routinely subjected to large volumes of laxatives and bone-chilling ice baths. Another grotesque invention was a rapidly spinning chair that would so disorient its "victims" that they became "tranquil." Psychosis was, at various times, dealt with by bloodletting, the near drowning of patients (quite like the waterboarding of war prisoners), and insulin shock treatments. A Portuguese neurologist named Egas Moniz conducted the first lobotomies. Moniz won the Nobel Prize in 1946 for his important "innovation." An American, Walter Freeman, presumably advanced the operation by inserting an ice pick through the patient's eye socket. Over 50,000 people were lobotomized before this terribly damaging brain surgery was largely discredited.[25] Whereas "scientists" surely believed passionately in the value of their treatments, they were also driven by the desire for fame. Such a history should make us more circumspect about current treatments for illness. Several recent critics,[26] for example, have argued that our present "antidepressant era" might well be viewed by future generations as another misguided medical experiment.

Although founded with good intentions, the hospitals were hardly comforting "asylums." Too few in number, without appropriate financial support, grossly overcrowded, and run by essentially untrained staff, these new institutions resembled prisons more than places of respite, emotional support, and helpful medical care. Unhappily, mental hospitals also mirrored prevailing social class and racial inequalities that negatively affected the daily treatment of "inmates." Under the auspices of staff acting fundamentally like guards, corruption and abusive maltreatment became the organizational norm. These negative processes were only compounded during the Great Depression and Second World War as social attention to the mentally ill virtually disappeared, further exacerbating the quality of care. You might not be surprised that such deplorable conditions were among the factors that gave rise to an "anti-psychiatry movement" beginning in the 1960s.[27] In its most extreme form those part of the antipsychiatry movement maintained that the idea of mental illness was simply a "social construction" that led to unwarranted medical intervention for "life problems." Consequently, proponents of the "myth of mental illness"[28] argued that mental hospitals and psychiatric treatments only contributed to the misery and ill health of patients.

The first half of the twentieth century could very well be termed "The Age of Psychotherapy." Of course, Sigmund Freud's theories were revolutionary and have been among the most historically influential intellectual ideas shaping our images of who we are as human beings and the internal psychic processes that propel our thoughts and behaviors. Freud's ideas led to the triumph of a therapeutic mentality in the United States and Americans' quest for greater self-awareness. Although there remained a flourishing belief in the efficacy of psychotherapeutic interventions between 1960 and 1980, optimism about psychoanalytic and other psychodynamic theories had been waning within the now burgeoning field of psychiatry. Partly, psychiatry's negative response to "talking cures" arose from the clear weaknesses of psychoanalytic theory. Equally important, though, were political and professional concerns. Psychiatry's continued embrace of talk therapy was keeping the field at the bottom of the medical hierarchy. Psychiatrists wanted recognition as full-fledged doctors who were treating clearly medical conditions. This could only happen with a decisive paradigm shift that claimed mental illnesses as plainly medical, biologically based, disorders.

In 1952, the American Psychiatric Association published its first manual of mental disorders called the *Diagnostic and Statistical Manual of Mental Disorders*. As might be expected, this first effort to list the range of psychiatric diagnoses reflected Freud's psychodynamic model of psychiatric illness. Moreover, the manual listed "only" 106 disorders or "reactions." The first revision of the DSM arrived in 1968. Still committed to a psychodynamic etiology of human mental distress, the number of diagnoses in this emerging dictionary of psychiatric disorders had jumped to 182. A critical turning point in this institutional history was the (accidental) discovery of such major tranquillizers as Stelazine and Thorazine. These new "wonder" drugs provided hope that even the most intractable mental illnesses could be controlled and that patients could return to their families and communities. The widespread use of these drugs also fueled two interconnected beliefs. The first was that the correct route for psychiatry was to clearly codify mental disorders so that psychiatrists would agree on proper diagnoses. The second was to accelerate the search for medications that would treat presumed biological dysfunctions.

The failures of the hospital system and the availability of new drugs that relieved people of their worst symptoms jointly fostered another dramatic social change—rapid deinstitutionalization. The hospital population nationwide decreased from over half a million at its peak to the approximately 50,000 individuals who are hospitalized today. Although conditions vary considerably in contemporary mental hospitals, we would be hard-pressed today to find institutions comparable to the "snake pits" so alarmingly described in documentary exposés like "Titicut Follies."[29] Still, we should not minimize how profoundly the history briefly described here continues to affect patients. Even those who do not require hospitalization still live in a society whose understanding of mental illness is shaped by the idea that the mentally ill ought to be segregated, spatially and emotionally, from the "sane." In this regard it might be argued that psychiatry, by defining mental illnesses as exclusively the product of biological dysfunctions, further marginalizes patients and thus actually promotes both social and self stigma.

The discovery of minor tranquilizers for anxiety such as Miltown, Librium, and Valium during the 1960s and 1970s fostered the routine acceptance of drugs as essential to emotional well-being. In retrospect, these drugs maintained the status quo by largely treating anxious women who, by the cultural standards of that era, were expected to remain in their suburban homes, raise children, keep everything sparklingly clean, and ensure that dinner would be on the table shortly after their husbands returned from work. It is no wonder that Valium, in particular, was described as "mother's little helper." Although it became clear by the late 1970s that these "minor" tranquilizers had created a very significant addiction problem, the die had been cast. Psychiatry was now fully committed to the discovery of drugs to ameliorate human distress. Of course, the pharmaceutical companies warmly welcomed psychiatry's new direction. They would, after all, eventually reap huge profits by producing drugs to combat the diagnoses "constructed" by the American Psychiatric Association.

The gradual movement toward a full embrace of "biological psychiatry" reached its most important moment with the publication of DSM-III in 1980. This version of the manual named 265 disorders. The critical change was that the DSM-III codified diagnostic criteria for each disorder listed. Now, presumably, psychiatrists could consistently agree on such diagnoses as major depression. Once it was established that a patient met a minimum of five out of nine depression criteria (But, we should ask, "Why five rather than four or six?"), for a period of at least two weeks they required treatment. The new DSM solved a number of conundrums for psychiatry. Now, the field had established much-needed consensus about a constantly expanding number of mental disorders. Conveniently, the new manual made it easier for psychiatrists to satisfy insurance companies who required affirmation that a patient clearly needed treatment. The new manual also coalesced the partnership between psychiatry and the pharmaceutical companies. Both psychiatry and "big pharma" were anticipating huge profits from the treatment of an ever-increasing population of mentally disturbed patients.

DSM-III established a high measure of "reliability" in the way that diagnoses were named and identified. However, as any student of research methods knows, there is a big difference between reliability and "validity." Simply measuring something consistently (reliability) does not mean that you are truly and accurately measuring what you think you are measuring (validity). Because the DSM helps psychiatrists to agree on a definition of depression, for example, does not mean that they are correctly diagnosing a genuine biological disorder. Simply put, classification is not explanation. Although it may be something of a harsh assessment, Gary Greenberg, in his evaluation of the DSM entitled *The Book of Woe*, remarks that, "The DSM is at best a clumsy and imperfect field guide to our foibles and at its worst a compendium of expert opinions masquerading as scientific truths."[30] And quite to the central point of this chapter, the psychiatrist Allen Frances offers this observation about DSM-III:

> DSM III was the victim of its own success – it became the 'bible' of psychiatry to the exclusion of other aspects of the field that should not have been, but were, cast beneath its shadow. Diagnosis should be just one part of a complete evaluation, but instead it became dominant. Understanding the whole patient was often reduced to filling out a checklist. *Lost in the shuffle were the narratives of the patient's life and the contextual factors influencing symptom formation* (my emphasis).[31]

Frances, the central architect of the DSM-IV, published in 1994, tried to introduce still greater rigor and transparency into the processes of diagnostic creation and to minimize the secret political processes that so often determined whether a researcher's pet diagnosis would be included in the volume. He also hoped to change the informal definition of the DSM from its "bible" status to a useful "guide" that could inform the diagnostic decisions of psychiatrists while requiring that clinical judgment and an intimate knowledge of the patient's life be central in making final judgments about diagnosis and treatment. However, in his book entitled *Saving Normal,* Francis acknowledges that despite his best intentions, the forces of professional expansion, personal ambitions, and economic interests led ultimately to continued "diagnostic inflation"[32] and an overreliance on the DSM.

The latest version of the DSM (DSM-5) was recently published in 2013. Rather than solving any of the problems recognized in the earlier versions, this volume has drawn heavy criticism. Now containing nearly 350 diagnostic categories, this edition continues to pile up new and controversial mental disorders. Since its appearance, doctors are now able to treat people for such "pathologies" as Minor Neurocognitive Disorder, Temper Dysregulation Disorder, Autistic Spectrum Disorder, Hypersexual Disorder, and Binge Eating Disorder. Readers need to understand that although designated committees certainly rely on research studies to inform the inclusion of new diagnoses, the decision is ultimately determined by a vote. Votes also determine whether previous diagnoses should be removed from the DSM. One famous example was a vote in 1973 to remove homosexuality as a mental disorder. In short, decisions about the existence of psychiatric disorder are as fundamentally political as they are scientific. Equally, each time a new and often controversial disorder is agreed on, such as the recent inclusion of Childhood Bipolar Disorder in the DSM-5, we witness a veritable epidemic of diagnoses and drug treatments.

A revealing example of the political bases for DSM entries involves the "bereavement process." The decision was made in the DSM-IV that bereavement should be an exception to the usual criteria for establishing and treating major depression. Consequently, those mourning the death of a loved one were seen as "normal" despite meeting the established diagnostic criteria for major depression. However, in the DSM-5, the bereavement exclusion was removed; and despite the clear circumstances of their profound sadness, mourners for longer than two weeks were now candidates for medical treatment. How are we to think about such a dramatic shift in the meanings attached to bereavement and its status as a mental disorder? One interpretation is that any exemption from the established DSM criteria creates a conceptual problem in sustaining the purely medical model of psychiatric illnesses. After all, if psychiatry were to acknowledge that certain forms of sadness were based on difficult life experiences, might this call into question its biological origin? If an exception was made for bereavement, why not exemptions for job losses, failed relationships, economic hardships, and the like? To preserve the image of scientific integrity, it must have seemed far safer to remove the bereavement exemption than to acknowledge a larger principle—that the same symptoms might be an illness in some social contexts and not in others.

Years ago, the author M. Scott Peck began his best-selling, Buddhist inspired book, *The Road Less Traveled*,[33] with the observation that "Life is difficult." Indeed, life is unfortunately filled with suffering; it is filled with the "normal" pain of living. This simple observation raises profound questions for psychiatry. If we can think of a continuum that extends from normal pain to pathological disorder, just how do we draw the line between normal and abnormal suffering? Psychiatry's critics worry that the field is dangerously blurring the line between normal and pathological distress. Many instances of normal sorrow may be inappropriately labeled as depressive disorders. A significant factor contributing to such "false positives" is psychiatry's methodological approach. The urge toward categorical checklists to increase diagnostic reliability has been accomplished by largely disregarding the personal accounts of patients and the cultural contexts of their lives. In their book entitled *The Loss of Sadness*, Allan Horwitz and Jerome Wakefield describe the problem this way:

> The recent explosion of putative depressive disorder, in fact, does not stem primarily from a real rise in this condition. Instead it is largely a product of conflating the two conceptually distinct categories of normal sadness and depressive disorder and thus classifying many instances of normal sadness as mental disorders.[34]

It is hard to imagine that a nearly fourfold increase in the number of psychiatric abnormalities since 1952 is simply the product of dispassionate scientific inquiry. The transition in the DSM has been from "disorders of the mind" to "diseases of the brain."[35] The proliferation of such diseases is, moreover, perhaps more a function of cultural, economic, and political processes than unbiased research. In fact, the sharpest critics of psychiatry's current stance maintain that except for a few major psychotic illnesses, there is no evidence that the hundreds of conditions listed as brain diseases in the DSM warrant that designation. Diagnostic disagreements and the extremely tenuous connections among symptoms, diagnoses, treatments, and therapeutic outcomes significantly undermine the validity of the disease model in psychiatry. Thomas Szasz puts it this way:

> Asserting that a particular person's problem is a disease because the patient or others *believe* it is a disease, or because it looks like a disease, or because doctors *diagnose* it as a disease, and treat it with drugs as if it *were* a disease, or because it *entitles the subject to be qualified as disabled*, or because it *presents an economic burden to the subject's family or society*—all that is irrelevant to the scientific concept of disease. (italics in the original)[36]

The DSM methodology underlying the naming of psychiatric disorder may currently be under fire, but it seemed unquestionable by the mid-1990s that although severe depression might be "influenced" by environmental circumstances, the root causes were biological, the result of faulty brain chemistry. I must note, however, that the dominant neurotransmitter deficiency "theory" was discovered quite accidentally. Researchers in the 1950s noticed that a drug being tested to treat tuberculosis had an ameliorative affect on patients suffering from psychosis. Further investigation showed that this, and later, similar drugs, increased certain neurotransmitters, especially serotonin, in the brain. Eventually, the production of drugs based on this theory multiplied, and television advertisements for these newest antidepressants showed cartoon-like images of neurotransmitters jumping across brain synapses. Then the commercial treated us to images of formerly depressed persons (primarily women) now happily dancing in open fields. By the mid-1990s, the biological narrative, repeated over and again, seemed unassailable.

Despite the widespread cultural acceptance of the new biological revolution in psychiatry, there have always been critical voices of dissent. After all, unlike conventional areas of medicine, psychiatry has not produced a single diagnostic test to affirm the biological dysfunction presumed to exist in the brains of depressed persons. Doctors might tell patients reluctant to take antidepressants that these drugs are equivalent to taking insulin for diabetes. The analogy breaks down, however, because the linkage between insulin deficiencies and diabetes has been definitively established. There is no scientific question about the biological bases of diabetes. In contrast, the connection between neurotransmitter deficiencies and depression remains a matter of faith rather than science. Doctors simply decide after briefly listening to patients' symptoms that such a deficiency exists and must be treated with brain-altering medications.

The legitimacy of psychiatry's biological revolution and the alleged miracles of drug treatments have recently been still further eroded. Within the last decade, a new chorus of voices has challenged the efficacy of antidepressant medications for the vast majority of consumers. Although there is evidence that the medications may have a palliative effect for the most severely depressed patients (approximately 12 percent of all those diagnosed and treated for depression), there is increasing experimental evidence that the drugs are statistically no more effective than placebos. Writers such as Stuart Kirk and his collaborators,[37] Irving Kirsch,[38] and David Healy,[39] have been provocatively "exploding the antidepressant myth." These authors provide evidence from a number of carefully controlled studies showing the negligible effects of antidepressants compared with "active" placebos (sugar pills with an ingredient that produces the equivalent of side effects). As long as patients believe they are being treated with a real antidepressant, they report a reduction in symptoms equal to those treated with a drug marketed for depression.

Perhaps even more devastating to current biological theories of depression, one study compared a French produced drug that *decreases* serotonin levels in the brain with conventional antidepressants, both SSRIs such as Prozac and an earlier generation of drugs called "tricyclic" antidepressants. If the serotonin theory is correct, a drug reducing levels of this neurotransmitter in the brain should induce depression symptoms. Instead, patients taking all three types of medication reported essentially equal degrees of relief from their symptoms. Describing these studies, Irving Kirsch concludes that "If depression can be equally affected by drugs that increase serotonin, drugs that decrease it, and drugs that do not affect it at all, then the benefits of these drugs cannot be due to the specific chemical activity. And if the therapeutic benefits of antidepressants are not due to their chemical composition, then the widely proffered chemical imbalance theory of depression is without foundation. It is an accident of history produced serendipitously by the placebo effect."[40]

A powerful factor in fostering a belief in the effectiveness of antidepressants has been the economic power and the highly questionable strategies of pharmaceutical companies. Shortly after the recognition that psychiatric medications would yield huge profits, the pharmaceutical companies formed what many deem an unholy alliance with the field of psychiatry. Drug company representatives flooded the offices of medical practitioners with persuasive information about their most profitable medications, lavished these doctors with gifts and free drug samples, and kept careful records on the prescribing practices of these same physicians. The drug companies also poured huge amounts of money into "educational" retreats, during which physicians were treated royally while listening to handsomely paid "opinion leaders" who spoke glowingly about "their company's" products. As well, the industry's lobby is among the largest in Washington. And many researchers who publish in the most prestigious medical journals have financial ties to certain companies, as do many experts who sit on the US FDA (United States Food and Drug Administration) panels that decide the drugs' futures. These practices have generated so many conflicts of interest that the quality of knowledge available to physicians, regulatory agencies, and patients has been tainted.

Even more problematic, the drug companies too often manipulate drug trial research to ensure that only favorable accounts of their products reach prescribing doctors. Exposés by such writers as Marcia Angell, John Abramson, and Jay Cohen[41] demonstrate the way drug companies slant research findings and limit damaging information to gain FDA approval for their pills. Among the "tricks of the trade," drug companies compromise the credibility of their research findings when they:

Commission multiple studies to assess a drug's effectiveness and then report only the research most flattering to their product.

Fire doctors who serve as well-paid consultants on effectiveness studies if they report negative findings, thereby putting pressure on doctors to search the data for positive results.

Hire multiple physician-researchers to publish slightly different versions of the same set of complimentary findings in several journals.

Compare their medication with competing drugs by giving control groups only the lowest effective dosage of the competing product.

Devise questions to measure their drug's symptom relief
in ways that maximize the likelihood of positive reports and
then use different measurement procedures to evaluate the effectiveness of competing drugs.

Fail to systematically ask study respondents about certain
side effects, thus ensuring that rates of adverse reactions are
greatly minimized.

Aside from the blatant dishonesty of such practices for economic gain, critics also maintain that the overconsumption of
pills of questionable medical value too often undermines patients'
health. In his recent book entitled *The Anatomy of an Epidemic*,[42]
the medical journalist Robert Whitaker provides a persuasive argument that the widespread use of psychiatric medications may
ultimately be permanently hurting patients. His book begins
with the observation that rates of disability for the whole range of
mental illnesses have skyrocketed since psychiatry's full embrace
of the drug paradigm as the primary medical response to human
suffering. He reports that in the two decades following the introduction of Prozac " . . . the number of disabled mentally ill on SSI
and SSDI rolls soared to 3.97 million. In 2007, the disability rate
was 1 in 76 Americans. That's more than double the rate in 1987
and six times the rate in 1955."[43] In addition, Whitaker reports on
data showing that the rate of remission from such major mental
illness as schizophrenia is significantly higher in third world
countries where individuals do not have easy access to psychiatric medications. Such data are the starting point for his argument
that pills meant to alleviate mental illnesses are actually fostering
"a modern plague."[44]

By systematically examining long-term outcome studies of
patients treated for such diagnoses as depression, schizophrenia,

anxiety, bipolar disorder, childhood bipolar disorder, and attention deficit hyperactivity disorder, Whitaker provides compelling evidence that although medications may alleviate symptoms
in the short term, their long-term use creates brain abnormalities
that ultimately lead to the chronic character of the illness treated.
When, for example, patients suffer horrible relapses after stopping
medications, the psychiatric perspective sees this as the return
of their mental illnesses and thus as evidence of the need to stay
on prescribed medications. Rarely entertained is the alternative
notion that such disabling results are iatrogenic illnesses caused
by the drugs themselves and their negative effects on normal brain
functioning. Near the end of his book, Whitaker summarizes his
position when he says that

> Our societal delusion about the benefits of psychiatric drugs
> isn't an entirely innocent one. In order to sell our society on the
> soundness of this form of care, psychiatry has had to grossly
> exaggerate the value of its new drugs, silence critics, and keep
> the story of poor long-term outcomes hidden. This is a willful,
> conscious process, and the very fact that psychiatry has had to
> employ such storytelling[45] methods reveals a great deal about
> the merits of this paradigm of care, much more than a single
> study ever could.[46]

It bears repeating that few critics of psychiatry's reliance on
medications would advocate that drugs never be used. They do,
after all, help severely ill patients to move more easily through
difficult periods. Rather, those who offer the kinds of criticisms
described in the last several pages are unanimous in their view
that mental disorders be treated in the least invasive, most conservative ways possible. They agree that diagnoses should be

made only after several meetings designed to establish a greater appreciation for the unique circumstances of patients' lives. Even after a diagnosis is made, physicians do well to "wait and watch" before prescribing powerful medications. Rather than quickly resorting to nearly ritualistic drug treatments, responses to suffering should be "case specific." They also suggest that the relationship between patients and healers be more collaborative and less hierarchical. Such prescriptions for more humane and less invasive treatments are all contingent on listening carefully to patients' stories.

Implicit in the expanding criticisms of biologically reductionist explanations of mental disorders is the call for yet another revolution. If the current paradigm of treatment is significantly a product of economic and ideological interests, we should be alert to political changes and social movements that are based on alternative images of mental illnesses and the proper responses to them. We need to listen to the otherwise marginalized mentally ill to better appreciate how the suffering of individuals may reflect pathological social structures. We need to adopt the kind of sociological perspective offered throughout *Speaking of Sadness* that mental illnesses are surely as much a product of "cultural chemistry" as of "brain chemistry." In the last section of this chapter,[47] I want to examine how an alternative set of voices, those part of a "psychiatric liberation movement," provide a counter-narrative to the one relentlessly pushed jointly by psychiatry and the pharmaceutical companies. I am persuaded that we must also listen to these alternative stories, not merely for the sake of the mentally ill but also to better understand how hurtful social structures potentially undermine everyone's emotional well-being.

VOICES FOR CHANGE

Social movements, by definition, seek structural changes that provide democratization, equal rights, autonomy, and full personhood to members of groups that have historically been subjugated, rendered powerless, stigmatized, and oppressed. Such movements, whether for racial equality, gay rights, equity for those with disabilities, women's rights, or the humane treatment of the mentally ill, require the development of a "class" consciousness rooted in commonly constructed narratives about shared conditions. Social movements, in other words, evolve from individual storytelling and the eventual recognition of commonalities in those stories. The sharing of individual accounts among those occupying marginalized statuses constitutes the nucleus for the construction of new "collective" narratives that challenge the legitimacy of those who exercise power and control over their lives. Social movements, in short, are rooted in what race, gender, and disability theorists, among others, call "counter-storytelling."

Counter-storytelling is a "method of telling the stories of those people whose experiences are not often told."[48] These stories typically stand in opposition to the ideological narratives that sustain the power and privilege of society's dominant groups—for example, whites; men; the middle and upper classes; heterosexuals; and here, those free of mental illness. As several sociologists have argued,[49] dominant groups maintain their hegemonic power by discrediting and silencing those who do not conform to their socially constructed norms. This is accomplished by labeling such groups as outsider, deviant, inferior, and dangerous. Although many groups are marginalized in any society, it is not surprising that those deemed mentally ill are so virulently stigmatized.

Because the line between "sanity" and "insanity" is so thin, those deemed mentally ill elicit particular fear among the vast majority of persons who must regularly question their own "normality." The psychological imperative to stereotype the mentally ill as uniquely different, deficient, and dangerous is well captured in the following observation:

> The banality of mental illness comes in conflict with our need to have the mad be identifiable, different from ourselves. Our shock is always that they are really just like us. This moment, when we say, "they are just like us," is most upsetting. Then we no longer know where lies the line that divides our normal, reliable world, a world that minimizes our fear, from the world in which lurks the fearful, the terrifying, the aggressive. We want—no, we need—the "mad" to be different, so we create out of the stuff of their reality myths that make them different.[50]

New movements and their motivating counter-narratives do not appear spontaneously on the social scene. Typically they evolve haltingly and intermittently, often plagued by internal dissent and uncertainty about goals. Sometimes groups protesting psychiatric hegemony have gained a measure of traction, only to later disappear as members become disillusioned by lack of progress in the face of all too powerful competing ideologies. Whereas movements may evolve in fits and starts, they are always built on earlier efforts to have similar voices heard. In this regard, we should briefly acknowledge how even the so-called "lunatics" in the earliest and most horrific asylums sometimes tried to speak about their lives.

Even during the latter part of the nineteenth century, women could become hospital "inmates" for such "insane" acts as

disobeying their husbands. Inmates were systematically deper-
sonalized, objectified, and largely ignored by both staff and physicians. Under such historically brutal conditions, individuals involuntarily committed to asylums had little opportunity to speak or
record their thoughts. In England during this period, any inmate
letters discovered by the staff were legally classified as "insane
literature" and confiscated. It was forbidden for those trapped in
the asylum to possess pen and paper.[51] Such tactics make it all the
more remarkable that inmates sometimes found ingenious ways
to record their experiences. In her book entitled *Agnes's Jacket*,[52]
Gail Hornstein describes how Alice Richter, a former seamstress,
sewed cryptic written descriptions into her institutional jacket,
discovered after her death. Rather than seeing this artifact as evidence of her insanity, Hornstein understands Agnes's creation as
a desperate effort to preserve a sense of dignity and identity in an
institution bent on destroying her humanity.

The powerful urge of ex-patients to recount their often tragic
hospitalizations is reflected in the fact that hundreds of written accounts, some disguised like Agnes's, and others appearing
as published memoirs or exposés, have been produced since the
very beginnings of psychiatric institutionalization. However,
establishing a coherent, organized, ex-patient effort to question
the unrestrained power of psychiatry, to assert human rights
against involuntary hospitalization and forced "drugging," to establish self-help groups run exclusively by former patients, and
to promote political change did not really begin until the early
1970s. In other words, the emergence of a psychiatric liberation
movement coincided with the general "radicalism" of the sixties
and seventies and paralleled movements for the rights of blacks,
women, homosexuals, and the disabled. The widespread voices for
change during this era synergistically provided the momentum

for consciousness-raising efforts among those who believed themselves to have been "psychiatrized."

All social movements are necessarily pushed along by certain individuals who provide a vocabulary for articulating the causes of a marginalized group's suffering and the proper responses for change. For example, Betty Friedan's book, *The Feminine Mystique*,[53] greatly accelerated the women's movement. In the same way, many credit the publication of Judi Chamberlin's book entitled *On Our Own: Patient-Controlled Alternatives to the Mental Health System*[54] as providing the language, in effect, that allowed those who felt injured by the mental health system to speak out more communally and coherently.

Chamberlin coined the term "mentalism" (like sexism or racism) to describe the kind of unquestioned discrimination, stigma, inequality, and abrogation of human rights exercised against those labeled as mentally ill. The word is meant to counter the prevailing idea that those deemed mentally ill are "out of their minds," totally irrational, and thoroughly unable to recover without the forced intervention of psychiatry. Chamberlin, in sharp contrast, maintained that she and other ex-patients could better thrive "on our own." Comparing the ex-patient movement with the women's movement, Chamberlin affirms that neither could come into being and then move ahead without the sharing of personal stories:

> The consciousness-raising process is one in which people share
> and examine their own experiences to learn about the contexts
> in which their lives are embedded. As used by the women's
> movement, consciousness-raising helped women to under-
> stand that matters of sexuality, marriage, divorce, job discrimi-
> nation . . . and so forth were not individual, personal problems

but were instead indicators of society's systematic oppression of women. Similarly, as mental patients begin to share their life stories, it became clear that distinct patterns of oppression existed and that our problems and difficulties were not solely internal and personal, as we had been told they were.[55]

Individuals are increasingly demanding a greater voice in the way their mental distress is managed. However, we should note that the patient liberation movement is quite varied, ideologically and structurally. Individual patient responses and those of groups range from very conservative, to those cautiously questioning psychiatric expertise, to those advocating absolute separation from the intrusive grasp of psychiatric professionals. These differences in the way emotionally troubled persons see themselves in relation to the mental health system are reflected in the words they employ to describe their status. The words that have been most thoroughly parsed by students of psychiatric movements are "patient," "consumer," and "survivor."[56] Each of these words reflects variations in the way illness stories are constructed. Those who label themselves, respectively, as patients, consumers, and survivors have different ways of talking about mental illnesses and the health care system.

On Wednesday nights at the DBSA meetings, the conversation typically begins with a "check-in" during which participants in the self-help group describe how they are doing and the issues they might like to discuss collectively. They also normally announce the diagnosis or diagnoses they have received. The different ways that individuals introduce themselves reveal the different illness identities that group members possess. A person might begin with a statement like, "My name is Joe and I am a depressive." On occasion, another member of the group might question that mode of self-identification. He or she may point out that saying "I am a depressive" discounts so many other aspects of personal identity that equally define who we are. The questioner might then gently suggest that it is more accurate to say, "I am Joe and I suffer from depression." Still others might say something like, "I'm stable at the moment but I have episodes of depression."

The way group members talk about themselves and often about their connections with psychiatrists and the mental health system suggests a continuum ranging from those who define themselves simply as a "repository of pathology,"[57] to those who question "official" diagnoses, to those who thoroughly reject explicit disease labels. Each of these responses to personal problems reflects a different narrative and, thus, different ideas about proper approaches to their problems as well as the prospects for living a "normal" life. Those who see themselves exclusively as "patients" accept psychiatry's diagnoses for their pain. They do not question the treatments proposed by their caregivers. Others, influenced by the arguments and counter-narratives of movement groups, think of themselves as "consumers." Consumers remain associated with mental health practitioners but expect to exercise greater autonomy in shaping the medical labels placed on them and the most reasonable treatments for their distress. Those who have embraced the "survivor" discourse reject the patient label altogether and do not accept psychiatry's medical model. The three narratives correspond, respectively, to responses of acceptance, negotiation, and resistance.[58]

The lived experience of those with emotional problems is still more complex because persons may sometimes shuttle back and forth among the available narratives. They may, for example, move from patient to consumer and then to resistance status. In my own case, influenced by the stories of others who have quit medications altogether, I embarked on the disastrous journey to quit Klonopin as earlier described in the chapter. I wanted to be a survivor, but my drug difficulties and ongoing bouts with depression and anxiety force me to remain reluctantly connected to psychiatric professionals. I feel trapped in the consumer role, uncomfortably conforming to a medical model of mental illness that I now seriously question. Consequently, when introducing myself during the DBSA check-in, I may say, "Hi, my name is David and I suffer from depression and anxiety, but my biggest problem may be habituation to psychiatric drugs."

The essential thread of this chapter has been to affirm the critical character of listening well to the perspectives of those who have been labeled mentally ill. The idea of "giving voice" appears over and again in these pages. It seemed correct to begin the chapter by hearing how readers of *Speaking of Sadness* have profited from the accounts of the fifty people whose words you will shortly encounter in the following chapters. I also added my own voice in describing how my experiences with depression and psychiatry have gradually reshaped my ideas about the potential friction between those who are experts by training and those who are experts by experience. Given my intentions, it feels at least slightly inappropriate that I have gone on at some length about the political goals of patient liberation movements without letting you hear how "psychiatric survivors" speak about their quest for autonomy and personal empowerment. Via a simple Google search you can read hundreds of psychiatric survivor testimonies that mirror comments like these:

> Meeting so many people who have fought through an oppressive mental health system, who have been forcibly electro-shocked and drugged, who have been treated as less than human—and who are now leading accomplished and fulfilling lives as

authors, directors of organizations, social activists, etc., has been inspiring and empowering. I just hope that eventually the general public will hear our stories and take them as their own.

I didn't get better because of anything that the clinicians did for me. I got better because I surrounded myself by people who showed that they cared about me.

We have to be witnesses for those millions who are not speaking up now for whatever reason. That's the role that I feel our movement needs to play right now in society—to speak up, tell the truth about what we have known, what we have experienced in our own lives.

Why did the doctors tell me—an intelligent, gifted person—that I would never work, would never get through school, would be on medications for the rest of my life, and should stay on social security disability indefinitely? I tend to excel at whatever I do, but I was told I'd never do anything beyond a social security check.

Sometimes I have this tremendous sadness because I think that I might be in a much bigger place than I am now. I'm happy with my life but I'm also 51 years old. I might have been where I am now twenty years ago had all this not happened. I figure I'm here in spite of the mental health system.

As powerful and poignant as these voices are, I want to add one more. I first talked to Laura Delano when she was an undergraduate at Harvard simultaneously struggling with emotional pain and completing an honors thesis. On her *Mad in America* web page Laura describes herself as a psychiatric liberation activist, writer, and community organizer. She recounts that her first encounter with the mental health system was at the age of thirteen. This was the beginning of multiple hospitalizations and many unwelcome treatments. As she describes it, reading Robert Whitaker's *Anatomy of an Epidemic*[59] motivated her recent five-year odyssey to escape psychiatric drugs. I want you to hear a representative excerpt from her Mad in America blog because of the power, elegance, importance, and courage of her writing. Here, at some length, is her piece entitled "I am Alive":

Of the many reasons I'll be in New York City this weekend to protest the American Psychiatric Association is this: I am alive.

Today, I feel this aliveness on the bottoms of my feet as they rest on the carpet below my desk, and on the right side of my face as the setting sun crosses it gently from where I sit to write these words. I feel it in the air that fills my nose and throat and lungs, in my belly as it rises and falls, in the beating of my heart that moves me if I'm still enough. I feel this aliveness in the surges of emotion in my gut and chest, in the joy and the pain and the fear and the sadness that fill me today, that remind me second by second that I'm here, that this life is real, that I'm connected, that I'm a human being. (Sometimes, I still feel the urge to pinch myself to see if it's all just a dream.) Most importantly, I feel this aliveness when I close my eyes and realize that I know myself deeper today than any word or label or category could possibly have known me, and that my life is full of meaning and connection and purpose, even on its darkest days. These are the beautiful facets of humanness that only a few years ago, to me, were nothing but my mental patient fantasy.

This—this moment—is a gift, just as every moment of my post-Psychiatry life is, and I view it as a second chance, this life I'm living on borrowed time. This is why I'll be protesting the APA, because Psychiatry took me as far from this life as I could possibly have gone, and it is my duty to use this gift to fight for the freedom of those still enslaved. . . .

I view opportunities like Sunday as a human obligation—we must speak out against this tentacled beast called the Psychiatric-Pharmaceutical Industrial Complex, whose voracious and unquenchable appetite for the human spirit is only growing by the day. We must take our gifts of freedom and integrity of mind, body, and spirit and use them as weapons and as tools. We must use our voices, which Psychiatry tried so desperately to take from us, to name this Industry for what it is: a powerful mechanism of social and behavioral control cleverly disguised by a façade of science and medicine. If we are to bring our collective human family closer to a future free from Psychiatry, it starts by taking every chance we have to stand up and fight for human liberation.[60]

APPROACHING THE FOLLOWING CHAPTERS

Having reached this point in the chapter, you hopefully appreciate why I have chosen to subtitle it "Voices and the Politics of Illness." Those of you who write no doubt understand what a mysterious process it is. In some respects, this chapter has moved in directions that I could not have fully anticipated when I began with the broad aspiration to affirm the importance of illness stories, to recount what has happened to me in the last twenty years, and to consider changes in the field of psychiatry. I did not anticipate that my reflections would assume quite such a critical political perspective. You will see that the tone of my analysis in the original edition of *Speaking of Sadness* is more neutral and moderate, although I repeatedly raise questions about the limitations of biologically reductionist explanations of mental illness. Almost unwittingly, the writing of this chapter has more fully sensitized me to the degree of my disenchantment with psychiatry's current direction.

While repeatedly editing this new introductory chapter, I have somewhat worried that it could be seen as an unbalanced, ideologically slanted treatment of psychiatry. Although I hope that you will agree that my evaluation of the politics surrounding psychiatric diagnoses and treatments is based on a careful reading of available literature, please understand that my goal has not been to proselytize. I understand that many will disagree with parts of my commentary in these pages. I welcome such disagreement. An important measure of the value of social science writing, in my view, is the degree to which it raises important questions about ongoing conversations. If our work does not provide readers with new frameworks for thinking about essential human matters, it has not succeeded. If our writing does not provoke a measure of critical questioning, it has not succeeded.

My largest aspiration is that you will find value in the angle of vision provided by my field—sociology. Too often different social science disciplines seem to be in competition. It is unproductive to quarrel about whether sociologists, psychologists, economists, anthropologists, historians, or political scientists have the most truthful or complete understanding of such fundamental human experiences as illness. Rather, these different fields provide complementary angles of vision to such essential human matters.

Sociology is most primarily committed to the idea that there is a dialectical connection between the "micro" worlds of our everyday interactions and the "macro" worlds of the social structures within which we must act.[61] Our perceptions, reflections, and actions are constituted by multiple, intersecting social positions. To borrow the title of George Herbert Mead's classic work, there are constant and ever-changing interactions among "mind, self, and society."[62] Moreover, we are not, for example, just men or women. We are, in addition, men and women of different races, social classes, ethnicities, and ages. Consequently, human distress encompasses an enormous array of hues, intensities, and responses depending on the combinations of our multiple social positions. Although not a sociologist by training, I will yet again turn to Judi Chamberlin who expresses so well how this perspective applies to the rehabilitation of those grappling with severe emotional distress. In an essay entitled "Rehabilitating Ourselves: The Psychiatric Survivor Movement," Chamberlin concludes with the following mandate:

> I urge you to look at rehabilitation in its broadest sense. It is not merely that we are broken and need to be fixed. We exist in a society that is broken and that affects our functioning and well-being. We are damaged by racism, by sexism, by classism, by heterosexism, by poverty and oppression. If our functioning is viewed in a vacuum, these factors are ignored, and we are seen as defective. If, instead, we are seen within the context of these factors, then efforts to help us will be more meaningful and much less focused on our individual defects and pathologies. It makes little sense to ignore the society in which we all must live.[63]

If you accept the validity of Chamberlin's words, you will likely feel unfulfilled by any paradigm for understanding depression and other mental illnesses that dismisses the voices, the subjective experiences, the interpretations, and the social contexts of those who too often suffer greatly. I hope that you accept the central premise of this chapter. It is that the willingness to listen carefully and respectfully to difficult, often confusing, illness accounts is a deeply moral act that humanizes both narrators and listeners. In this regard, I also hope you will agree that the voices in the following chapters, first presented twenty years ago, remain cogent, instructive, and even personally transformative.

Chapter 1

Living with Depression

Nothing so concentrates experience and clarifies the central conditions of living as serious illness. . . . Illness narratives edify us about how life problems are created, controlled, made meaningful. They also tell us about the way cultural values and social relations shape how we perceive and monitor our bodies, label and categorize bodily symptoms [and] interpret complaints in the particular context of our life situation. . . .

Arthur Kleinman, *The Illness Narratives*, p. xiii

In greater or lesser degree I have grappled with depression for almost 20 years. I suppose that even as a child my experience of life was as much characterized by anxiety as by joy and pleasure. And as I look back, there were lots of tip-offs that things weren't right. I find it difficult to remember much of my early years, but throughout high school and college I felt uncertain of myself, feared that I could not accomplish what was expected of me, and had plenty of sleepless nights. At college one of my roommates nicknamed me "weak heart," after a character-type in Dostoyevsky novels, because I often seemed a bit of a lost soul. During all those years, though, I had no real baseline for evaluating the "normalcy" of my feelings. At most, I had defined myself as more anxious than other people and as a "worrier." None of this seemed to warrant treatment of any sort. Even though I was muddling along emotionally, probably like having a constant low-grade fever, I was achieving well enough in school to presume that underneath it all I was okay. It wasn't until my early thirties that I was forced to conclude that something was "really wrong" with me.

People who have lived with depression can often vividly remember the situations that forced them to have a new consciousness as a troubled person. One such occasion for me was a 1974 professional meeting of sociologists in Montreal. By any objective standards I should have been feeling pretty good. I had a solid academic job at Boston College, had just signed my first book contract, and I had a great wife, beautiful son, and a new baby daughter at home. From the outside my life looked pretty good.

During the week I was in Montreal I got virtually no sleep. It's true, I was staying in a strange city and in a borrowed apartment—maybe this was the problem. But I had done a fair amount of traveling and never had sleeping difficulties quite as bad. Then, I thought, "Maybe I'm physically ill. It must be the flu." But again, it was unlike any flu I'd ever had. I wasn't just tired and achy. Each sleepless night my head was filled with disturbing ruminations and during the day I felt a sense of intolerable grief as though somebody close to me had died. I was agitated and sensed a melancholy qualitatively different from anything in the past. I couldn't concentrate because the top of my head felt as if it would blow off, and the excitement of having received the book contract was replaced by the dread and certainty that I wasn't up to the task of writing it. It truly was a miserable week and the start of what I now know was an extended episode of depression. It was also the beginning of a long pilgrimage to figure out what was wrong with me, what to name it, what to do about it, and how to live with it. It has been a bewildering, frustrating, often deeply painful journey.

Despite a progressive worsening of the feelings I first experienced in Montreal, it took me quite a while before I fully connected the word depression to my situation. Being depressed was not yet part of my self-description or identity. It was another prolonged and even more debilitating period of insomnia, compounded with anxiety and sadness, that pushed me to a doctor's office (an internist, not a psychiatrist). For the first time, I heard someone tell me that I was clinically depressed and that I needed "antidepressant medications." This too was a decisive moment in my growing self-definition as a troubled person.

Over the years I have taken a large number of prescribed medications in what now seems like an absolutely trial and error fashion. The first of these was a drug called Amitriptyline (which, indeed, was a real "trip"). I began the drug just before a family vacation (now it was 1978) to Orlando, Florida, to "enjoy" Disney World, SeaWorld, and Circus World. Even as I boarded the plane, I knew something was desperately wrong. My head was in a state of fantastic turmoil and, as anxious as I had been in the past, it didn't compare in intensity to what I felt then. The feelings were so awful that I should have known that the drug was a disaster, but I had no experience with these things. Maybe this was supposed to happen before I became accustomed to the medication. Things only got worse in Orlando. No sleep. I couldn't pay attention to anything and an extraordinary panic overwhelmed me. The worst moment, though, came late in the week as we were driving back to our hotel after one of the longest days of my life.

The contrast between what you are supposed to feel at Disney World and what I felt was so enormous that it engulfed me. I was often on the edge of crying, but as we drove away from Disney World I lost it altogether. I told my wife to stop the car in the breakdown lane and that's actually what happened—I got out of the car and "broke down." Somehow we reached the hotel and I got in touch with a doctor in Boston who told me to get off the medication. Stopping the drug helped, but that experience was unforgettable and pivotal in my developing "career" as a depressed person.

I returned to Boston, badly shaken but resolved about two things. I would never again take medication and I would get to the bottom of my difficulties. And so I became a kind of mental health explorer. Initially, I felt that only deeply disturbed people saw therapists and since I wasn't that bad off I would look for other routes to comfort and cure. Self-help books seemed a good place to start, but I could not easily identify with the vignettes usually provided and the seven (or eight or nine or ten) sure-fire steps to happiness necessary for a bestseller always seemed silly to me. I began scouting around for some kind of therapy short of seeing a "shrink." One of my most memorable involvements was with something called co-counseling.

I heard about co-counseling from a colleague in another department. He was a guy I respected intellectually and was refreshingly forthcoming about the life problems that had gotten him to try co-counseling. It may even be that he claimed co-counseling had saved his life. In any event, he had been going to meetings for several years and gave me the name of a person to call. It turned out that you had to be interviewed before being allowed to join one of the groups. I never learned whether the purpose of the interview was to determine if I was sufficiently off balance to warrant membership or too crazy to be helped. The young woman who interviewed me was extremely appealing. She was physically attractive, warm, and empathetic. She was instantly likeable and made me feel confident in her and her group.

It was called co-counseling because along with the meetings of the whole group we were expected to work independently with a "partner." The idea seemed to be that in both the wider group and with your partner, therapeutic success was measured by the amount of tears shed as you told your "story." The theory, I guess, was that the tears somehow released all the negative energy that was keeping you down and low. I happened to be linked with a woman in her early twenties. We dutifully met a few times at her apartment and along with the discomfort I think we both felt because of our age difference, neither of us ever succeeded in doing too much "discharging," as the group leaders described it. Although it was compelling to hear the range of problems of those in the group, I could never "get with the program" by weeping and quit after about six months.

Like everyone who suffers with depression, I spent a lot of time during these years considering its causes. Throughout the early 1970s I thought I had a pretty good explanation. I was a young assistant professor struggling to do enough publishing so that I would not lose my job. As they say in the academic business, 1977 was to be my "up or out year"; I would either be promoted or "terminated." In short, I was under enormous pressure for six years, juggling the tasks of teaching, counseling students, serving on departmental and university committees, presenting papers at professional meetings, and writing two books that had to be done before I was evaluated for tenure.

I thought for sure that my depression was rooted in these situational demands and that once I got tenure it would go away. I was promoted in 1977 and found that the depression actually deepened. Of course, this meant that my "tenure theory" was wrong and I needed to construct a new one. However, discarding it was no easy thing. The theory's failure suggested a wholly new and more frightening interpretation of depression's locus. Now I had to confront the possibility that my sickness might not arise from social situations, but somehow from my self.

By 1980 my sleeping, which has always been the key barometer of my psychic state, had become just awful. I might get a reasonable night's sleep here and there, but most nights followed a similar and tortuous pattern. Feeling totally exhausted, I began each night with the hope that sleep would relieve me of the misery generated by dragging myself through the day. By now I had tried everything short of prescribed medication to sleep—L-tryptophan from the local health food store, warm baths, meditation, a glass or two of wine, changing bedtimes in an effort to reset my biological clock. Nothing helped. Sometimes I might get to sleep, but even on my best nights I was up every hour or so. On my worst nights I got no sleep. I remember those nights especially well because they were so distinctly horrible.

The loneliest moments of my life have been in the middle of the night while, as I imagined it, everybody else was sleeping. Since I teach and often needed to be standing in front of 80 students in the morning, many nights were spent obsessing about how I would pull it off "this time." Although there was some comfort in knowing that it had always been possible to get through my classes before, one of the insidious things about depression is the feeling that each moment in it is the worst yet. I felt angry toward those who were sleeping, especially my wife who was right there so visibly and easily doing what I couldn't and desperately needed to do. Whatever bad feelings I had were intensified in the middle of the night. It was as though the volume of my personal agony had been turned to a deafening pitch.

The two central feelings typifying my depression were frantic anxiety and a sense of grief. These feelings coupled to generate a sort of catastrophic thinking about events in my life as concrete as the next day's lecture and as amorphous as the quality of my relationships. None of these thoughts were productive. They were just insistently there, looping endlessly in my brain. Sometimes, as though God were serving up a particularly ironic punishment, I would drift off to sleep only shortly before I had to begin my day. The day did follow, filled with obligations that seemed burdensome and often impossible. Each day was spent struggling to appear competent, constantly feeling amazed that I had gotten through the last test and that I would certainly "shut down" in the face of the next.

Some of the people whom you will hear speak in later chapters experience depression primarily as a kind of mental misery. My own feelings have always had a physical component as well. As I saw it, my mind made a choice each day about how to torment my body. One day it might be a terrible "grief knot" in my throat. On another it might be chest pains that could easily be mistaken for a heart attack. Other days it might be an awful heaviness in my eyes, pressure in my head, feelings of sadness in my cheeks, shaky hands and legs, or even some combination of all these. On my most difficult days I was constantly aware of my body, monitoring from minute to minute whether things had become better or worse.

During all of this I felt deeply alone. Everyone else seemed to be moving through their days peacefully, laughing and having fun. I resented them because they were experiencing such an easy time of it; I felt utterly cut off from them emotionally. I was angry because there was no way they could understand what I was going through. Their very presence seemed to magnify my sense of isolation. I never felt seriously suicidal, but the combination of those days and nights often led me to feel that my life was not worth living. Although some days were far better than others, raising the elusive hope that I might be emerging from my difficulty, I basically dragged along, feeling barely alive.

I am leaving out of this narrative all the therapeutic avenues I tried, ranging from seminars in holistic health to weekends spent learning the "relaxation response." I should mention, though, that I saw a number of therapists. The first was a woman with a Ph.D. in clinical psychology. Since I am an academic and greatly value intellectual journeys of all sorts, I found it interesting to do an archeological excavation of my biography. I also did it with the hope that by understanding the early life circumstances that had created my distress, I would be healed. With her direction, I did some interesting exercises like browsing through old picture albums to stimulate reflection on various aspects of my childhood. In the end, none of this relieved my bad feelings and I stopped going. I tried other therapists, thinking that the key to turning things around was to find the "right one." After several attempts to discover a savior, I became tired of recounting my biography and fundamentally dubious about the efficacy of talking as a solution. Each new therapeutic venture began with hope and ended with disillusionment.

During one of my worst periods I read an advertisement in the *Boston Globe* asking for volunteers for a drug study at McLean's Hospital in Belmont, Massachusetts. Although I had sworn off the drugs some time back, my family and friends urged me to try the program, and a sense of desperation overcame my reluctance. Participation in this program, like my experience with co-counseling, required a preliminary interview, this time with the psychiatrist in charge of the study. I remember arriving at McLean's, often referred to as the Harvard of mental hospitals. In fact, with its mixture of old and new buildings and extensive greenery, McLean's Hospital has the feeling of a college campus. Still, it was a mental hospital and I couldn't escape the sense that by showing up there I had crossed an important identity threshold.

I passed a basketball court on the way to the interview and re-member thinking how strange that seemed since any kind of sig-nificant physical effort was impossible in my state. Could it be that the in-patients were in better shape? The answer to that question was partially answered as I climbed the three flights of stairs to the psychiatrist's office. On each level I passed a door with a small rectangular window that let me look into what must have been a "locked ward." I saw some attendants, identified by their full key rings and white uniforms, but didn't observe any patients. It was sort of eerie. Everything was totally quiet, with no visible patient life. Where were they? What was being done to them? Why was I here? Could I end up in such a place? At that moment I felt like a mental patient and, as much as I wanted to get out of there, I imag-ined I had no choice. What else was left for me to try?

I met the psychiatrist in a familiar looking office since it could easily have belonged to a professor. Dr. Rosen[1] was a pleasant look-ing man in his mid-thirties who continuously puffed on a pipe and displayed a relaxed demeanor thoroughly fitting someone totally in charge of his life. I assumed that I would once again be asked to give the shortened version of my biography. I was surprised, therefore, to learn that Dr. Rosen was not at all interested in my relationships with my parents, my siblings, my wife, my children, or my job. He simply asked a series of questions about my symp-toms. Did it feel the worst in the morning? Did I feel an elevation in mood in mid-afternoon? Did I fall asleep quickly only to wake an hour later? Did I often finally fall asleep between 5:30 and 7 in the morning? And so on. The experience was unnerving because the questions seemed to cut to the center of my feelings and expe-riences. I was like a disbeliever going to a psychic who said things in so pertinent a way that it melted skepticism. At the end of my 25 minute interview Rosen said the magical words, "I think I can help you." His question-asking performance, presumably based on the accumulation of scientific knowledge and a wealth of clinical evidence, filled me yet again with new hope.

I could not clearly have realized at the time that my association with Rosen and McLean's marked the beginning of a new phase in my illness journey. By now, I had entered a socialization process that entailed commitment to a medical model of depression. After all, Rosen's judgment was that a trial with Imipramine, then one of the most widely used and effective antidepressant medications, would set me on the right course. In addition, the whole process seemed so clearly premised on my having a biological disorder. The purpose of the medication was to increase levels of norepinephrine in my brain and the frequent blood tests I took somewhat assured me that the treatment was essentially equivalent to the way diabetics keep careful watch over insulin levels. As a study participant, I filled out a questionnaire once a week to determine if the depression was lifting. At the same time, the lab carefully watched my levels of this and that. The Imipramine, as the doctor told me it would, made my mouth feel as if it was filled with cotton. This and other side effects were troublesome, but I did begin to feel better. Even a slight respite in my bad feelings had a profound influence in accelerating my belief that if only I could get my neurotransmitters working correctly I would be home free.

I stayed on the Imipramine for well over a year. However, I had to come to grips with the fact that although it diminished my symptoms, Imipramine was not going to be my ticket to normality. I also learned that psychopharmacologists are very keen on trying each of a new generation of drugs that might finally do the trick for you. As a result, I took a bewildering array of medications over the course of the next few years, sometimes experiencing terrible side effects like those in Orlando. By now, though, I knew enough not to tolerate a drug that seemed to separate me, as though behind a glass wall, from everyone else, or that made me impotent, or gain weight rapidly, or a number of other very unpleasant things.

All the while I had to contend with the apparent contradiction between my training as a sociologist and my drug-taking behavior. One of the central messages of my discipline is that culture, rather than biology, is destiny. This was the message I preached in my introductory sociology class. I was also familiar with the argument made by a number of sociologists writing in the 1960s that the idea of mental illness is a myth.[2] Their claim was that mental illness is nothing more than a political category; that everyone has "problems with living" and that we ought to do away with the arbitrary and destructive illness label. Sociologists are professionally inclined to look for the source of personal "disease" within social structures rather than as a result of biology gone awry. I knew all this and often felt confused about the interplay of nature and nurture in making me depressed. It did not help to read that antidepressant medications might work by doing damage to people's brains. Intellectual debates aside, I felt dependent on medicines that sometimes helped me to sleep and which I thought allowed me to live life somewhat more easily than in the past.

The concrete details of my story leave off in about 1986. However, exactly as I write these words I am struggling emotionally after another typically lousy night's sleep. About eight months ago I tried still another medication, once more out of a sense of desperation. Doxepin was magical at first. Shortly after swallowing the first pill my anxiety noticeably decreased. Within a few days my sleep patterns changed. I began to have a few experiences of sleeping throughout the night and waking up anxiety-free, refreshed, and eager to get going with my day. It was marvelous and a glimpse into feelings of normalcy I had long forgotten. Certainly I am grateful for those nights and days, but the miracle has been short-lived. Perhaps the biochemical revolution in psychiatry will eventually yield a pill—some currently believe it is Prozac[3]—that will permanently solve problems like mine. That would be fantastic, but I think it unlikely.

By some standards I have been fortunate. Even though depression has periodically made me feel that my life was not worth living, has created havoc in my family, and sometimes made the work of teaching and writing seem impossible, I have not lost my family, my work, or, for that matter, my life. At age 51 I have surrendered myself to depressive "illness" in the sense that I do not believe I will ever be fully free of it. For me, depression has a chronicity that makes it like a kind of mental arthritis; something that you just have to live with. My aim is to live with depression as well as I can. I continue to take medication, although it is never clear to me whether it "works," and my hope is that depression never cripples me to the degree it did in Orlando and during the years immediately following that trip.

One way to deal with a personal problem is to write about it. Writing has, I believe, a truly significant therapeutic value. As a sociologist I have always felt privileged to be able to work on topics and problems that matter in my own life. Sociology has been a means for working on personal puzzles and doing research that might contribute to a broader understanding of human behavior. The idea of looking inside oneself for important research problems was well put by C. Wright Mills[4] who advocated in his book *The Sociological Imagination* that social scientists "translate private troubles into public issues." If you are going through a divorce, that's a private trouble. When half the marriages in

America are failing, divorce is a public issue. If you happen to be unemployed, that is your private trouble. Once again, though, when the unemployment rate reaches double digits it has surely become a public issue. This book is motivated by my personal trouble and the hope that I can provide for sufferers, and for those close to them, a sociologically informed perspective on depression.[5]

To be sure, depression is very much a public issue. The American Psychiatric Association[6] estimates that over 10 million Americans suffer from anxiety disorders and nearly 10 million suffer from depression. Newspapers routinely report that as many as 15 percent of America's population will need to be treated for an "affective disorder." According to these numbers, depressive illness is rising at an epidemic rate. As a sociologist I'm inclined to look at such figures with a critical eye. In fact, depression has in a sense been "discovered" in the last two decades. A glance at the *Readers Guide to Periodical Literature* indicates that 20 years ago few stories existed on depression. Since then, the number has exploded. Such media coverage coincides with a revolution in psychiatry that defines depression as a biochemical disorder best treated with drugs. In this respect, the numbers appearing in the newspapers may be a product of what some social scientists[7] have termed the "medicalization of society." The number of people suffering from depression may be partly an artifact of the way that a powerful group—medical doctors—defines depression in the first place. Such a caveat aside, huge numbers of Americans are indeed in mental misery.

Given the pervasiveness of depression, it is not surprising that both medical and social scientists have tried to understand its causes and suggest ways of dealing with it. When I first considered writing about depression I did a computer search that turned up nearly 500 social science studies done in just the last few years.

Researchers have tried to link the incidence of depression to every imaginable social factor. For example, since the rate of depression is twice as great for women than for men, studies have been conducted seeking to relate depression with gender roles, family structure, powerlessness, child rearing, and the like.[8] Studies can also be found trying to link depression with, among other things, age (especially during adolescence and old age), unemployment, physical illness, disability, child abuse, ethnicity, race, and social class.[9] Another focus of the literature is on the efficacy of different social programs or intervention strategies for reducing the impact of depression. Of course, the medical literature alone contains hundreds of studies on the use of different drugs for treating depression.

As valuable as these studies might be, something crucial is missing. My view is that to really understand a human experience, it must be appreciated *from the subjective point of view of the person undergoing it*. To use the language of social psychology, it is necessary to "take the role" of those whose behaviors and feelings we want to fathom. Underneath the rates, correlations, and presumed causes of behavior are real human beings who are trying to make sense of their lives.

The essential problem with nearly all studies of depression is that we hear the voices of a battalion of mental health experts (doctors, nurses, social workers, sociologists, psychologists, therapists) and never the voices of depressed people themselves. We do not hear what depression feels like, what it means to receive an "official" diagnosis, or what depressed individuals think of therapeutic experts. Nor do we learn the meanings that patients attach to taking psychotropic medications, whether they accept illness metaphors in assessing their condition, how they establish coping mechanisms, how they understand depression to affect their intimate relationships, or how depression influences their occupational strategies and career aspirations.

The absurdity of this omission was dramatically called to my attention when I came across a periodical called *The Journal of Affective Disorders* that has been in the Boston College library since 1987. In all twelve volumes available there is *not one word* spoken by a person who lives with depression. Someone once described social statistics as human beings with the tears washed away. Nowhere is such a characterization more apt than in trying to grasp what depression is all about. There is something dehumanizing and distorting about social "scientists" reducing an extraordinarily difficult human experience to indices, causal models, and statistical correlations. Certainly such research has its place, but an empathetic understanding of depression can only be accomplished by bringing human beings back into the picture. Research about a feeling disorder that does not get at people's feelings seems, to put it kindly, incomplete.

This book is primarily directed at letting people speak about how their lives, feelings, attitudes, and perspectives have been influenced by depression. Some writers such as Sylvia Plath, Nancy Mairs, William Styron, and Elizabeth Wurtzel have attempted to record their battles with depression.[10] As instructive as these accounts are, they are not based on systematically collected data nor are they directed at discovering underlying patterns in the depression experience. I have elected to do in-depth interviews with 50 people who have been "officially" diagnosed as depressed and who consequently became involved in a therapeutic world of psychiatric experts.[11] I approach in-depth interviews as a directed, artful conversation requiring a sensitivity about when to ask certain questions, when to prod respondents, and when to respect people's need for privacy. Each of these interviews both tells a unique story and reveals common themes in the lives of depressed people. Each interview caused me to marvel at the courage depressed people display in dealing with extraordinary and debilitating pain.

I used several avenues to solicit interviewees. Initial interviews were done with personal acquaintances whom I knew had long histories with depression. Advertisements were placed in local newspapers—this strategy yielded a number of responses. Finally, after each interview respondents were asked to describe my study to friends whom they knew had histories of depression and to refer names of willing participants. As with any project based on in-depth interviews, no claims can be made for the statistical representativeness of the sample. However, I feel confident that what my sample gives up in breadth is more than made up for by the depth of insight respondents provide.

Each of the taped interviews typically lasted between one and a half and three hours. In several cases two interview periods were required to capture the complexity and richness of the individual's experiences. Each interview began by asking the person to trace the history of his or her experience with depression from "the first moment you realized that something was wrong with you, even if you did not initially define the problem as depression." This broad opening question normally led to conversation that provided information in the following areas: description of what depression is like, the experience of hospitalization, views on whether depression should be considered an illness, feelings about therapeutic experts, depression's impact on relations with family and friends, the influence of depression on work, feelings about using psychotropic medications, and coping strategies. While the goal was to obtain information in all these areas, the time given to each topic was dictated by the particular contingencies of each person's life.

Although it is impossible to know what information people might have withheld, I found it remarkable how candidly most of those interviewed appeared to speak about their experiences, including such difficult topics as child abuse, drug addiction, work failures, broken relationships, and suicide attempts. Several times, interviews were punctuated by tears as people recounted especially painful incidents. In every case, I reserved time at the end of the interview for respondents to "process" our conversation and to communicate how they felt about the experience. Nearly everyone expressed gratitude for the chance to tell their story, often saying that doing the interview gave them new angles on their life. Several also indicated that they were motivated to participate in the study because they wanted others to hear what depression is all about. They expressed sentiments similar to the 41-year-old baker who told me why she responded to my newspaper advertisement:

> I thought maybe I could say something that might help people who are depressed. ... [I want] to encourage us as human beings to make more of an effort to respond to each other. [I want others] to see ... the connection we have with each other and the effect we can have with each other. I want people to hear that part of the predicament of depression is isolation and that anybody can do something about that. [I want people to feel] that they are empowered ... that everybody can do something, that every person probably knows someone who is depressed, and everybody can do something; you know, be a little kinder or something. It can really make a difference. [female baker, aged 41]

This comment also points out that depression is a disease of isolation. One of those you will again hear in later chapters described depression as "a radical constriction and narrowing of the self. . . . A balling up inside yourself. It's an imploding almost." During periods of depression people feel terrible because they are cut off from others, and yet they feel the need to isolate themselves. A paradox of depression is that sufferers yearn for connection, seem bereft because of their isolation, and yet are rendered incapable of being with others in a comfortable way. I hope this book diminishes isolation and loneliness (1) by letting those who suffer from depression realize how similar their experiences often are, (2) by helping professionals to see the world as their clients do, and (3) by giving family and friends of depressed people a better sense of their plight.

So far, I have argued that a subjective, experiential, or person-centered approach to depression has been neglected and that such a gap provides one motivation and justification for this study. Valuable sociology, however, requires more than an important topic and the goal of informative description. That's a good start, but the value and vitality of a piece of research depend on its providing *theoretical* illumination of the topic under investigation. Like any piece of social science, insight into a process or situation requires having a perspective to order facts and thinking.

My analysis throughout this book is informed by "symbolic interaction theory."[12] A basic principle of symbolic interaction is that all objects, events, and situations acquire their meanings through processes of human interpretation. The meanings attached to objects, events, and situations are not built into them. Instead, they are products of our *responses* to them. In this regard, all human experience is an ongoing exercise in sense-making. Social psychologists allow, however, that some social situations are inherently more ambiguous than others and, consequently, require more extensive interpretive efforts. As studies of multiple sclerosis, childhood leukemia, and epilepsy have illustrated,[13] chronic illnesses of uncertain origin and outcome pose particularly difficult problems of meaning attribution.

Aside from the personally compelling nature of the subject matter, the case of depression almost demands reflection on questions of identity and self-transformation. Questions about the origins of self, its consequences for behavior, and its changes over time are among the most central of social psychology. Because depression is often defined precisely as an illness of the self[14] it constitutes, in effect, a case study for considering how individuals arrive at illness definitions and then reconstruct their identities accordingly. Thus, the underlying question animating my thinking in this book asks how depressed individuals make sense of an intrinsically ambiguous and seemingly intractable life condition.

As I see it, efforts to authoritatively uncover the causes of depression are doomed to failure. Depression is simply too complicated for that. However, it is a reasonable sociological project to discover how depressed people try to give order to their lives. As the contours of my own biography illustrate, it is impossible to live with depression without theorizing about its causes and what one might do to cope with it. Therefore, what can be accomplished here is an analysis of meaning-making as people themselves speak about the intersection of illness, identity, and society.

All of life involves periodic assessments of who we are and where we are heading. Kierkegaard is reported to have said that life is made sense of by looking backwards, but must be lived by looking forward. While we all constantly recreate ourselves, dramatic emotional problems call forth special efforts to figure out how the past has shaped us and what our prospects for the future might be. The data analysis in later chapters illustrates that much of the depression experience is caught up with interpreting past selves, coping with present selves, and attempting to construct a future self that will "work" better. Depression, like other life altering illnesses, is characterized by critical turning points in identity. The sociologist Anselm Strauss[15] talks about identity turning points as those life moments when we come to see ourselves in a thoroughly new light. They are moments when "critical incidences occur, forcing a person to recognize that 'I am not the same as I was, as I used to be.'" Depression, as my short autobiography suggests, repeatedly generates just such self-recognitions.

I have already disclaimed the possibility of solving the riddle of depression. In addition, no single book can hope to illuminate all features of the depression experience. In large measure, the boundaries of my writing are determined by the accounts of my informants. I have tried to organize my materials to best capture the range of things they have told me. Let me conclude this first chapter by briefly describing the blueprint I have in mind for conveying their experiences.

In Chapter 2, "The Dialectics of Depression," my goal is to let you hear how people talk about the depression experience itself. From the first moment I considered studying depression I resolved to write about the essential character of depression, about what depression feels like. One of the dilemmas of depression arises from the incomprehension of those who have never experienced it. A great frustration for people with clinical depression is the expectation that they can (and ought to) "shake it off," "pull themselves up by their bootstraps," "just think more positive thoughts," and so on. I want to convey to those who say such things what the experiences of depression are "really" like. Such an impulse is consistent with a general goal of sociology to provide a forum for those whose voices are either stilled or not well understood.

While the main goal of Chapter 2 is to hear how depression is described, I have, as in all chapters, a conceptual agenda as well. My analysis in this chapter turns on the most insistent theme in my conversations with depressed people. It is that depression is an illness of isolation, a disease of disconnection. As with much of social life, and consequently with much compelling sociological analysis, it is irony that captures the complexity of things. The irony to be explored in Chapter 2 is that depressed persons greatly desire connection while they are simultaneously deprived of the ability to realize it. Much of depression's pain arises out of the recognition that what might make one feel better—human connection—seems impossible in the midst of a paralyzing episode of depression. It is rather like dying from thirst while looking at a glass of water just beyond one's reach.

Chapter 3, "Illness and Identity," picks up on the central idea that depression is a condition of the self. Since self-consciousness as a depressed person unfolds in a predictable fashion, we can speak of a depression *career* with discernible stages. Sociologists have made good use of the career idea to refer to a range of human processes. I find especially congenial to my purposes Everett Hughes'[16] definition of career as "the moving perspective in which the person sees his life as a whole and interprets the meanings of his various attitudes, actions, and the things which happen to him." Consistent with earlier comments, this definition calls attention to the subjective, evaluative aspects of depression and to the ways individuals impose meanings onto their situation over time.

While the experiences of the respondents suggest regularities in the sequencing of the depression experience, people differ considerably in the length of time they spend in any particular phase. For instance, some individuals, like myself, describe years of discomfort before they arrive at the definition of themselves as depressed. Others reach that conclusion much more quickly. Such variations depend on whether the onset of "acute" depression first occurs in childhood or later, and whether the depression is characterized by plainly defined episodes or a more chronic pattern of disease. These differences aside, all the respondents in this study described clear identity turning points in the evolution of a depression consciousness.

These days, virtually everyone diagnosed with clinical depression is treated with antidepressant medications. Chapter 4, "The Meanings of Medication," explores the symbolic meanings attached to taking antidepressant medications. As my own story intimates, the decision to embark on a course of drug taking is not a simple matter of unthinkingly following a doctor's orders. In fact, a patient's willingness to begin a drug regimen and stick with it involves an extensive interpretive process that includes consideration of such issues as the connection between drug use and illness self-definitions, the meanings of drug side effects, attitudes toward physicians, evaluations of professional expertise, and ambiguity about the causes of one's problem. Most respondents are initially resistant to taking drugs, but are eventually induced to use them and then to accept biochemical explanations for their problem. Chapter 4 thus describes the socialization process through which people are transformed into patients who ultimately adopt a medical version of depression's reality.

Chapter 5 is on "Coping and Adapting." This chapter parallels and extends the discussion in Chapter 3 of the stages involved in the construction of an illness identity. If the focus of Chapter 3 is on patterned changes in *consciousness and perception* as people try to make sense of their psychic discomfort, my attention in Chapter 5 turns to *action*, to what individuals *do* about the pain they eventually label as clinical depression. Depression totally envelops those who suffer from it and emotional pain, like all pain, insistently demands that something be done to relieve it. In effect, each of the 50 interviews conducted for this study constitutes from beginning to end a story of adaptation. From the first moment people recognize that something is wrong, they begin efforts to diminish the problem. How individuals try to cope with and adapt to depression's pain depends on how they understand its meaning at a given moment in time.

The issues raised in Chapter 5 provide the platform for my discussion in Chapter 6, "Family and Friends." In a very real sense depression is a contagious illness. It "infects" those who are close to depressed people. Part of understanding the experience of depression depends on appreciating the reactions of "normal" individuals to family members or friends who are depressed. Certainly, a critical aspect of depression for me has involved its effects on my wife and two children. I have worried a great deal over the last two decades about the influence on my children, a son now 23 and a daughter 20, of growing up in a household with a father who was often unreasonable, crazily irritable, and too often inaccessible. It is also nearly astounding that my wife has not left me. Since depression is equally their story, I elected to interview ten individuals whose lives are intertwined with depressed persons. Chapter 6 tries to capture the phenomenology of depression from their standpoint.

My more specific analytical concern in Chapter 6 is to consider the limits to sympathetic involvement with a depressed person. Those who are close to a sick friend or family member have the difficult task of negotiating the degree of help, concern, and sympathy they should offer. Too little and they have failed to honor their commitments, too much and they become contaminated by the gloom and pain of the ailing person. I also pursue the idea that the character of sympathy negotiations will be different depending on the social statuses of those involved. Departing from the mode of data presentation in earlier chapters, I present four "case studies" in Chapter 6. These four accounts of caring and commitment will help to reveal the different demands made on the spouses, parents, children, and friends of someone who suffers from depression.

Years ago, C. Wright Mills[17] maintained that most people in society had difficulty linking their personal malaise to the big historical changes and institutional contradictions within which they act out their daily lives. Indeed, my respondents plainly located the source of their personal troubles only within the daily milieus of their immediate experiences and, in a still more limited way, within themselves. Their consciousnesses about the source of depressive illness rarely extended to the ways in which society is organized as a whole or how broad cultural changes influence their psychological well-being. The last chapter goes beyond the words of my respondents in an effort to link depression to the character of modern society.

We would be hard-pressed to explain such a sea change in the incidence of a major illness in terms of frail selves alone. If our selves are, in fact, becoming more easily sickly, we need to consider the larger social conditions that serve as the context for this burgeoning "psychological" problem. Many Americans are becoming unmoored from society's institutions and from each other. America's inner cities, for example, are characterized by a hyper-ghettoization[18] that results in a far deeper isolation of poor people and minorities than has ever before been the case. Traditional families are disappearing and now serve far fewer as a "haven in a heartless world."[19] The occupational structure is increasingly made up of disposable workers to whom companies feel no obligations.

Moreover, the ethic of individualism, celebrated as the cornerstone of freedom in America, has taken a radical turn that erodes social attachments. As Robert Bellah[20] has put it, "the freedom to be left alone is a freedom that implies being alone."

Although most respondents in this study made no equation between the kinds of social transformations noted previously and their affective disorder, there were some who seemed to grasp how such forces might be implicated in their troubled lives. One respondent depicted his life in terms of fundamental disconnections. Al is a custodian in a warehouse on Boston's waterfront. He described himself as a lifelong loner who has always been estranged from his family, has no friends to speak of, has had difficulty in establishing relationships with women, and has spent much of his life drifting from job to job while living in single room welfare hotels. Although Al has little formal education, he viscerally understands marginality and its consequences. Unlike most of those I interviewed, Al seemed more inclined to blame society than himself for his difficulties.

> A big thing about depression in the United States is a lack of a sense of community. . . . We aren't a people. We are a collective . . . and nobody feels like they owe anyone. . . . It's like a tough shit society. You know, if you're homeless, tough shit. If you get AIDS, tough shit. They say in England "I'm all right, Jack." You know, "I've got mine, Jack." And to that degree I find the United States a pretty uncivilized society. There is just a dreadful shallowness that promotes sociopathic thinking in even normal people. [male custodian, aged 33]

Al's words suggest the need for a research agenda that links the depression experience to the structural factors responsible for loosening social connections—those among individuals and those between individuals and society. Chapter 7 argues that only through such analysis can we hope to grasp the relationship between personal discomfort and the social forces operating "behind our backs," as it were.

Some readers will feel let down by this book because I am simply not interested in providing The Theory that finally explains the cause(s) of depression and a sure-fire way to get rid of it. This book is not focused on causes and cures. As already indicated, I feel that the scores of books on emotional dilemmas found in the self-help sections of bookstores do a disservice by offering ridiculously simple injunctions for solving enormously complex problems. I doubt that there will be a solution to the enigma of depression; that we will ever fully sort out the interplay of nature and nurture that sometimes makes people desperately unhappy. In this book, centered as it is on the consciousnesses of those interviewed, cause and cure enter into the analysis only in so far as *they* have theories about this.

Although my primary goal seems relatively straightforward—to understand the phenomenology of the depression experience—my personal pilgrimage and a lifetime spent reading about human behavior make me feel that even that aspiration might be too immodest. It is said that the more you learn, the more you realize what you don't know. My working life as a sociologist powerfully confirms this idea. The more I read about people's behaviors, attitudes, and emotions, the more awestruck I am by the extraordinary diversity and complexity of most things human beings do, think, and feel. The failure of social scientists to produce definitive laws about social life is not from lack of trying, inadequate methods, or enough brain power. The problem lies in having to contend with the paradox of culture that people create their social worlds and then are refashioned by their own invention. Societies and individuals are involved in an ongoing, never-ending process of mutual transformation.

To respect the complexity of social life and human behavior requires seriously entertaining the theoretical view, mentioned earlier, that nothing human comes with meaning built into it. Human beings live in a world of symbols in the sense that they are the ones who endow everything in their lives with meaning. Ernest Becker[21] put it nicely when he said that "Nature provides all life with H_2O, but only man could create a world in which 'holy' water generates a special stimulus." Such an enormous symbolic dexterity means that all human experiences—illness being a perfect example—take different shapes in different cultural worlds. I am hardly surprised by the finding of anthropologists that depression carries quite different meanings in different societies.[22] I begin with the premise that comprehension of any illness experience requires looking at the intersections of body, mind, self, and society. On the face of it, this is a daunting task.

You might now understand my difficulty with the way depression has been discussed in the United States recently. Newspapers regularly carry stories or advice about depression. Many communities support medical screening for depression at shopping malls. Joan Rivers narrated TV spots, saying that depression is a curable disease if only you will call a certain telephone number when you feel hopeless. The biggest event, however, in the last few years has been the arrival of Prozac. Last year I saw Bette Midler perform at Radio City Music Hall in New York and among the one-liners that got a good laugh during the show's first few minutes was "time sure goes by fast when you're on Prozac." Jokes like that can only be told when a drug reaches into the public's consciousness through cover stories in national magazines like *Time* and *Newsweek*.[23]

These media stories often claim that the cure for depression is just around the medical corner. They describe depression as clearly a biological disease best treated with antidepressant medications like Prozac and virtually promise a "brave new world" in which we will be able to choose our personalities, like selecting clothing off a department store rack. Prozac and other drugs do wonderful things for some people, but the claim that depression is wholly a matter of biology is overblown and represents a form of determinism I find unacceptable. It is appealing to have simple recipe theories because they offer neat and tidy explanations. The problem is that social reality is a very messy thing and can rarely be understood with such easy prescriptions. In fact, I see this book as an antidote to overly pat biological explanations about the meaning of depressive illness. Plainly, there is a biology to bad feelings. To assume, therefore, that bad biology constitutes the explanation for depression is specious thinking. As a sociologist writing about depression, one of my messages is to be very careful about jumping on a bandwagon that locates the source of illness in any single thing.

Before I commit the error of communicating that all medical people have capitulated to biologically reductionist theories of depression, I want to quote one of the anonymous reviewers who looked at the plans for this book in its early stages. Although publishing companies sent my sample chapters primarily to fellow social scientists, one reviewer was a psychiatrist who fully shares my reservations about the direction of current medical thinking on depression. This is what he said about the "long overdue" importance of looking at the subjective experience of depression.

Psychiatrists often lose track of the fact that neurotransmitter research is merely a heuristic tool. The knowledge about medications it affords enables us to intervene in the most extreme cases of human suffering with the goal of palliating its worst aspects. This partial relief may then allow patients to discover more truly powerful responses to their condition in the world of social and personal meanings and relationships. The profession's mistake is not that it emphasizes biological research and the use of helpful drugs to treat, for example, major depression, but that it is gradually reducing the accepted understanding of what depression *is* exclusively to biological and pharmacological elements. I do not mean to dispute that many forms of depression will one day be found to have common biological signatures (for example, reduced serotonin levels in certain brain cortical areas). But I do believe that this is only a "sign" of depression and not a "meaning." In order to find meaning we will have to look at the ever-changing interplay of lived experience, which is always socially developed, and which will come to include as only one among its many creative sources those very discoveries of neuroscientists.

I have one final thought about my role as a researcher and writer. I see my primary responsibility as letting those interviewed speak for themselves—their thoughts, feelings, and experiences are the heart of this book. Obviously, I can present only a portion of what they have told me. I am forced by the volume of data to be selective in determining which parts of their accounts are most worth telling. In making my choices I have tried to respect the rich, varied, complex, and finely textured quality of their lives. I know that the wisdom in each of their stories has helped me to live my own life more easily. For that reason I owe those who have shared their time, thoughts, and experiences much more than the usual debt of scholarly gratitude.

Chapter 2

The Dialectics of Depression

Depression is an insidious vacuum that crawls into your brain and pushes your mind out of the way. It is the complete absence of rational thought. It is freezing cold, with a dangerous, horrifying, terrifying fog wafting throughout whatever is left of your mind.

Unemployed female administrator, aged 27

Nina was among the 30 people who read about my study in the newspaper and came to talk with me at my Boston College office. At exactly the appointed time, an attractive woman, dressed in a conservative business suit appeared. If ever there was a person who could destroy the stereotype that only occupational unsuccessful individuals, or those from severely dysfunctional families, suffer from depression, it would be Nina. Nina's parents, it turned out, were successful professional people. While she described her father as "somewhat odd and eccentric," her mother and father were, she thought, good and loving people. Both Nina and her sister had been identified as gifted children and from the age of three Nina was placed in exclusive private schools where her talents might be nurtured. Nina's otherwise positive childhood was, unfortunately, deeply marred by an unusual illness that still often requires several operations a year. She has an auto-immune condition that causes frequent cancers, especially in her mouth and jaw area. As a result, she constantly needs attention to detect the potentially deadly cancers and then to remove them once they appear. In fact, shortly before we spoke, Nina learned that her problems would require yet another hospitalization. Because of this condition, she was frequently absent from school as a child. And because of changes in her physical appearance occasioned by the surgeries, Nina was often the brunt of the kind of venomous attacks of which children seem uniquely capable. In response she "read voraciously, cultivated unusual interests and hobbies, and avoided large social gatherings."

As we talked I was thinking to myself that Nina's depression was certainly understandable in light of this medical difficulty. However, as she told her story and theorized about the causes of her depression, she claimed that it had little to do with her difficult medical history. Rather, she believed, it was precipitated by a sexual attack experienced in the home of her brother and sister-in-law while visiting them in Europe. The attacker had been a family friend and when Nina reported it to her parents, as well as to her brother and his wife, she was disbelieved. She was told by everyone that the close family friend could not have done this and perhaps she was misinterpreting what actually happened. Nina and I explored the meaning of this event to her. She described in detail how the event has affected her relations with family members.

About a month after we talked I received a letter from Nina. I had given her a draft of one of this book's chapters and in the letter she shared her thoughts about it. She also indicated that, in retrospect, she felt she had not provided a clear enough answer to my interview question "How would you describe what depression feels like to someone who has not experienced it?" With an artistry that affirms her status as a gifted person, Nina tried to convey what depression feels like. In the spirit of retaining her narrative in complete form, the body of her letter to me is reproduced as follows:

As I related to you, things began falling apart after my disastrous experiences in Europe. I was beginning to realize everything I had missed as a child and my own emotional limitations as an adult. I used the phrase "something dropped" to describe my recognition that something was wrong.

A better image would use an ubiquitous "little red wagon." My wagon lost a cotter pin somewhere in Europe. I knew it had fallen out, didn't know what to do, didn't know how to fix it. Just knew it was gone and that I needed it back. I was still rolling along, but one wheel was starting to wobble.

When I completed my MBA and was laid off from [names company] two years later the vital structure that held my world together collapsed, and my wheel fell off. I had nothing to do any more, I had nothing to *be* [her emphasis]. Professional and academic responsibilities could no longer shield me from my emotions or my memories. I fell into depression.

Depression is an insidious vacuum that crawls into your brain and pushes your mind out of the way. It is the complete absence of rational thought. It is freezing cold, with a dangerous, horrifying, terrifying fog wafting throughout whatever is left of your mind. In the beginning I tried to ignore it, to force my eyes and mind to read or get dressed or make breakfast in spite of the encroaching monster. Then I got tired—or it got bigger—and I stopped trying. The warp and woof of my mind disintegrated before me and I could do nothing to stop, ameliorate, or affect the vaporization.

When you are in it there is no more empathy, no intellect, no imagination, no compassion, no humanity, no hope. It isn't possible to roll over in bed because the capacity to plan and execute the required steps is too difficult to master, and the physical skills needed are too hard to complete. For me, the loss of academic skills—reading, writing coherently, basic math—was particularly hard to deal with since I had excelled in all of those areas throughout my life and I took pride in my intellectual capacity.

Depression steals away whoever you were, prevents you from seeing who you might someday be, and replaces your life with a black hole. Like a sweater eaten by moths, nothing is left of the original, only fragments that hinted at greater capacities, greater abilities, greater potentials now gone. Nothing human beings value matters any more—music, laughter, love, sex, children, toasted bagels and the *Sunday New York Times*—because nothing and no one can reach the person trapped in the void. You have no idea of what will happen next, when it might be over, or even where you are now. Suicide sounds terrific, but much too difficult to plan and complete.

No one around you understands what you're going through and tells you you're a "party pooper" for not socializing or taking a shower or going to work. I was laying around feeling sorry for myself when I should have recognized my great good fortune (I am white, single, no children, well-educated and professionally competent) and gone out and found another job instead of moping around. I was in no position to explain myself since I didn't trust my local friends enough to try and tell them and wasn't even sure what was going on. Nor did I have any idea what was going to happen next, or when it would go away.

It was far and away the worst experience of my life. The worst phase lasted only a few weeks in "real world" time, but in my own mind it filled an eternity. I'm not sure why I got through it alive, and don't know when or if it will ever come back. Nor do I know what I would do if it does.

Your article discusses how people view themselves and their condition after they come out of deep depression. Some speak of "life after depression." Based on my own research and experiences I am not sure it is possible to use the word "after" because I think I will always be susceptible to it. My experiences have also affected me so deeply, so profoundly, I'm not sure I will ever be "over" or "beyond" them. That period is a part of who I am, and it can't be sloughed off like a bad case of the flu.

I'm not sure what I should/can do to avoid falling into depression again. I am trying to maintain a sense of perspective on my life and my objectives, trying not to expect too much of myself.

Recognizing the moments or events that make me sad and letting myself feel sad when they occur rather than bottling them up. Trying to learn to rely on friends on occasion, remembering that though they cannot understand many parts of my life that doesn't mean they don't care about me. Trying to avoid put-downs and circuitous derogatory thoughts. Making sure I take "down time" to read the Sunday paper or play with my cats and recharge my batteries.

Since my recent lay-off from [names company] I am deeply concerned I will go down into that purgatory again. If I do I'm not sure how I will cope. I've made lists of reasons why I shouldn't give up (e.g., my cats, grandmother, etc.) and remind myself that—whatever happens—it does get better again. I can empathize with the subject in your paper who had believed he would never be depressed again, and the loss of faith he experienced when he went under the second time. I am not always sure the quality of my life warrants the kind of repeated psychological abuse that depression brings, so am trying to make sure it is high enough to sustain me if I ever want to crawl under a mattress and die again.

Will this work? I don't know. In more pessimistic moments I doubt it. However, I also don't have much choice. If nothing else, depression has taught me perspective and forced me to concentrate on this second/minute/day, ignoring both past and future.

I hope the previous pages have been of some help to you, and would appreciate receiving a copy of any paper that may come out of your current efforts. I paused a long time before I first contacted you, trying to identify what I hoped to gain from our meeting and what I was willing to give up in my efforts to try and improve the academic realm's understanding of depression.

The one thing that seems to be missing in all of the academic/clinical data I've read is how it actually feels. No one seems to care about the experiences of the people affected by the disease, their needs (outside of drugs) while they are going through it, their feelings once they come out of the worst phases, and the ramifications depression will have on their lives.

I have searched and searched for articles or studies focusing on the perceptions of depressed people and have found very few. I think it would help me if I had access to someone else's descriptions of their own trip through this private hell, and how they managed to continue on in spite of it. Something like

Styron's *Darkness Visible* without the need for a nice, neat, totally improbable "happy ending." I don't think there is a happy ending with depression, at least not yet.

I do think that depressed people need access to the very real experiences of others who have survived it. You can't get that from psychologists, psychiatrists, drugs, or hospitals. The stories provide perspective, they provide balance to all the hype about drugs and "cure," they provide information and background that may help other depressed people get a handle on their experiences, they prove that you're not alone with this monster. And they give hope.

SOCIOLOGY AND SOCIAL CONNECTION

Nina's letter is a valuable document because it so beautifully conveys some of the features of depression shared by all the people in my sample. The remainder of this chapter builds on her comments by offering a sociological interpretation of the phenomenology of clinical depression. My analysis proceeds from the fundamental premise of the sociology of medicine that there is a dialectical relationship between illness and social experience,[1] an articulation especially intimate in the case of depression. As Talcott Parsons observed several decades ago,[2] people with illness are expected to withdraw from normal social obligations during their recuperation, but may come to be seen as deviant, as malingerers, if their disinvolvement from work and family expectations extends too long. Affective disorders represent a unique category of illnesses since social withdrawal is both a consequence of the condition and one of its chief defining characteristics. To dramatize the point, those suffering from, say, cancer might very well find social interaction difficult, but it is not the difficulty of interaction that provides a clue to cancer's presence. Social withdrawal is not a relevant observation for diagnosing cancer. In contrast, social withdrawal is a central observation in diagnosing depression since the inability to remain socially connected is a chief consequence of the illness.

An insistent theme raised in every interview centers on human connection. Each person's tale of depression inevitably speaks to questions of isolation, withdrawal, and lack of connection. The pain of depression arises in part because of separation from others; from an inability to connect, even as one desperately yearns for just such connection.

The related themes of disconnection, isolation, and withdrawal coincide with the most basic issues of sociology itself. Classical sociological theorists shared a common interest in the changing nature of social integration as agrarian societies were being transformed into urban, industrial societies. Nearly all were disturbed by the progressive weakening of our ties to society, and the theorist Emile Durkheim, writing on issues immediately central to this research, explored the linkage between integration and suicide.[3] Following this tradition, recent sociologists have considered the ill effects of a society characterized by radical individualism.[4] In all of this, the presumption is that the emotional health of individuals— and ultimately society itself—is related to how firmly individuals feel embraced by and connected to communities large and small.

Durkheim and his nineteenth-century colleagues wrote about the large institutional structures of society and how they were changing. On a more social psychological level, it has been an enduring sociological perspective that our very humanity is a product of social connection. George Herbert Mead, Charles Horton Cooley, and W. I. Thomas, among others, are justifiably famous for establishing the idea that we are transformed from biological to social human beings through interaction. We are all made human through a socialization process that increasingly links us to others and to social structures. Sociologists generally argue that if children are deprived of interaction—kept away from human connection—they cannot acquire the traits we generally recognize as human. The flip side of this idea is that our humanity can easily erode if we are denied human contact. To be sure, research on isolation testifies to the relationship between social integration and psychological well-being.[5] Studies detail how such isolation relates to a range of affective disorders.[6] In short, there is a long and continuing history in sociology on the importance of strong social ties.

The words of the respondents suggest the dimensions of the social bond most badly frayed, eroded, or absolutely severed during episodes of depression. Although depression alters perceptions in multiple ways, the social world seems to lose its normal temporal dimension for most sufferers. Their present bad feelings so thoroughly capture them that the sense of hope and security normally framing images of a future is destroyed. For some, the world loses its very dimensionality, appearing flat, lifeless, and colorless. Most fundamentally, however, the self is itself the bond between the person and the social world. Thus, when the pain of human association leads to withdrawal and isolation, the self loses its social foundation, begins to wither, and in that process the social world comes to appear even more alien. It is in depression's vicious feedback loop—the downward spiral of hopelessness, withdrawal, the erosion of the self, the still more powerful feelings of hopelessness, the even greater impulse to withdraw, and so on—that we witness, in its most negative form, the dialectic of self and society.

The foregoing paragraphs preview the fundamental observation that animates my thinking here. As with much of social life, and consequently with much compelling sociological analysis, it is irony and paradox that capture the complexity of things. The paradox I explore throughout the remainder of this chapter is that depressed people greatly desire connection while they are simultaneously deprived of the ability to realize it. Much of depression's pain arises out of the recognition that what might make one feel better—human connection—seems impossible in the midst of a paralyzing episode of depression. As a first step in providing a more nuanced elaboration of this idea, we should hear how others try to articulate the feelings associated with depression.

DESCRIBING DEPRESSION

Part of what makes depression difficult to comprehend is its intrinsic ambiguity. Unlike most illnesses that we either do or do not have, everyone feels "depressed" periodically. Most people who feel "blue" from time to time would not describe themselves as clinically depressed. Others can't get out of bed in the morning and deny they are depressed. In contrast, the sports fan whose favorite team has just lost an important game might truly mean it when he or she declares that the loss has precipitated a major depression.

Because the diagnostic categories associated with mental disorders are questionable and culture-bound[7] researchers have properly given significant attention to the social/political processes through which these categories are created and used.[8] With the recognition, therefore, that depression submits to multiple meanings, there are still clear regularities in the way that respondents struggle to convey their experience of depression. As with literary prose writers whose art depends on translating ineffable emotions into written words, several of those interviewed, like Nina, explored metaphors as their medium of expression. Indeed, it was striking how many people independently equated the depression experience with drowning, suffocating, descending into a bottomless pit, or being in a lightless tunnel. These images hint at the intensity of hopelessness, despair, and just plain terror experienced during the worst moments of depression. Consider this sampling of metaphorical thinking.

If you were trying to convey to somebody what the feeling of depression is about, how would you try to do it? I mean, I know it's difficult.

Yeah. Well, I've done it before. I've referred to it as a dark storm at sea. The sea would, like, relate to the insecurity. You're going to sink. You're going to lose yourself, your life, your everything, and then sink to death. I guess, maybe the sea is death. And the dark storm is, I think, hopelessness. The sea is below you. There is a storm above you. It's a dark storm between your ears. That's how I see it. . . . I mean it's doom, it's hopelessness, down the water is death, and up is just a dark storm that you want to get away from, but can't. . . . That's why the sense of doom. And that causes a paralysis, you know. . . . The sense of doom actually paralyzes you. . . . It incapacitates you. [male custodian, aged 33]

One of my big things is don't lose touch with [depressed people]. They can't reach out to you after a certain point. The darkness, the gray fog and then the black hole. That's all one set of images. The other is drowning. And that's in succession— You know, now I'm up to my knees, the waves are washing over me, I'm treading water, and then I'm drowning. [female librarian, aged 43]

How would you go about describing it?

A sense of being trapped, or being caged, sort of like an animal, like a tiger pacing in a cage. That's sort of how I feel. I feel like I'm in a cage and I'm trapped, and I can't get out and it's night time and the daylight's never going to come. Because if the daylight came, I could figure out how to get out of the cage, but I can't. . . . Sometimes I feel like I'm being smothered in that I can't breathe. I am being suffocated. . . . And it's like falling down a well, like I'm free-falling. That's what it is. And I have nowhere to grab onto to stop it. And I don't know what will happen when I land. Sort of being down a well, and how do I climb back up? [female nurse, aged 37]

I would say it kind of feels like somebody is holding a match that's lit and just the flame is really hot and you're trying to stand it, and it's just consuming you more and more and then it just gets down to the end and there's no more, and the consuming part is just complete hopelessness. You start off as a whole person and then little by little things that you care about start floating away and they're not important anymore and they get harder to hold on to. They just become less and less important and harder to try to do and the easiest thing to do is to just to lie down and let it consume you. [female nanny, aged 22]

The best analogy [between everyday blues and serious depression] I can think of is like, you know, people have colds, where you get the sniffles and the raspy throat. And of course, I've had like super bad colds where I'd lose, you know, a week or more of school. But then you have like death-feeling pneumonia which lays you out for the entire week and where you can barely make it to the bathroom and you go back and fall in bed. You've had that kind, maybe. Well that's about the relationship, you know, between the sniffles and the flu that [makes] you figure you might as well die. [unemployed male, aged 58]

Sometimes respondents try to equate feelings of depression with colors including, as might be expected, blackness. One woman, though, told of "waking up in the middle of the night and literally everything was white." She went on, "I can never explain this [to anyone]. I was definitely awake and everything was white. It was all one color. It was a terrible whiteness." And another person described a "sort of depressed yellow without light." In other cases, individuals depicted a world that suddenly seemed flat and two-dimensional. The words death and dying came up frequently as with the person who said, "I was dead. You could actually say I was dead at that point." While people struggled to communicate with a variety of images, there was near consensus that depression, during its bleakest moments, utterly robs them of concentration, motivation, and energy. Even the simplest acts can become impossible.

[W]hen you're really depressed, you know, if you're in your bedroom and someone said there's a million dollars on the other side of the room and all you have to do is swing your feet over the edge of the bed, and walk over and get the million, you couldn't get the million. I mean you literally couldn't. [male professor, part-time, aged 48]

My therapist, and the people in the hospital, they always said "If you feel bad, call somebody." [But] I'm like, "When I feel bad, I can't even get off the bed." I'm like, "The phone is way over there." (laughs) And I just look at it. I think about the conversation that I could have with somebody, but no way am I going to pick up the phone. [Now] I might actually take the phone with me to bed, and call somebody from bed and say just very vaguely, "Help!" [female nanny, aged 22]

Moreover, sufferers are often exquisitely aware of their progression downward. They know where they are heading and there is nothing they can do about it.

What happens [is] my head, I feel kind of light-headed, and it just kind of shuts off. And it can be very frustrating, especially if you're working and trying to do something. The whole head, it's just . . . awful. What happens [is] I can tell when I'm starting to get depressed. When I begin to have some depression [I begin to have] dark thoughts, something bad is going to happen. . . . You're going to die. It doesn't matter how you're going to die. You're just going to die. These are the thoughts. That type of thing, you know. Isn't it sad that you're going to, you know, [die]. It's kind of like a black thought process that just begins to kind of take over, and then the anxiety, light-headed, don't feel like eating. These are all symptoms. . . . But when those initial thoughts start to come in regularly, they basically take over. Then it's like life is worthless, and why even bother to get out of bed. [male salesman, aged 30]

The last several comments illustrate the common theme of a downward spiral that people feel powerless to stop. It is, one person said, a kind of "downward slide and there is no way I can turn it around." Those who have episodic depressions eventually recognize the symptoms that accompany the beginning of the slide. Insomnia is often a sign. Other signs might be increased anxiety and agitation, or insistent ruminations of self-blame. After repeated depressions, they inevitably begin to theorize about the causes of their problem, about the situations or stimuli that apparently precipitate it, and then they speculate on how to prevent depression from happening again.

Anyone who takes a basic course in sociology or psychology learns about the nature/nurture debate. For most people the debate remains at an abstract level, removed from the stuff of daily life. For those suffering from depression, however, efforts to appreciate whether their condition is explained by biology or environment is an ongoing puzzle. In the end, nearly everyone comes to favor biochemically deterministic theories of depression's cause. As we will more fully explore in Chapter 4, this is partly a result of their gradual commitment to a medical version of reality. It is also a result of the intrinsic nature of depression itself. Over and again, respondents described in nearly identical ways how once the "slide" had developed a momentum, it was beyond their will to control it. The following comments illustrate one of the signal features of the depression experience—a sense of helplessness.

What is most terrible about my illness is sometimes having to be dependent. . . . The illness cripples you. It can really cripple you. It's disabling. And it's hard to accept, for me anyway, that some things are just out of my control. Some things are going to happen to me that are out of my control. [They are things] that I have no influence over, that I have no way of stopping, preventing [or] slowing down. That's the really scary thing about it. [unemployed female, aged 23]

You know, if you say to someone when you're depressed, "You lose your pleasure in things" they think of something like eating a cookie and find that insipid. And that's not what anhedonia really is. Anhedonia is when . . . you name things to yourself that you used to love to do. Eating! Sex! Even reading a book. Going for a walk in the woods. You can't . . . even remember what it's like to go and do something and feel pleasure from it. You look at the world, the array of things that you could do, and they're completely meaningless to you. They're as meaningless to you as if you were an earthworm. Because if you can't get any pleasure or satisfaction from something you have no reason ever to do it. And you come to this terrible still point where there's no reason to move because there's nothing out there for you. [female software quality control manager, aged 31]

It's that feeling of unpredictability and lack of control over something that has a life of its own that contradicts my feeling of mastery. And I know that now. I've had this experience for so long that [I know] I'm going to be up and that I'm going to be down and I suppose it makes it a little bit easier. I mean, I know that it's going to happen. It is out of my control and therefore I shouldn't feel so dreadful when it does happen because it's just part of the rhythm of my life I suppose. [male professor, aged 48]

[There is a] difference between just sadness and depression. There's a real strong element of despair [to depression]. I mean it was like so overwhelming that [despair] was all that I felt. And . . . when I got myself admitted [to the hospital] this last time I just had this incredible sense of despair [with] no end to it. You know, just a constant ocean of it. . . . Also, after a while it takes on a life of its own. You don't have any control [over] your thinking or how despairing you feel or how morose you start feeling. It just takes off. And you need some intervention or some relief because you can't deal with the pain anymore. [unemployed disabled female, aged 39]

When I'm flat out nothing helps. [female librarian, aged 43]

Erik Erikson once suggested that the essence of being human is "hope"; that even in the most dire circumstances human beings are, remarkably, able to retain hope. Accounts of such seemingly unbearable circumstances as life within concentration camps[9] show that hope may be necessary for survival. Of course, we can debate whether hope truly distinguishes us from other animals. There is no debate, though, that depression simultaneously erodes hope and makes ongoing involvement with others difficult and uncomfortable, if not impossible. At its worst, the experience is so powerful and encompassing that no matter how many times one has emerged from depression in the past, it is impossible to believe that a resurrection will be possible *this time*. The word "never" often came up in my conversation with respondents as in "I can never get back to the plateau of feeling on top of everything" or "I'm in it. I can't believe I'm really in it again. It's here, it's back. It always comes back. And I don't know when I'm going to get out of it. And maybe this time I'll never get out of it." Contributing to the perception of hopelessness is the unremitting character of depression's pain.

For all those years I was depressed the whole time. There wasn't like a let up of a good day or a bad day. In fact, when I look back on all those years I can't even remember events that stick out. It seems all black, a lot of it. You know, it's not one day I have a good day, one day I have a bad day. It was . . . constantly feeling depressed and [at] other times feeling really depressed and suicidal, nothing beyond that. [female graduate student, aged 24]

Depression is always there. People don't realize that I do these things (traveling, going to parties), but I'm still suffering within myself. That's what they can't understand. I suffer every minute of every day. I don't think I've had one happy moment in seven years. Not one happy moment. I mean, I travel. I go to Europe, but I'm miserable and they don't understand. This is what is so awful. I mean, all these nice things and I hate every one of them. It's just an agony. It's agonizing to me. [female travel agent, aged 64]

I guess for me . . . the ongoingness of it was what was fundamental about the depression . . . the unrelieved quality of it, the monochromatic quality of it. [male therapist, aged 45]

The first time I heard a guy at Mclean's say he'd been depressed for two years I nearly fainted. I figured there's no way in God's name I could [stand that]. And I really couldn't have. I got to the point, not too long after I got down there, [where] I became really suicidal. I mean, I wrote a note and got a piece of metal. I was going to go off into the woods and cut my throat. And I used to go there before appointments and stand there with the thing and I really fully intended to do it. Well, the only thing that stopped me was that I was afraid I wouldn't do a proper job; that I'd just partially cut my throat and end up in some back ward for the rest of my life. And that was a worse fate than death. I just wanted an end to the pain. I was willing to gamble that there may be hell on the other side or whatever. I'd just settle for nothingness. Just stop the pain. I would have settled for that. If there was a heaven and forgiveness after that, fine. I wasn't even thinking about it. I was just thinking it's either going to be nothing or more hell. You know, I'll hope for nothing. Just switch off the lights. [unemployed male, aged 58]

The descriptions offered in the last several pages only capture part of the dilemma of depression. I began with theoretical observations about the importance of human association for our personal well-being. It was impossible to listen to depressed people without being struck by the frequency with which themes of "isolation," "withdrawal," and "disconnection" came up. As with all feelings and emotions, isolation is experienced in different degrees and hues. Some individuals feel obliged to withdraw from virtually all arenas of social life. Most people though, unless they become hospitalized, struggle through their daily obligations, sometimes heroically maintaining a facade of "normalcy." Others may continue to associate with friends and family while nevertheless feeling disengaged, uncomfortable, marginal, and profoundly alone. Indeed, as everyone knows, sometimes being in the presence of others and ritualistically moving through the motions of interaction can dramatically magnify a sense of loneliness and isolation. The following section amplifies on the depression experience by drawing out the features of its central paradox: the need to withdraw and the distress of isolation.

THE PARADOX OF DEPRESSION

The discussion thus far does something of an injustice to the complexity of depression because it disassembles the feelings associated with it. People do not feel emotions one at a time. More typically, depression simultaneously engenders multiple feelings: grief, loneliness, anxiety, marginality, and danger. Nevertheless, a hierarchy of feelings is intimated by the frequency with which they are mentioned and the intensity used to describe them. One common feeling related to the matter of social connection is *safety*. To live comfortably, people must trust that they will be protected by the individuals and structures making up their daily worlds. A culture provides its members with a set of guiding principles for living, for making life's uncertainties and ambiguities manageable. However, many of my interviewees do not feel protected by a group's embrace. Instead they feel unsafe. This feeling, I should add, is disproportionately expressed by the women interviewed.

> I totally felt unsafe in my house. I felt unsafe everywhere. I felt unsafe at school. . . . It's the kind of thing like which came first the chicken or the egg. But I was feeling very unsafe. It was just an underlying feeling. [unemployed female, aged 22]

> I'm sure that I've had a lot of agitated depression without knowing that you call it depression, and . . . I've probably been depressed most of my life. . . . [But] I grew up in such a destructive environment that I don't think I had the luxury to be depressed. The agitated depression may be the form that the depression would take, but I think you've got to be in a safe environment to afford to be depressed. In my house if you got depressed you got killed. I mean, you had to be able to move fast (snaps fingers in quick succession) and think fast to stay alive. And I don't mean killed actually, literally, but it was a very destructive environment and I was always insecure, I never had anybody to support me, I had to depend on myself. [female college professor, aged 49]

> I thought I was going crazy [at home]. I thought there were nights that if a person could, I mean even physically, go insane, I thought that's what would happen to me. If my parents didn't stop fighting, or whatever was going on, that I probably would

go crazy. And I wondered if that's how it happened. Like if people could just physically sit there, you know, and go crazy. [So now] I look at the world differently. Like I look at things sort of as gloomy and very precarious. The world is a very precarious place, and very hostile place, and so I tread very . . . carefully. [female nurse, aged 37]

Such quotes tempt theorizing about the causal relationships among early family arrangements, basic trust or distrust, chronic feelings of disconnection, and the eventual onset of depression. That difficult family lives would be related to depression has a common sense validity and it is no surprise that numerous studies demonstrate the association.[10] However, the linkage between family dysfunction and depression is neither simple nor invariable. A number of individuals insistently made the point that it would be impossible in their cases to trace the evolution of depression to an unhappy childhood or poor parenting. Indeed, the extraordinary variation in experience among even the 50 persons represented here suggests the unlikelihood of ever establishing *invariable causes* for depression. There do, though, seem to be *invariable consequences*. Chief among these is social withdrawal. Depressive feelings make interaction arduous and sometimes the need to withdraw from others overrides the realization that self-isolation will only deepen one's anguish.

It's this real catch-22 because you feel bad and you feel that if you see your friends you're going to make them feel bad too, or you're not going to have a good time. Or you're just going to complain. You're going to whine. So then you want to stay by yourself, but if you stay by yourself it just gets worse and worse and worse. [female graduate student, aged 32]

I would just withdraw from people and places and things that were going on around me. I would end up just sitting in front of a TV or sitting at home in bed. ... I just got to the point where I just wanted to be alone and withdrawn from other people. All I can say is that I would find myself uncomfortable being with other people. [male office clerk, part-time, aged 37]

I was exceptionally isolated to the point where I was eating alone in the cafeteria. I was living on a dormitory floor and by the second semester I had given up talking to anybody. [unemployed male, aged 26]

Are there physical things that happen to you, body feelings?

What occurs to me in relation to the physical is . . . the inability to sleep, the inability to function through the day as a result of not having slept well. Feeling groggy, unable to concentrate, unwilling to answer the phone sometimes, or see anybody, feeling withdrawn. Those are the physical manifestations of feeling the way I do. You know, and at times it even extends to my family, although certainly I feel closer to them than to anyone else. My wife complains a lot about my withdrawal. She perceives me as going into my little study and closing the door and being unavailable. And, rightly so, she's very critical of that tendency in my own behavior. [male professor, aged 48]

I avoid the phone. When it rings, I'm like, "Shit! Who's calling? I don't want to talk to them." But you have to, because of normalcy and . . . you're bummed when somebody else comes into the room. You don't want to be disturbed. I'd rather just have my TV and my soda. You can't maintain a relationship anyway, you know. You can't. You don't want to go out. You don't want to see her friends. You don't want to see your friends. It's like you're not there. It doesn't matter if you have a relationship or not. And it's almost like you're breaking up to relieve her of the burden of me. That's part of the thought process. [unemployed male waiter, aged 33]

Immediately, the urge to withdraw, to be alone, seems sensible when "it hurts even to talk," as one person described the difficulty of interaction. However, withdrawal eventually turns out to be a false emotional economy. Although providing momentary respite from social obligations that seem impossible to carry out, withdrawal's long-term costs are negative. Like drugs that have good short-term effects and debilitating long-term consequences, social withdrawal becomes part of a crucible melding fear and self-loathing, a brew that powerfully catalyzes hopelessness. Hopelessness, in turn, makes the urge to withdraw still more powerful. And so it goes—a truly vicious cycle. The paradox of the process I am describing is that its victims are well aware of the double bind they are creating for themselves. They withdraw and isolate themselves while realizing that this response to the feelings of depression will only make them worse.

Oh, I was so alone. I played basketball. I was a member of a team. I had a roommate, but I was so alone. I had a lot of friends, but I was completely isolated. And that's what, like, I believe depression is—a disease of isolation that tells you to withdraw, stay away, don't be a social person. *Stay away from the people who are going to make you better* [my emphasis]. Yeah, the need to be alone, to withdraw. That's one symptom. But I was like, just so alone. I can remember walking around, walking around in the rain one day, just like, "What the hell? What was wrong with me? What is wrong with me?" [male salesman, aged 30]

Thus far depression has been characterized as though it had a course independent of social processes. To sufferers it does appear to have a life of its own that demands certain behavioral responses, especially withdrawal and isolation. Such a description catches part of the "truth" about the character of depression. Yet to think about isolation and disconnection as inevitable and "natural" outcomes of depression is to construct, at best, only half the picture. It is impossible to understand how individuals attach meanings to their own behaviors apart from the *responses of others* to those behaviors. Along these lines, Morris Rosenberg[11] has astutely commented that it takes at least two persons to make a psychotic—one to act in a particular fashion and a second to label it as psychosis. The sections to follow focus on the interactions between those with depression and others. These interactions will reveal the social processes deepening the isolation of depression.

DEEPENING DISCONNECTION

Establishing human connection is plainly linked with empathy. Social psychologists would say that we remain apart from others who will not or cannot "role-take" with us; who are unable to put themselves in our place and see the world as we do. All role-taking, of course, is imprecise because we can never actually be another person; we can only try to put ourselves in another's place and imagine how he or she is seeing and experiencing things. We all necessarily make distinctions among people in terms of their capacity to appreciate our inner life. Thus, the decision to keep the pain of depression private casts others into the status of strangers, persons who are near and distant at the same time.[12] They may be proximate in an immediate physical way, but they are perceived as distant because we do not share with them the perceptions and emotions that most centrally define our experience of the world. Since depression utterly dominates one's "lived world,"[13] keeping it secret dramatically distances sufferers from everyone, including family and friends with whom they might have a significant volume of daily conversation.

In early 1994, America was shocked by the suicide of Vincent Foster, one of Bill Clinton's "closest" aides. People asked, "How could he have been so distressed without anyone knowing about it?" The press speculated on who to blame for "not seeing the signs." In all likelihood, no one is blameworthy since depressed people often strategically keep their turmoil to themselves and any signs of a troubled self that do "leak out" cannot be clearly associated with a life-threatening mood disorder. Of course, secrecy becomes impossible if individuals experience a crisis, a "breakdown," that makes their difficulty immediately visible. However, especially during the early stages of their experience with depression, individuals normally elect to keep their feelings private for three reasons: (1) they do not themselves have an adequate vocabulary for naming their trouble, (2) they believe that others simply cannot comprehend their circumstance, and (3) they are aware of the stigma attached to having a "mental illness." In what follows, I trace through how these three social factors conspire to deepen the sense of isolation that defines the depression experience in the first instance.

Naming Depression

The shape, predictability, and duration of different career paths vary considerably. For example, those following organizational careers may be provided with very clear formal and informal time clocks detailing where they "ought" to be in their careers at different ages. While the experiences of the respondents suggest regularities in the sequencing of the depression experience, individuals differ considerably in the length of time spent in any particular phase. Relevant for my immediate purpose is the observation that several respondents describe years of distress before they arrived at the definition of themselves as depressed. All the respondents in this study described a period of *inchoate feelings* during which they lacked the vocabulary to label their experience as depression.

The ages of respondents range from the early twenties to the middle sixties. Everyone described a period of time during which they had no label for their problem. Many traced feelings of emotional discomfort to ages as young as three or four, although they could not associate their feelings with something called "depression" until years later. It was typical for people to feel different, uncomfortable, marginal, ill at ease, scared, and in pain for years without attaching the notion of depression to their situations.

Most of those reporting bad feelings from an early age could not conclude that something was "abnormal" because they had no comparative baseline of normalcy. As indicated earlier, several interviewees came from what they now describe as severely dysfunctional family circumstances, often characterized by alcoholism and both physical and emotional abuse. The individuals whom we earlier described as feeling unsafe at home often devised strategies to spend as much time as they could elsewhere. Some took refuge in the homes of friends, and one man described school as a haven. In fact, he made a point of becoming friendly with the school custodians so that he could extend the school day in their company rather than returning home. These children knew they were uncomfortable at home but did not have wide enough experience to see their lives as unusual.

I tell you, I could not think in terms of "something isn't right" because I had nothing to judge it against. I've always been a

loner pretty much all my life. . . . I just reacted or didn't react to
the situation I was in. I never thought in those terms of something isn't right here and comparing it to a norm. I had no idea
of what a norm was. . . . It was a kind of naturally unnatural
state to me. [male custodian, aged 33]

For most of the respondents, the phase of inchoate feelings was
the longest in the eventual unfolding of their illness consciousness. Particularly salient in terms of personal identity is the fact
that initial interpretations of their problem focused on their situations rather than on their selves. Their emerging definition was
that escape from the situation would make things right. Over and
again individuals recounted fantasies of escape from their families
and often from the community in which they grew up. However,
initially at least, they felt trapped without a clear notion of how the
situation might change.

I felt sort of overwhelmed by the situation, and I was kind of sad
that I was living the way I was living, and I didn't quite know
how to get myself out of it . . . I guess a sense of feeling trapped.
I think it was a recognition that this was not the way I wanted
to live, but also the fact that I did not know how to get myself
out of it. So it was feeling kind of trapped and kind of panicky.
Now what do I do? [female nurse, aged 37]

The dilemma posed for persons at this stage is that they clearly
feel that something is wrong, but that it is impossible to make sense
of their personal trouble until they possess the conceptual apparatus to give it meaning. Somewhere along the line people make
the connection between their difficulty and depression. They may
read about depression, see a list of symptoms in the newspaper

that describes their feelings, or, more usually, have a crisis that lands them in a doctor's office, and sometimes a hospital, where their trouble is diagnosed as depression. Before that happens, they live in a state of frustrating bewilderment and consternation. As one young woman recounted the onset of her first depression at age 10, she told how the quality of the pain was related to the un-availability of a label for it.

> What was so bad about it [was that] I had no words for it. I didn't understand [what it was]. It was definitely like a total abyss, you know, where everything that I'd ever counted on was gone some-how. Yeah, it was terrifying to me. I was, you know, incapacitated. I'd never been incapacitated before. You know, and the pain is really kind of raw just because you have no vocabulary for it, and you'd never experienced it before. I mean, you're not jaded at all at the time. [female mental health worker, aged 27]

In whatever way people arrive at the definition of their bad feelings as depression, we might suppose that feelings of isolation could be reduced with the announcement to family and friends, "I suffer from depression." However, such a declaration/explanation is rarely forthcoming because the depression label alone cannot accurately convey their inner experience. Depression is still only a code word that cannot bridge the chasm of feelings separating their world from that of friends and family who they believe, in contrast to themselves, are "normal."

The Incommunicability of Depression

Completely "successful" communication would entail the indi-viduals in an encounter exactly attributing the meanings to each other's gestures (words, demeanor, behavior) as were intended. In virtually all interactions, however, there is "meaning slippage" between the motives that generate words and deeds and the way they are encoded by an observer. In every encounter, of course, we are simultaneously actor and audience, both observer and observed, continually constructing our own "performance" in terms of the ongoing interpretations we give to another's behaviors. Such a view of interaction implies the inevitability of transmission noises causing individuals to miss much of the intended meaning in each other's communications. Nevertheless, social life would be impossible unless we proceeded "as if" others were getting our meanings. That is, most of the time we presume to share "enough" of an intersubjective common reality for others to fundamentally comprehend what we mean. However, as any marriage counselor, labor negotiator, or diplomat knows, people's realities can sometimes be so disparate that meaningful communication breaks down altogether.

Negotiating daily life requires carefully monitoring what we talk about with different audiences. To minimize misunderstanding we reserve certain domains of conversation for certain audiences. We need to assess which individuals or groups are most able to role-take with us on particular issues and then to practice a corresponding conversational segregation. Parents talk animatedly with each other about their children's first steps or words, but avoid such conversation with single friends lest they be seen as boors. Members of the same occupation may endlessly "talk shop" when alone, but run the risk of alienating spouses and friends with their narrow and parochial conversation. Sometimes young people do not trust their parents to understand important pieces of their lives.

Communicating with others who have no firsthand knowledge of the life experience one is trying to convey is difficult enough. However, problems of communication are dramatically

compounded when individuals themselves have only partial comprehension of the feelings and emotions they want others to understand. It does not take long to figure out that people who have
never been badly depressed simply don't "get it."

It's the worst feeling in the world. It's right where my heart is.
I don't know if you can feel . . . yuh, you can feel emptiness. Like
there's a black hole there. I'll tell you, it's the scariest thing . . .
I lived with that, you know, for a couple of years, from the ninth
grade until the eleventh grade, with that feeling, with the depression. But it was all very private . . . I kept it quiet. It was
something inside. I didn't really talk about it. I might have
talked about it with one of my friends, but no one understood.
You can't talk about your depression with people who don't
experience it. They don't understand. How are you going to
bring it up? Everyone's so happy. You are going to start talking
about this deep dark secret, deep dark hole? [female graduate
student, aged 24]

My mother's words [always were] "Why can't you snap out of
it?" I was calling her a few years ago when I was really sick, and
I said "I feel like killing myself, I don't want to die, but I just
can't take it anymore." And I spoke to my brother and he said,
"Why don't you do yourself a favor and everybody else, do it
already. I'm sick and tired of hearing about this from you every
few years. Just do it." And so I told him also where to go and
I said, "I really need to hear this." You know, here's my family.
My mother begged me to come home. "Please come home. I'll
take care of you." I said, "Mother, you have no idea what I'm
talking about." And until she lost my father, she had no idea
what depression was. For the first time in her life, she said "I'm

depressed." It took her two years to say it. I said "Thank God, you finally said it." She said, "Now I know what you mean." [female lab technician, aged 49]

My best friend. She understands. She doesn't judge me. She treats me the same. She said, "I'm not going to treat you any different" and that's what I want. But my other friends ... It's taken some getting used to. I mean, this is a hard thing to accept. Over the past three years I've been in five hospitals and I've had some serious problems. And I've stopped trying to force them to understand. I accept the fact that they don't understand. [unemployed female, aged 23]

The people that have really had it, they know what you're talking about. You don't have to try to explain it. You really can't [understand it] if you've never been to the point where it's more than you can do to get your ass out of bed and get in and take a shower. I mean, to take a shower is a major production. You can't even think, "What do I need to do [to take the shower]?" How do I need to do this? A normal person just goes and does it. You don't even think about it. You just do it. But this is a major production [for a depressed person]. My brother put up with me this last time and he helped a lot, but he didn't understand. He really couldn't. [unemployed male, aged 58]

Perhaps we should not be surprised that those who have never experienced depression can't "get it." They can't get it for the same reason that male senators just could not get what Anita Hill was saying to them, that whites don't really get the pain and frustration of blacks, that heterosexuals can't get the militant stance of some gays, or, for that matter, that even the most well-intentioned middle-class Marxists can't fully get the pain of the poor. The only way anyone can ever get something is to be it and experience it exactly as those who live it do. Cognition alone of a human condition always falls short of complete understanding. Moreover, when it comes to human pain and suffering, why would anyone be emotionally predisposed to truly get it? Were it somehow possible to willfully experience the kind of unbearable pain that leads thousands to suicide, would even those social scientists most ardently committed to what Max Weber called "meaningfully adequate explanation" put themselves in that circumstance?

While the inability to share feelings of depression with family and friends unhappily deepens a sufferer's sense of isolation, at least their incomprehension is understandable. Alternatively, when society's professional listeners—therapists of all sorts— seem unable to appreciate the depth of their problem, people are likely to respond angrily.

> I was freaking out. I just couldn't do anything. It was just petrifying. And I remember the psychologist at [name of college]. . . . I felt like "I can't function." I'd be like hysterical and she'd say something like, "Well, you know you've got to learn how to handle the lions in the forest as well as the bunny rabbits or something." And I'd be like, "Oh Jesus Christ, help me, you know. God, don't you get it?" I was telling her like "I've got to be hospitalized. I can't go on like this." She just didn't get it. [unemployed female, aged 22]

In her engaging book entitled *The Managed Heart* Arlie Russell Hochschild explores America's transformation from a production to a service-based economy.[14] She argues that the emergence of a "post-industrial" society has created new forms of alienation at work. Hochschild studied two occupational groups—airline stewardesses and bill collectors—that require high degrees of "emotional labor." Airline stewardesses are trained to cater to the needs of passengers and treat them with friendliness and esteem however rudely they might behave. Bill collectors, on the other hand, are required to collect on services and must, therefore, behave in a nasty fashion toward debtors. Hochschild estimated that about 33 percent of men and 50 percent of women have jobs that require such emotional labor and that the number is growing. Whereas Karl Marx argued that factory workers, as mere instruments on the assembly line, became alienated from their own labor, the workers in the emerging service economy who must suppress their true emotional feelings suffer a new form of alienation— alienation from themselves. Jobs that require workers to "manage their hearts" by suppressing their true feelings and acting insincerely produce an emotional exhaustion and alienation as destructive and debilitating as the physical exhaustion and alienation in the emerging factories of the industrial era.

All of us are regularly required to behave in a fashion that stands in contrast to our subjective inner feelings. In the face of an uncomprehending world, those with depression experience an abidingly deep emotional alienation. Unable to communicate their feelings, sometimes even to psychiatrists, they must move through daily life engaging in a heightened form of impression-management. However, unlike Hochschild's airline stewardesses who can, after all, leave work at the end of the day, sufferers of depression, who elect to keep their feelings private, experience chronic, unremitting emotional alienation. Each moment spent "passing" as normal deepens the sense of disconnection generated by depression in the first instance. In this regard, depression stands as a nearly pure case of impression-management. For depressed individuals, the social requirement to "put on a happy face" requires subjugation of an especially intense inner experience. Yet, nearly unbelievably, many severely depressed people "pull off the act" for long periods of time. The price of the performance is to further exacerbate a life condition that already seems impossibly painful.

> One of the things that has gotten me into some trouble at times is because I have this capacity to be incredibly competent, and I can sit here [and be] incredibly uptight. I could sit here and have a discussion with you and then I could go home and feel extraordinarily suicidal. . . . I could go to a dance in the evening and you know, do a whole social thing, and then just go home and just drop right to the bottom of a pit. [female baker, aged 41]

> It just got to a point when I was in college where I was just like, "I can't keep this up anymore. I hate it. I'm so sick of trying to be happy all the time when I'm not." And people asking me "How are you?" and I'm just like "Great!" when I really want to say, "Life is really biting the big one right now" (laughter), you know. So it took almost dying to say "This is it. I've had it. I can't keep up with the facade anymore, and people are going to know what's been going on." [female nanny, aged 22]

> Every few years, since I was about 17 or 18, I've had relatively very bad depressions. And it seemed to me that my entire life was falling apart, and that I had no control over any of it, and that it was all so awful that I didn't even think I could care about it. And what I would do to try to get through these [depressions] is just pretend that everything was okay, and just go on like normal. But it would take an enormous amount of energy just to do that, just to go to work and do the things that I had to do, and I wouldn't do things that would take any more energy than that. I would just do what I had to do. The last time

that it happened, I was afraid that I would lose my job because it seemed more than I could take. I just didn't know how I was going to manage to continue doing what I had to do. [unemployed female, aged 35]

When I was going to school I was playing in this band and the first week the band played this great show. It was probably the best fun, the most fun I had in college. For about the first week I was the big hero on my [dorm] floor. But then it turned out that I wasn't that kind of person at all. I was very introverted, very self-conscious and so I had to live with this contrast [between] the person I presented when I performed and the person I really was. [unemployed male, aged 26]

As the theme of Michael Douglas' movie *Falling Down* portrays it, American society may be pushing the limits of people's capacity to maintain public postures deeply at odds with their private feelings. At some point, the discrepancy between inner subjectivity and outward performance becomes untenable, and, as a result, socially acceptable facades begin to melt under the psychic heat created by the contradiction. This is what happens to Douglas' character who finally "goes crazy." Similarly, most of those interviewed eventually reach a point where they cannot sustain normal appearances. When that happens they experience a "breakdown." Twenty-nine of the 50 respondents in this study spent time in hospitals. In several cases, hospitalization was precipitated by suicide attempts. Their words suggest that suicide attempts may sometimes be a final effort to communicate to an uncomprehending audience the intensity of one's dysphoria. It is a last try to "get through."

I think that first suicide was . . . really my way of saying, "Look, you're not getting it. Something is really wrong, but it's not what you think." And that's what I was hoping to get. I was hoping for them to stand back and be sort of like, "There is something deeply deeply wrong here." [female freelance writer, aged 41]

Several individuals confirmed the line of analysis on these pages by describing how their "nervous breakdowns" reflected their inability to sustain normal appearances. Over and again, I heard some variation of "I just got really crippled, just emotionally not able to function." Hospitalization freed them from the struggle of appearing and acting normally. It is important, though, to keep the meaning of hospitalization in proper context. As helpful as it sometimes was to "safely crash," most persons agreed with the individual who said "the experience of hospitalization was devastating to me" and the several who reported that being hospitalized made them feel like "damaged goods." Whether people entered the hospital gladly or reluctantly, the experience was a pivotal "turning point in identity"[15] because "institutionalization" undeniably persuaded them of the seriousness of their condition and fostered a new self-definition as a "mental patient." Here, the point is that regardless of their overall assessment of hospitalization, respondents did find others who understood their experience. One respondent spoke for many when she commented that with others who are depressed "It's like [you] don't have to explain how [you're] breathing. Like [you] don't have to explain the smallest activity. They just got it. They understood."

The kind of empathy that is possible when someone is with fellow sufferers helps to explain the appeal of "self-help" groups. In some respects, the self-help revolution reflects the full-flowering of what Philip Rieff has termed the therapeutic culture.[16] In self-help groups people turn to others afflicted with the same personal troubles and try, through conversation, to heal themselves of what they perceive to be their shared problem. An illness rhetoric (often implying biological causation) is sometimes joined with a spiritual vocabulary (as in programs like Alcoholics Anonymous) positing that "recovery" requires surrendering to a higher power. Thus, the self-help phenomenon derives its allure, in part, by combining elements of therapy with elements of religion and science. Beyond this, a critical part of the appeal of self-help groups is the opportunity to be understood, to be with people who both comprehend each other's plight and remain nonjudgmental.

Stigma, Secrecy, and Self-Hatred

Beginning with Erving Goffman's[17] path-breaking formulation of the problem of stigma, social scientists[18] have studied how groups as diverse as divorced persons, those missing limbs, dwarfs, and the elderly manage information and adopt behavioral strategies that afford maximum protection of already tainted identities. Despite all the public education that has recently surrounded depression, sufferers know they have a condition that is conventionally defined as a mental illness. Thus, they fall into a category with a range of "others" who have what Goffman terms "blemishes of individual character." Possessing feelings that are simultaneously incomprehensible and unacceptable to others provides a powerful stimulus to secrecy. It is, therefore, not surprising that depressed people typically adopt "passing" strategies similar to others whose stigmatized conditions are not immediately visible.

> Of course, you could never tell anybody, because [of] the stigma. . . . Depression is a mental illness, Sssssh! Don't talk. Don't tell anybody. . . . Nobody talked because of the stigma attached, depression being a mental illness. [male salesman, aged 30]

All I know is that I could never run for political office (laughter). [male office clerk, part-time, aged 37]

I'm still afraid of people. I feel if I don't tell them [about my depression] I can never really become close to them. If I do tell them, then I feel further away. I'm really bogged down with it, and what happens is that I can't even make just fun friends because I need so much to talk to people and let everyone know about it, but I can't because it's just too damaging. [female house cleaner, aged 23]

I was just carrying it around. It never occurred to me to talk to anyone about it. . . . Yeah, I never told anybody what I was thinking then. I had this idea that it just wouldn't be acceptable (laughter). . . . I think that there's something of a taboo against talking about bad things or bad feelings. . . . I had this sense that if I told someone how I felt—what was going on— they'd take advantage of me. Or they'd try telling me that I was crazy or something like that. I had to maintain a facade so that people would treat me with respect. They wouldn't [treat me with respect] if they knew. [unemployed female, aged 35]

While self-management may simply take the form of keeping one's unacceptable identity secret, sociological literature is replete with examples of how stigmatized individuals attempt to foster more positive definitions of their situation. Certainly, one general function of subcultures among disvalued groups is to provide support for alternative, non-stigmatizing, definitions of their common circumstance. Such subcultures function minimally to sustain positive self-evaluations (sometimes self-pride) in the face of others' negative labeling. In addition, many groups have the larger agenda of responding to negative definitions with the aim of changing them.

To be sure, even individuals practicing behaviors considered utterly reprehensible by the vast majority in a society may collectively find ways to create a positive self-image and justify their life styles.

Although those with a range of mental illnesses have also entered the arena of "identity politics,"[19] depression is a unique case since the most critical assaults on self come from within. Those with depression may collectively want a greater public understanding of their "illness," but in the midst of an episode of depression individuals feel a self-hatred far greater than could possibly be expressed by others toward them. We have already seen that depression assumes a momentum as persons spiral downward into ever more profoundly difficult emotional feelings. In this process the dialectical intersection of self and society is most plainly seen.

The process begins with a range of bad feelings. Chief among them is that one possesses a deeply problematic self, a self that feels socially uncomfortable. At a point, it becomes a self deemed wholly unworthy of public presentation. Such feelings lead, as we have seen, to social withdrawal. Withdrawal, in turn, makes the performance of social functions difficult and sometimes impossible. The inability to meet social obligations expands the disdain and hatred people feel toward themselves, thus sustaining and extending the felt need to withdraw. In this way, depression is characterized by an ongoing and mutually reinforcing double stigmatization—by self and society. Nearly every respondent expressed the feelings of self-hatred that initially foster disconnection and are then exacerbated by isolation.

> [There was] a lot of self-monitoring, and a lot of self-doubt, and at its worst, self-hatred, sort of self-blame. If I was only such-and-such, then I wouldn't be feeling this way. [female physical therapist, aged 42]

And when I'm feeling shitty I think half the deal was that I felt so ashamed of myself that I couldn't do all these things that I should be doing to get out of this funk. That was half the battle. That was half the depression also. Like I should be able to go to a dance class, because I know that a dance class would get me out of it. But I can't get out of bed [and] so I'm a shit. This total self-hatred stuff. [unemployed female, aged 22]

I'm trying to remember now for you how it was. [It was] the inner self critic. The inner self-hatred. Depression is a lot about not having energy. [But] one place in my life where there was loads of energy was in the self-hatred. There was endless energy for that and it was a powerful energy. . . . I couldn't make contact with people. I was blaming myself, re-evaluating my whole life in the most negative kind of context. There was endless energy [for self-criticism]. I would just wake up doing it . . . [and] I would spend ten hours a day at it, just blaming myself. [male therapist, aged 45]

CONCLUSION

As the last several quotes illustrate, feelings about the nature of one's self are at the epicenter of the depression storm. Depressive feelings seem to emanate from and then reflect back on a self that is seen as somehow inadequate, improper, disliked, or damaged. For this reason alone, depression is a critical topic for social psychologists who are professionally interested in the social origins of selves and how they influence us in an ongoing way. The last phrase "in an ongoing way" is important because human selves are not fixed, determined, or static. Instead, they are constantly being revised as a result of our encounters with others.

I have shown that a large part of depression's isolation arises from the real or imagined responses of others. Once we conceive of the self as a process rather than a thing, we necessarily view illness identities as emerging over time. My account in Chapter 1 and the data in this chapter suggest that coming to see oneself as a depressed person may take several years. In fact, it has been estimated that only one in four persons suffering from clinical depression is ever diagnosed. Huge numbers of people are likely trudging through their lives with only the dimmest comprehension of how to think about their malaise. This book, of course, recounts only the histories of those who have come to label their trouble as depression. Readers ought, therefore, to keep in mind that my interviews constitute individuals' *reconstruction* of the past from the perspective of the present. Chapter 3 will show, however, that these histories reveal clear patterns in the evolution of an "illness identity."

I also meant for this chapter to display the value of a sociological approach to depression; that is, the utility of a perspective emphasizing how subjective illness experiences are shaped by one's embeddedness in various social worlds. The ability eventually to say "I am a depressed person" is often the product of a long journey aimed at discovering the kind of self one is. The acquisition of such an identity, moreover, has critical implications for how individuals decide to respond to their pain. In the next chapter I describe how the persons participating in this study came to the realization that they possess a sick self requiring medical treatment. The materials in Chapter 3 begin to explain how individuals come to accept medical versions of depression's cause and cure. In particular, I use the concept of "identity turning points" to think about the socially constructed character of depressive "illness."

Chapter 3

Illness and Identity

You know, I was a mental patient. That was my identity. . . .
Depression is very private. Then all of a sudden it becomes public
and I was a mental patient. . . . It's no longer just my own pain.
I am a mental patient. I am a depressive. *I am a depressive* [said
slowly and with intensity]. This is my identity. I can't separate
myself from that. When people know me they'll have to know
about my psychiatric history, because that's who I am.

Female graduate student, aged 24

At the time we spoke, Karen, whose words open this chapter, had
been doing well for more than two years, but described being
badly frightened by a recent two-week period during which the all-
too-familiar feelings of depression had begun to reappear. Aside
from the terror she felt at the prospect of becoming sick, Karen
realized that if depression returned, it would mean recasting her
identity yet again. After two years with nothing but the "normal"
ups and downs of life, she had started to feel that it might be possible to leave behind the mental patient identity she earlier thought
she never could shed. By the time of our interview, only her family
and a few old friends knew of her several hospitalizations. Her current roommates thought of her simply as Karen, one of about eight
students in the large house they shared. She told me, "No one in

my life right now knows . . . I'm so eager to talk to you about it [in this interview] because I can't talk about it with people." I said, "It must be hurtful not to be able to talk about so critical a part of your biography," and Karen responded, "Yes, but I don't want to test it with people. . . . [If I told them] they might not say anything, but their perception of me would change."

Karen was willing to be interviewed because I was one of those who knew about her history with depression. Years previously, while taking one of my undergraduate courses, she had confided that she was having a terrible time completing her course work. After much tentative discussion, the word depression finally entered the conversation. She seemed embarrassed by the admission until I opened my desk drawer and showed her a bottle of pills *I* was taking for depression. With this, we began to trade depression experiences and thereby formed the kind of bond felt by those who go through a common difficulty. As her undergraduate years passed, Karen came to my office periodically and during these visits we often spoke about depression. Our shared identity as depressed persons blurred the age and status distinctions that otherwise might have prevented our friendship. Like Nina's account in the last chapter, Karen's story is worth telling in brief because it so well reflects the more general process through which most of those interviewed eventually come to define themselves as depressed and then interpret the meaning of that identity.

Although we had shared thoughts often, my interview with Karen was the first time I heard her depression biography in a complete way. As the interview moved along, Karen also commented on the fact that it was the only time she herself had ever "recited the history." She occasionally had to pause, explaining "It is very hard [to recount these things]. It chokes me up. And when I recite the history [I realize] it's so fucked up." After another pause, she restated with emphasis, "What an awful history!" My interview with Karen was only the second for this project and I was, in fact, shocked by her account. Since the worst of my own depression did not happen until my early thirties, I was unprepared for descriptions of a childhood so pained that it included suicide attempts by early adolescence. Unfortunately, by the time all 50 interviews were completed, such stories no longer seemed unusual.

Like nearly everyone with whom I talked, Karen could pinpoint the beginning of her depression career. Although she described a "home filled with feelings of sadness" for as long as she could remember, it was, she said, "the beginning of the ninth grade that touched off . . . ten years of depression." She elaborated with the observation, "I was always sad or upset, but I was so busy and social [that the feelings were muted]. You know, things were not doing so well at home, but at school no one knew how much of a hellhole I lived in." She described a home life that was fairly stable until her father became ill when she was a sixth grader. "When he came back from the hospital," she said, "he was very different, unstable [and] extremely violent." Till then Karen had been able to keep the misery of her home life apart from her school world, which served as a refuge. By the ninth grade, however, she "could no longer keep the two worlds separate" and in both places the same intrusive questions, feelings, and ruminations colonized her mind. Now she didn't feel safe anywhere in the world and had these relentless thoughts: "I'm miserable. [There is] such a feeling of emptiness. What the hell am I doing? What is my life all about? What is the point?" "And that," she said, "basically started it."

In the ninth grade Karen had no word for the "it" that had started. When I asked whether she recognized her pain as depression then, she replied, "Did I say this was depression [then]?

Did I know [what it was]? It was pain, but I don't think I would have called it depression. I think I would have called it *my* pain." There was another factor that contributed to the anonymity of her misery and kept her pain from having a name—Karen was determined to keep her torment hidden. She said, "I lived with that for . . . a couple of years, from the ninth grade until the eleventh grade. [I lived] with that feeling. . . . But it was all very private. I kept it quiet. It was something inside. I didn't really talk about it. I might have talked about it with some of my friends, but no one understood."

During this time, though, a subtle transformation was taking place in her thinking about "it." Previously, Karen felt that her pain came exclusively from her difficulties at home, but by the eleventh grade she was beginning to suspect that its locus might be elsewhere. She told me, "My family life might have been hell, but it was always, 'Oh [I feel this way] because my father is crazy. It's because of something outside of me.' But it was the first time I'm feeling awful about myself." By the eleventh grade Karen's new consciousness was that there was something really wrong with *her*. Now, her feelings about the pain took a critical turn when she began to say to herself, "I can't live like this. I will not survive. I will not be here. I can't live with the pain. If I have to live with the pain I will eventually kill myself." Despite such a shift in thinking Karen still succeeded in keeping things private until she experienced a very public crisis. It was, moreover, a "crash" that she understood as a major "turning point" in her identity. Here's what she said:

> My whole family life just fell apart. There was no anchor. There was no anchor. . . . [Now] I was able to label it and say it was depression when I crashed in the eleventh grade and was hospitalized. You know, in ninth grade I told you about an experience

where I was conscious of feeling pain, or whatever, but no one else knew about it. . . . It is sort of like what my life is like now. I couldn't tell people about it. How can you tell people about it? What do you say? . . . But then it was like the two worlds just crashed in the eleventh grade. I did not want to be hospitalized because that meant for me [that] I could no longer deny that I was depressed. Everyone knew it. Everyone in my class . . . And I was a mental patient. . . . And I'll tell you, that depression in the eleventh grade . . . it came to a head and I have never crashed so much. First of all, landing in a hospital, going into a hospital, in a way it was a relief because I didn't have to have that pretense. I really could crash. For three days I didn't even get out of that bed. I just remember being like in the fetal position. I wanted to die. It was like dying.

Then the interview turned to a lengthy discussion about psychiatric hospitals, doctors, and power—all of it negative. She expressed hostility toward doctors who wanted her to "open up" and toward institutional rules that seemed authoritarian and arbitrary. She said, "Psychiatrists and mental health workers have the power to decide when you are going to leave, if you're going to leave, if you can go out on a pass, if you're good, if you're not good." This first hospitalization (eventually there would be four) also started a long history with medications of all sorts. When I asked whether she was treated with medications she replied, "Yup, always medication. That's the big thing. . . . Oh my God, I've had so many. . . . I don't think they really affected me that much. By the time I left I was doing okay. Did I have these problems solved? No, [but] I had an added one. Now I felt crazy." I used Karen's observation about "feeling crazy" as a cue for asking if she had a disease. I said, "Did you now think of yourself as having an illness in the medical sense?" and her answer reflected the ambivalence and confusion I would later routinely hear when I asked this same question of others.

> I think of it less as an illness and more something that society defines. That's part of it, but then, it is physical. Doesn't that make it an illness? That's a question I ask myself a lot. Depression is a special case because everyone gets depressed. . . . I think that I define it as not an illness. It's a condition. When I hear the term illness I think of sickness . . . [but] the term mental illness seems to me to be very negative, maybe because I connect it with hospitalization. . . . I connect it with how people define people who have been hospitalized. I see so many people in psychiatric facilities . . . that are just like you and me. What makes them any different is just a diagnosis. Sometimes the diagnosis can make people sicker. Sometimes the diagnosis can keep people there, you know. Yuh, I had a physical problem. Yuh, it affects my emotions. It's something that I can deal with. It's something that I can live with. I don't have to define it as a problem. But the thing about mental illness is that it lasts. . . . Once a diagnosis always a diagnosis. And that's what I was saying [earlier] that it has only been within the last two years that I have been able to say, "I'm something beyond being mentally ill."

Before it ended, my interview with Karen covered other difficult emotional terrain, including a major suicide attempt, additional periods of hospitalization, stays in halfway houses, a traumatic college experience, failed relationships with therapists, job interviews that required lies about health history, and a personal spiritual transformation. As indicated at the outset, things had gotten better by the time of our interview and Karen believed she was pretty much past her problem with depression. She told me, "A couple of years ago, three years ago, four years ago, I would feel a need to tell people about it because I still felt depressed, because I still felt mentally ill. But now I no longer see myself in that way. I'm other things. I'm Karen the grad student. I'm Karen the one who loves to garden, the one who's interested in a lot of things. I'm not just Karen the mentally ill person." Still, such optimism about being past depression was sometimes distressingly eroded by periods of bad feelings and the ever-present edge of fear that "it" might return in its full-blown, most grotesque form.

THE SOCIAL CONSTRUCTION
OF ILLNESS IDENTITIES

Karen's illness biography, even briefly documented, previews many of the issues that, as a sociologist, I find conceptually interesting and practically significant about illness in general and depression in particular. Especially insightful is her comment that depression is something of a "special case" because, as she put it, "everyone gets depressed." Indeed, the phrase "I'm so depressed," is so common in everyday discourse that one might presume depression to be a normal rather than a pathological condition. Sigmund Freud himself raised the question of "normal pain" with his often quoted observation that the purpose of psychotherapy was to "transform hysterical misery into everyday unhappiness." While no one can doubt that Karen suffered greatly, her experience, like my own and everyone else's in this study, raises the very difficult question, "Just when does the discomfort inevitably a part of living become acute enough to call it a disease?" As a sociologist inclined to see reality as a "social construction,"[1] I assume that the answer to the question is surely as much political and cultural as it is medical.

In the first chapter I mentioned, nearly in passing, that during the 1960s and 1970s there was an "anti-psychiatry movement" in the social sciences that saw mental illness as essentially an arbitrary political label. Those who made the argument were plainly committed to a radically relativistic epistemology. Their view, similar actually to those who today call themselves postmodernists, was that what we accept as social fact—in this case the factuality of mental illness—is nothing more that the result of one or another powerful group successfully instituting its particular version of reality. Such a view led to the claim that mental illness is an illusion; that there is no such thing as mental illness.

Certainly the Russian government's definition, until the breakup of the Soviet Union, that anyone who publicly disagreed with the state's version of communism was *insane* and properly confined to a Siberian prison, shows the intimate connection between definitions of sanity and political ideology.[2] I am also persuaded by the demonstrated arbitrariness of the diagnostic categories in the medical "bible" of psychiatric disorders, *The Diagnostic and Statistical Manual of Mental Disorders* (DSM-IV), that much of what we call mental illness is nothing more than a political designation sold as science.[3]

Attention to the connection between definitions of illness and power is more than an interesting theoretical issue since illness labels can have profound consequences for individuals. Even when there is no dispute about the presence of disease, as in the case of AIDS, the treatment of those afflicted is inseparable from fears, prejudices, and moral evaluations that have an exclusively social origin. The role of social expectations and

human judgments is, of course, even greater when there is no demonstrable biological pathology for the human conditions and
behaviors termed illness. This is what makes the case of mental
illness so especially fuzzy and warrants deep concern about the
exclusive legitimacy of psychiatry to decide who shall be labeled
mentally ill and how they ought best be treated. Such reservations seem well-advised in light of what has been justified historically in the name of science and psychiatric medicine. Those
deemed mentally ill have, at different moments in history, been
subject to castration, involuntary incarceration, bloodletting,
brutal "electric shock" treatments, mind-numbing drugs in-
ducing permanent neurological damage, and a variety of brain
surgeries.[4]

My own view is that sociological critiques of psychiatry have
merit. At the same time, I think the anti-psychiatry theorists un-
dercut their credibility by taking their argument too far. To flatly
claim that mental illness does not exist seems nonsensical when
people are catatonic, visibly psychotic, or otherwise unable to understand or carry out even the most rudimentary behaviors necessary to function in a society. But my purpose in this chapter is
not to resolve debates about the reality of mental illness. I would
rather stick with verifiable lines of analysis that arise out of my
interview materials. Narratives like Karen's allow me to trace the
way individuals eventually perceive they have a "problem" with
something called depression. In other words, I can describe how
depression became a reality for those who spoke to me.

The remainder of this chapter is about how people come to
decide that their pain is pathological; that they suffer from a level
of misery requiring medical intervention. Put differently, this
chapter is about the way in which a depression identity comes
into being and evolves over time. As Karen's story suggests, and

other data will illustrate, a depression consciousness arises in an extraordinarily patterned way. It is, therefore, possible to analyze the depression experience as a "career" sequence characterized by distinctive identity transformations.

A CAREER VIEW OF THE DEPRESSION EXPERIENCE

As in many areas of social life, the notion of career seems an extremely useful, sensitizing concept. In his voluminous and influential writings on work, Everett Hughes showed the value of conceptualizing career as "the moving perspective in which the person sees his life as a whole and interprets the meanings of his various attitudes, actions, and the things which happen to him."[5] Hughes' definition directs attention to the subjective aspects of the career process and the ways in which people attach evaluative meanings to the typical sequence of movements constituting their career path. Here I shall be concerned with describing the career features associated with an especially ambiguous illness—depression.

Hughes' definition also suggests that each stage,[6] juncture, or moment in a career requires a redefinition of self. The depression experience is a heuristically valuable instance for studying the intersection of careers and identities. The following data analysis illustrates that much of the depression career is caught up with assessing self, redefining self, reinterpreting past selves, and attempting to construct a future self that will "work" better. Although all careers require periodic reassessments of self, illness careers are especially characterized by critical "turning points" in identity. In his discussion of identity transformations, Anselm

Strauss[7] comments on the intersection of career and identity turning points:

> In transformations of identities a person becomes something other than he or she once was. Such shifts necessitate new evaluations of self and others, of events, acts, and objects. . . . Transformation of perception is irreversible; once having changed there is no going back. One can look back, but evaluate only from the new status. . . . Certain critical incidences occur to force a person to recognize that "I am not the same as I was, as I used to be." These critical incidents constitute turning points in the onward movement of persons' careers.

The shape, predictability, and duration of different career paths vary considerably. For example, those following organizational careers may be provided with very clear formal and informal time clocks detailing where they "ought" to be in their careers at different ages.[8] Consequently, those pursuing such organizational careers can clearly feel that they are "on time," "off time," or even "running out of time." While the experiences of the respondents point to clear regularities in the sequencing of the depression experience, people differ considerably in the length of time they spend in any particular phase. For instance, some respondents describe years of discomfort before they even arrive at the definition of themselves as depressed; others move through the sequence described below in only a few years. To a large degree, of course, such variations depend on whether "acute" depression first occurs in childhood, as it did for Karen, or later, as in my life, and whether the depression is characterized by plainly defined episodes or greater chronicity. In my analysis, some attention is paid, as well, to the social and structural features of peoples' lives that influence their ability to recognize, to name, and to respond to their "problem."

While there is considerable variation in the timing of events, all the respondents in this study described a process remarkably similar to the one implicit in Karen's account. Every person I interviewed moved through these identity turning points in their view of themselves and their problem with depression:

1. A period of *inchoate feelings* during which they lacked the vocabulary to label their experience as depression.
2. A phase during which they conclude that *something is really wrong with me.*
3. A *crisis stage* that thrusts them into a world of therapeutic experts.
4. A stage of *coming to grips with an illness identity* during which they theorize about the cause(s) for their difficulty and evaluate the prospects for getting beyond depression.

Each of these career moments assumes and requires redefinitions of self.

Inchoate Feelings

As mentioned in Chapter 2, the ages of respondents in this study range from the early twenties to the middle sixties. All these people described a period of time during which they had no vocabulary for naming their problem. Many traced feelings of emotional discomfort to ages as young as three or four, although they could not associate their feelings with something called "depression" until years later. It was typical for respondents to go for long periods of time feeling different, uncomfortable, marginal, ill-at-ease, scared, and in pain without attaching the notion of depression to their situations. A sampling of comments indicating an inchoate, obscure experience includes these:

> Well, I knew I was different from other children. I should say that from a very early age it felt like I had this darkness about me. Sort of shadow of myself. And I always had the sense that it wasn't going to go away so easily. And it was like my battle. And so, from a very early age I felt okay, "There's something going on here, [but] don't ask me for a word [for it]." It hurts me. I feel sad. My parents can't give me as much as I [would have] liked them to. And there was a feeling of helplessness in some ways. I knew that I was too young to understand what was going on. And I knew that when I got older I would understand things. There was always that sense that I would. [female travel agent, aged 41]

> An awareness that was more intellectual was apparent to me about my sophomore year in high school, when I'd wake up depressed and drag myself to school. . . . I didn't know that's what it was. I just knew that I had an awful hard time getting out of bed and a hard time making my bed and a hard time, you know, getting myself to school. . . . I kind of just had the feeling that something wasn't right. . . . [It was] just like a constant knot in my stomach. But I didn't think that that was anxiety. I just thought I wasn't feeling good, you know (laughing). [unemployed disabled female, aged 39]

> If I think about it, I really can't pinpoint a moment [when I was aware that I was depressed]. . . . It was just something I felt I was living with or had to live through, and maybe that goes back as far as graduate school. [male professor, aged 48]

Most of those reporting bad feelings from a early age could not conclude that something was "abnormal" because they had no baseline of normalcy for comparison. As might be expected, several respondents in this sample came from what they now describe as severely dysfunctional family circumstances, often characterized by alcoholism and both physical and emotional abuse. These individuals described feeling unsafe at home and often devised strategies to spend as much time as they could elsewhere. Some took refuge in the homes of friends. One man, described in Chapter 2, made a point of becoming friendly with the school custodians so that he could extend the school day in their company. Another woman went to the library every day after school where "the librarian got to know me . . . and started to look out for me." These children knew they were uncomfortable at home but still did not have wide enough experience to see their lives as unusual.

For most respondents the phase of inchoate feelings was the longest in the eventual unfolding of their illness consciousness. Particularly salient in terms of personal identity is the fact that initial definitions of their problem centered on the "structural conditions" of their lives instead of on the structure of their selves. The focus of interpretation was on the situation rather than on the self. Their emerging definition was that escape from the situation would make things right. Over and again individuals recounted fantasies of escape from their families and often from the community in which they grew up. However, initially at least, they felt trapped without a clear notion of how the situation might change.

> I remember from like five, starting to subtract five from eighteen, to see how many years I have left before I could get out [of the house]. So, I would say the overwhelming feeling was that I felt powerless. I felt a lot of things early. And I felt that

I was stuck in this house and these people controlled me, and there wasn't anything I could do about it, and I was stuck there. So I just started my little chart at about four and a half or five, counting when I could get out. [female baker, aged 41]

The only thing that I thought about was, "Well, my family's got problems and the stress of that is getting to me. So I've got to get myself out of bed, make my bed, get dressed, have breakfast, and get to school. And then at least I can escape this and I don't have to deal with it until I come home. And I just kind of concentrated on "I have to get to college because if I go to college that means I can get out of here." [unemployed disabled female, aged 39]

I felt sort of overwhelmed by the situation, and I was kind of sad that I was living the way I was living, and I didn't quite know how to get myself out of it . . . I guess a sense of feeling trapped. I think it was a recognition that this was not the way I wanted to live, but also the fact that I did not know how to get myself out of it. So it was feeling kind of trapped and kind of panicky. Now what do I do? [female nurse, aged 37]

When I was in college I moved up to the third floor in our house. It was the attic, but it had always been an apartment and we painted it up. And that was literally very good, but I think it was also symbolic. Since I commuted to school, this was still a way that I was away. I could close that door downstairs and when I was very young I would go to my grandparents for the weekend. . . . And I think that is one of the ways I coped then. [female librarian, aged 43]

Not everyone, of course, described his or her childhood as unhappy. However, even when ill feelings did not emerge until later in life, individuals initially chalked up their difficulty to their immediate life circumstances. A professor viewed his struggle to gain tenure as the source of his malaise. A 27-year-old man at first saw his bad feelings as resulting exclusively from an unstable occupational situation. Another woman thought that her feelings of depression would go away once she got over a failed relationship. A business deal gone sour was defined as precipitating depression in another case. And so on. In each of these instances, people held the view that as soon as the situation changed their discomfort would also disappear.

Therefore, a decisive juncture in the evolution of a "sickness" self-definition occurs when the circumstances individuals perceive as troubling their lives change, but mood problems persist. The persistence of problems in the absence of the putative cause requires a redefinition of what is wrong. A huge cognitive shift occurs when people come to see that the problem may be internal instead of situational; when they conclude that something is likely wrong with *them* in a manner that transcends their immediate situation.

Something Is Really Wrong with Me

In 1977, Robert Emerson and Sheldon Messinger published a paper entitled "The Micro-Politics of Trouble"[9] that analyzes the regular processes through which individuals come to see a personal difficulty as sufficiently troublesome a problem that something ought to be done about it. The materials offered in this chapter affirm the general process they describe. The process begins with a state of affairs initially "experienced as difficult, unpleasant, irritating, or unendurable."[10] At first, sufferers try an informal remedy, which sometimes works. If it doesn't, they seek another remedy. The decision that a consequential problem exists warranting a formal remedy typically follows a "recurring cycle of trouble, remedy, failure, more trouble, and a new remedy, until the trouble stops or the troubled person forsakes further efforts."[11] Here, then, is their description of the transformation from vague, inchoate feelings to a clearer sense that one is sufficiently troubled to seek a remedy.

> Problems originate with the recognition that something is wrong and must be remedied. Trouble, in these terms, involves both definitional and remedial components. . . . On first apprehension troubles often involve little more than vague unease. . . . An understanding of the problem's dimensions may only begin to emerge as the troubled person thinks about them, discusses the matter with others, and begins to implement remedial strategies.[12]

Despite the difficulties they have in naming their feelings as a problem, all of the respondents eventually conclude that something is *really wrong* with *them*. To be sure, many used identical phrases in describing their situations. The phrases "something was really wrong with me" and "I felt that I could no longer live like this" were repeated over and over. Respondents commented in nearly identical ways on the heightened feeling that "something is really wrong with me."

> When it really became apparent that I was just a mess was in January of 1989. I made the decision really quickly at the end of 1988 to go to school at [names a four year college] and live with my father and my stepmother and commute. And I packed up all my stuff in my car and went. I was miserable. I cried every day. Every single day I cried. I think I went to two classes [at the new school] and lasted there only a month. I was absolutely

miserable. There was a lot of different factors that were involved with it [but] I just didn't feel right. There was something wrong with me, you know. [unemployed female, aged 23]

I guess it's the fall of 90 when I had done the family therapy. I felt great about that. I was back at Harvard. My work was going okay. I loved myself. I loved my husband. Everything was great. [But] I wanted to die. I had no pleasure in anything. What finally got me [was that] I looked at the trees turning and I didn't care. I couldn't believe it. I'd be looking at this big flaming maple and I'd look at it and I'd think, "There it is, it's a maple tree. It's bright orange and red." And nothing in me was touched. At that point I went back to my therapist and said, "There's something really wrong here." [female software quality control manager, aged 31]

Well, you know, you sort of get immobilized. You can't go to work. That's when it starts hitting you [that something is really wrong]. You're not sleeping or you're sleeping all the time. That kind of says something to you. [unemployed male waiter, aged 33]

As mentioned earlier, a professor who had struggled to get tenure no longer had an account for his bad feelings:

Getting tenure was a big struggle and, you know, in a way it sort of muffled over these other things. Now [after getting tenure] I no longer had a crutch. I couldn't justify my feelings to myself. I had nothing to worry about in a sense. These feelings, their origin, must have been something else than the need for tenure. [male professor, aged 48]

And others observed:

I felt vaguely responsible for my mother and my brother and I guess I knew there was something wrong. ... Something was just really wrong and I guess that was the beginning of the struggle ... *the recognition that something was wrong with me ... it wasn't just my mother.* [female college professor, aged 49, my emphasis]

Probably my experience at that time was that there was something not right with me. As I look back on it, basically, you know, one of the struggles is like, *is it really me or is it them?* I mean, that's still a struggle, really *knowing in your gut that there is something wrong with me.* ... Definitely something is not right, you know. [female physical therapist, aged 42, my emphasis]

These quotes suggest a fundamental transformation in perception and identity at this point in the evolution of a depression consciousness. Respondents now located the source of their problem as somewhere within their bodies and minds, as deep within themselves. Such a belief implies a problematic identity far more basic and immutable than those associated with social statuses. If, for example, someone has a disliked occupational identity, the possibilities for occupational change exist. If the occupational identity becomes onerous enough, it is possible to quit a job. Similarly, without minimizing the difficulties of change, we can choose to become single if married, to change from one religion to another, and, these days, even to change our sex if the motivation is great enough. However, to see oneself as somehow internally flawed poses substantially greater problems for identity change or remediation because one's whole personhood is implicated. Getting rid of a sick self poses far greater problems than dropping certain social statuses. The important point here is that the rejection of situational theories for bad feelings is a critical identity turning point. Full acceptance that one has a damaged self requires acknowledgment that "I am not the same as I was, as I used to be."

Another important dimension of the career process that becomes apparent at this point is the issue of whether to keep the problem private or to make it public, especially to family and friends The private/public distinction was a dominant theme in respondents' talk throughout the history of their experience with depression. The question of being private or public is, of course, central to one's developing self-identification. As Peter Berger and Hansfried Kellner[13] point out in describing the "social construction of marriage" and Diane Vaughan[14] indicates in analyzing the process of "uncoupling" from a relationship, the moment a new status becomes public is a definitive one in solidifying a person's new identity. In the cases of both creating and disengaging from relationships, people are normally very careful not to make public announcements until they are certain they are ready to adopt new statuses and identities. The significance attached to public announcements of even modest shifts in life style is indicated by the considerable thought people sometimes give to making public such relatively benign decisions as going on diets or quitting cigarettes.

Decisions about "going public" are, of course, greatly magnified when the information to be imparted is negative and, in the case of emotional problems, potentially stigmatizing. As Emerson and Messinger note, the search for a remedy necessarily involves sharing information with others. Still, at this early juncture of dealing with bad feelings, most respondents elected to keep silent about their pain. As discussed in Chapter 2, both the stigma attached to mental illness and what respondents perceived to be the inherent incommunicability of their internal experience kept them quiet. In one case, however, silence was the only politically acceptable choice. A man who spent many years as part of the resistance movement in South Africa said:

> I didn't have the chance to talk about it [feeling depressed] because people around me were so occupied and absorbed in the struggle. I always felt that if I articulated all these problems . . . they would sort of ridicule me; that I'm just panicking or sort of a nervous wreck. So these thoughts kept me from expressing the feelings. . . . They noticed my nervous tension, especially in the face of police questioning. I often broke down easily. It was unbecoming of a revolutionary, as they put it. [unemployed male bookkeeper, aged 51]

Whether or not they made their feelings public, this second phase of their illness career involved the recognition that they possessed a self that was working badly in *every* situation. Although everyone continued to identify the kinds of social situations that had caused their bad feelings in the past and precipitated them in the present, the qualitative change at this juncture was in the locus of attention from external to internal causes. At this point respondents were struggling to live their lives in the face of debilitating pain. This stage ended, however, when efforts to control things became impossible.

At some point everyone interviewed experienced a crisis of some sort. For the majority (29) the crisis meant hospitalization. At the point of crisis, whatever their wishes might have been, they could not prevent their situation from becoming public knowledge to family, friends, and co-workers. Whether they were hospitalized or not, everyone reached a point where they felt obliged to rely on psychiatric experts to deal with their difficulty. Receiving an "official" diagnosis of depression and consequent treatment with medications greatly accelerated the need to redefine their past, present, and future in illness terms. The crisis solidified the emerging consciousness that the problem was within themselves. More than that, it was now a problem beyond their own efforts to control.

Crisis

Nearly everyone could pinpoint the precise time, situation, or set of events that moved them from the recognition that something was wrong to the realization that they were desperately sick. They could often remember in vivid detail the moment when things absolutely got out of hand.

> So I went to law school in the fall. I was at Columbia and in the best of times Columbia is a depressing place. I mean, it's a shithole. And you know, I was pretty messed up when I got there . . . I remember Columbia was a nightmare. . . . So, I was getting to the point where I was paranoid about going to class and so someone talked to the dean and said, "Hey, you've got to do something about this guy, he's off the deep edge." [male administrator, aged 54]

> I think the significant moment was when I got stage fright in high school. There were earlier moments when I felt something was wrong. I can remember feeling real dizzy when I was on the stage in the 8th grade. But the significant moment was in high school and I was seized by just pure terror. And the fear was so horrible that I couldn't tell it to anybody. I couldn't share it. It was something beyond my ability to communicate. It was so horrible that no one could understand it. [male professor, aged 66]

> I'll never forget it as long as I live, when I got fired and I went and picked up my last paycheck. I was looking at it and I could just

feel my pupils were dilating. I could feel the physiological difference in who I was. What is this? What is this? And I remember calling my parents. I remember telling them I had lost my job and I just started crying there. [unemployed male waiter, aged 33]

There was this horrifying moment when I realized the back [problem] would get better, but that would not necessarily lift the depression. It had a life of its own. And what I saw basically recast my whole life until that moment. [male therapist, aged 45]

Well, when it came on so strong was . . . about the second week of school, my senior year. . . . I had this pain in my head like an ice cream headache that I'd developed when I was about a sophomore in high school. You know, when you get too much ice cream and you get this sharp pain. And nobody could find anything. I thought it was my eyes. And then they took out wisdom teeth thinking that might be it. Nothing. And just the bottom fell [out]. It's like I was catching pneumonia. You know, I just went right down the slide into depression. It was like an agitated depression. I couldn't eat. I couldn't sleep. You know, [I was] just crying uncontrollably. I had no idea what the hell [was going on]. [unemployed male, aged 58]

My husband would drive, we'd drive together, and he would be ready to drop me off on his way into to work. . . . I would sit in the car and try to nerve myself up to get out the door and force myself up the stairs [to work]. . . . Like I would freeze, and be unable to move. And I'd say "Okay, I'm going to open the door now," and I'd look at my hand, and say "I'm going to make my hand move to the door handle and open it," and it wouldn't go! And so I'd actually have to pick it up with my other hand and put it on the door handle. . . . And then I'd force myself up the stairs. And I couldn't do it everyday. So I'd just start to scream and rock back and forth. So things got very bad at that point. I began to want to try to hurt myself [female software quality control manager, aged 31]

At the crisis point, people fully enter a therapeutic world of hospitals, mental health experts, and medications. For many, entrance into this world is simultaneous with first receiving the "official" diagnosis of depression.[15] It is difficult to overstate the critical importance of official diagnoses and labeling. The point of diagnosis was a double-edged benchmark in the illness career. On the one hand, knowing that you "have" something that doctors regard as a specific illness imposes definitional boundaries onto an array of behaviors and feelings that previously had no name. Acquiring a clear conception of what one has and having a label to attach to confounding feelings and behaviors was especially significant to those who had gone for years without being able to name their situation. To be diagnosed also suggests the possibility that the condition can be treated and that one's suffering can be diminished. At the same time, being a "depressive" places one in the devalued category of those with mental illness. On the negative side, respondents made comments like these:

I kept going to doctor after doctor, getting like all these new terms put on me. . . . My family was dysfunctional and I was an alcoholic with an eating disorder and bulimia and depression and it was just all these labels. "Oh my God!" [unemployed female, aged 22]

My father went to his allergy doctor who referred us to a guy who turned out to be a reasonable psychiatrist. I'll never forget. He said, "Your daughter is clinically depressed." I remember sitting in his office. He saw us on a Saturday like at six o'clock. He did us a favor. And I remember I just sat there. It was a sort of darkened office. It was the first time I ever cried in front of anybody. [female social worker, aged 38]

And on the liberating side:

> They gave me a blood test that measures the level of something in the blood, in the brain. And they pronounced me, they said "Mr. Smith [a pseudonym], you're depressed." And I said "Thank God," you know. I wasn't as batty as I thought. It was like the cat was out of the bag. You know? It was a breakthrough. . . . [Before that] depression wasn't in my vocabulary. . . . It was the beginning of being able to sort out a lifetime of feelings, events . . . my entire life. It was the chance for a new beginning. [male salesman, aged 30]

> It [getting a diagnosis] was a great relief. I said, "You mean there is something wrong with me. Its not some sort of weird complex mental thing." I was like tying myself up in knots trying to figure out what strange mechanism in my mind was producing unhappiness from this set of circumstances. . . . It's like, "No, you're sick! (sigh) There was an enormous relief. [female software quality control manager, aged 31]

It is impossible to consider the kinds of profound identity changes occasioned by any mental illness without paying special attention to the experience of hospitalization. It is one thing to deal alone with the demons of depression, or to privately see a psychiatrist for the problem, but once a person "shuts down" altogether and seeks asylum or is involuntarily "committed," he or she adds an institutional piece to their biography that is indelible. Social scientists have properly given a great deal of attention to the identity consequences of hospitalization for mental illness.[16]

A dramatic experiment that speaks directly to the matter of labeling in psychiatric hospitals is D. L. Rosenhan's study entitled "On Being Sane in Insane Places."[17] To find out whether the sane can be distinguished from the insane, he had eight colleagues pose as "pseudopatients" and apply for admission to 12 different mental hospitals. None of the eight had any history of mental illness, but they were told to present themselves at the hospital admission offices complaining that they had been hearing voices. With the exception of that one lie, they were to tell the truth about all other aspects of their lives. Once admitted, they were to say they were feeling fine and no longer experiencing the symptoms. They were to arrange their own releases by convincing the staff, through their behaviors, that they were sane.

The experimenters were easily and immediately admitted, all but one with the diagnosis of schizophrenia. Their subsequent show of sanity could not convince the staff that these "patients" were fakes, however. The only ones who ever questioned their status as real patients were the other patients on the ward. Once they had been officially diagnosed as schizophrenic, there was nothing the experimenters could do to shake the label. In fact, the staff interpreted everything they did in terms of the label. The social scientists made written notes on what they were seeing and experiencing, for example. After they were discharged, they learned from the nurses' records that their note-taking was considered "obsessive," and "engaging in writing behavior" had been interpreted as evidence of their illness.

After hospitalization periods ranging from 7 to 52 days, the pseudopatients were discharged with a diagnosis of schizophrenia "in remission," but in the institution's view they were not sane and had not been since they applied for admission. Rosenhan concluded that "once a person is designated abnormal all of his other behaviors and characteristics are colored by that label."[18] He offers this conclusion about "the stickiness of psychodiagnostic labels":

> A psychiatric label has a life and an influence of its own. Once the impression has been formed that the patient is schizophrenic, the expectation is that he will continue to be schizophrenic. . . . Such labels, conferred by mental health professionals, are as influential on the patient as they are on his relatives and friends, and it should not surprise anyone that the diagnosis acts on all of them as a self-fulfilling prophecy. Eventually, the patient himself accepts the diagnosis, with all its surplus meanings and expectations, and behaves accordingly.[19]

A few interviewees described the hospital as truly an asylum that provided relief and allowed them to "crash." Being hospitalized enabled them to give up the struggle of trying to appear and act normally. One person, in fact, described the hospital as a "wonderful place" where "I was taken care of, totally taken care of." Another was relieved "to go somewhere where I won't do anything to myself, where I can get in touch with this." Someone else explained, "I was glad to be there, definitely. It was a break from everything." Sometimes people were glad to be hospitalized since it provided dramatic and definitive evidence that something was really wrong with them when family and friends had been dismissing their complaints. More usual, though, were the responses like that of the person who said that "the experience of hospitalization was devastating to me" and the several who reported that being hospitalized made them feel like "damaged goods."

Of all the tough things associated with depression, nothing would frighten me more than hospitalization. Along with the social science ethnographies that have been done over the years describing the deplorable and dehumanizing character of mental hospitals, I have seen Frederick Wiseman's incredibly distressing documentary, *Titicutt Follies,* which portrays the brutally awful conditions in a Massachusetts State Hospital during the 1960s. No doubt things have generally improved since the years when Hollywood could portray asylums as "snake pits" run by mean-spirited, authoritarian personalities like Big Nurse in *One Flew Over the Cuckoo's Nest.* As well, the "deinstitutionalization" process beginning in the 1970s resulted in the closing of many of the country's worst hospitals. Still, recent books on the hospitalization experience[20] and the sometimes gruesome stories I heard during interviews greatly strengthen my resolve never to go into a hospital.

I found particularly chilling Sam's account. Sam was a person I first met at a depression support group. At age 58, he seemed anxious to recount what hospital treatment was like "before they even had antidepressants." I knew from our previous casual conversation and his distinctive accent that Sam had grown up in the South. During the interview I learned more about his religious upbringing. His father had been a minister and his mother, although a stern figure, "was dependable." Sam first became sick enough to be hospitalized when he was a high school senior. He remembers that after his two-month stay, "You went back with the stigma on you because people who went off their rocker went to [names a state hospital]. You know how kids are. They make jokes about crazy people. . . . The cops also knew about this and had me marked down as a crazy person from then on." However, it wasn't remembrance of his return home that startled me. I could barely listen to his description of the hospitalization itself. Although Sam did not blame anyone for his treatment, saying, "It's not that they were cruel or anything. They just didn't know," I could not imagine being a 17-year-old and living through an experience like Sam's. Here, in some detail, is what he told me.

When were you first hospitalized?

You know, I'm looking back on it. I had never even heard the word (depression). In 1952 there was no literature. There were no medications. You got ECT and CO_2 treatments and insulin shocks.

What's CO_2?

It's when they put a mask on your face and give you carbon dioxide. . . . You're not getting enough oxygen, so it causes you to go into some sort of shock.

God, I never heard about that one before.

It's like suffocating. That's the first thing they did to me. I remember thinking, "My God, they're trying to kill me for being sad." This is at [names a university hospital]. Not pleasant. . . . And I had ECT before they put you out. . . . They gave it to you straight. No anesthesia.

No anesthesia?

You lie there and they put the electrodes on your head. . . . It's like waiting to be electrocuted. I can't put it any other way. You're leaning back, looking, and they got the machine over there and they throw the switch and I don't think you feel anything or know anything. It just knocks you out instantly. But, waitin' for it. . . . I'm not a scared person. There's not too many things that I'm afraid of, but that's one. I'll admit to that. And the woman who held the electrodes had a face that Dracula would kill to get. Ooh, she looked a lot worse than Elsa Lanchester in the *Bride of Frankenstein*. I'll never forget that. And you'd see the guy next to you getting it, and the grand mal seizure, and snorting, and they'd turn blue and purple. You'd see them go by in the beds right after they had it, and believe me people looked like a drowning case. And you're next, you know. It was not good. It's pretty awful. I remember waking up and you just had been talking to some nurse or something, but you can't remember her name for the life [of you]. You wake up and see them, but you don't know what things are. And then it eventually comes back . . . "Oh yeah, its the ceiling." And stuff starts to come back, short-term things come back. But, you know, you have to work hard for the names.

I don't want to recreate this for you . . .

Oh, yeah! I finally just couldn't take it anymore and I finally said "I'm not going to take anymore" after I had, I don't know, ten or eleven of these. These days you get about three a week. But [then] they had treatment days and I was a mess.

We're talking about the first time you got this treatment now?

No, I'm talking about the second time now. The first time wasn't as bad. The second time was worse. And it was beginning to look, you know, like this was going to be my lot for awhile. They had this extra long bed for me since I was so tall, and it had like chunks out of the wheel, so when they'd roll this bed down the hall the wheel would go "clunk, clunk, clunk, clunk." I'll never forget that [sound]. So anyway, one day I finally said, "I'm not going to take these." I knew they were going to get a bunch of people and make me do it anyway. But I just couldn't . . .

It must have been hard in those days to say no. Patients had to submit?

Yeah, you didn't do that [say no]. So, I was coming back from playing Ping Pong with this black orderly I was close to and there was a door off to the side. I didn't even know where it went to. But it was a little three-room suite where the hard cases went. And they like opened that and surrounded me. Well, I could have fought, you know. But I didn't have anything against this guy. He was just doing his job. So, I went in there and they gave me a treatment right there. [unemployed male, aged 58]

Although Sam's story was the most disturbing I heard, many of the 29 people who spoke of their time in hospitals spontaneously acknowledged the extraordinary impact of the experience on the way they thought about themselves. Sometimes they were themselves shocked that they had landed in a hospital. Several mentioned that hospitalization caused them to confront for the first time just how sick they were.

I remember being put onto the floor that was probably for the worst people of the sickness, because it was one of those floors where everything was really locked up. So I guess I was in pretty bad shape. [male administrator, aged 54]

So I went to [names hospital] and I remember praying that I would get out. To me it seemed at the time as if the door would close—It was a secure facility—and I would never leave. I know I'm a basket case at this point. . . . The experience of having that severe depression, going to the hospital, and most of all being given shock treatments. . . . It made me feel . . . like damaged goods, impaired in some way that I was just not normal. It did make me feel impaired. [male professor, part-time, aged 48]

Among the identity-related comments about the hospitalization experience, one set of observations, although made by only a few individuals, caught my attention. Once in the hospital these persons surveyed their environment, both the oppressive physical character of the place and the sad shape of their fellow "inmates," many of whom seemed to them destined for an institutionalized life. However awful their condition, these respondents made a distinction between their trouble and patients who were overtly psychotic. Unlike those unfortunates, they had a choice to make, as they saw it. Either they would capitulate completely to their depression and possibly, therefore, to a life in the mental health system or they would do whatever necessary to leave the hospital as quickly as possible.

Giving up completely did have some appealing features. Full surrender meant relief from an exhausting battle and absolution from personal responsibility. One woman said, "I saw these people going back and forth [in and out of the hospital] for their whole lives [and] that I could be one [of them]. If I went in that direction, it somehow absolved me from responsibility. And I teetered on the edge for a long time. It involved a conscious decision . . . [about whether] I'm going to become a [permanent] part of the system because it's safe and where I belong." Another person described giving up as seductive because "you don't have to go out there and live by the rules of life. You never have to go out and risk things because you're in a safe environment." In effect, hospitalization posed for these individuals a consequential identity choice; a kind of "to be or not to be" moment in which they would see themselves as either hopelessly mentally ill or as salvageable. The starkness of the choice is caught in the following comment.

> I spent a month there. . . . I saw people who really were insane. People who wanted to live their lives but had their lives constantly interrupted by having to come back here. And I saw what it was like to have my life taken away from me. Because for the first week or two they always keep you on a secure floor to make

sure you're not nuts enough to hurt yourself. Which at that time I wasn't. But, the unsecure floor where I was supposed to be promoted almost immediately was full up. I spent about ten days to two weeks on a secure floor with my sharps taken away from me. And having to be let in and out of the unit to go to lunch and dinner. And I think it sort of sank in that . . . I was going to have to redefine my choices. And that's what it took. It took being up against what it would be like to be an insane person. . . . [It was] seeing what being mentally ill was like, and saying, "This is not for me." [female software quality control manager, aged 31]

Another critical feature of this career juncture was the recommendation that as "patients" they ought to begin taking antidepressant medications. The meaning of taking medications will be the subject of Chapter 4. Right now, though, it should be noted that one outstanding uniformity in the interviews was the initially strong negative reaction people had to taking drugs. One person was "leery of it" and others variously described the idea of going on medications as "revolting," "certainly not my first choice," and "embarrassing." Others elaborated on the recommendation that they begin drug therapy in ways similar to the nurse who said: "I didn't want to be told that I had something that was going to affect the rest of my life and that could only be solved by taking pills. And there was sort of a rebellion in that: 'No, I'm not like that. I don't need you and your pills.'" Underneath these common responses was the shared feeling that taking drugs was yet another distressing indication of the severity of a problem they could not control by themselves. The concurrent events of crisis, hospitalization, and beginning a drug regimen worked synergistically to concretize and dramatize respondents' status as patients with an illness that required ongoing treatment by therapeutic experts.

Coming to Grips with an Illness Identity

Whether people are hospitalized or not, involvement with psychiatric experts and medications is the transition point to a number of simultaneous processes, all with implications for the reformulation of identity. They are (1) reconstructing and reinterpreting one's past in terms of current experiences, (2) looking for causes for one's situation, (3) constructing new theories about the nature of depression, and (4) establishing modes of coping behavior. All of these activities require judgments about the appropriate metaphors for describing one's situation. Especially critical to ongoing identity construction is whether respondents approve of illness metaphors for describing their experience. A few individuals were clearly willing to define their condition as a mental illness:

> I know I have a mental illness. I'm beginning to feel that. [But] actually, there is a real relief in that. It's a sense of "Whew! Okay, I don't have to masquerade." I mean, sure I'll masquerade with work, because, listen, I've got to get the bread and butter on the table. But I don't have to masquerade in other ways. . . . It's sort of like mentally ill people in some ways . . . are my people. There is a fair amount of really chronically mentally ill people at [names hospital where she works]. They're all on heavy-duty meds and I figure like "I know what it's like for you." I mean, I can imagine what it's like. I know some of that pain. I'm sure I don't know all of it, because, you know, I'm not that bad off, but there is sort of a sense like they could understand me and I could understand them in something that's really, really painful. [female physical therapist, aged 42]

> I do think of it now very much . . . as an illness. I don't know what its base is, what its origin is. . . . Is it because I have a

fucked-up family, or is there a screw up in my synapses? But I think, you know, I have an illness. . . . It's something that I see myself living with for the rest of my life. And it's something I see myself having to construct my life around, as opposed to being able to flush it down the drain, and say, "Okay, got rid of it." And because of that, I see it as an illness and not in any way related to my will or wants. [female mental health worker, aged 27]

Most, however, wanted simultaneously to embrace the definition of their problem as biochemical in nature while rejecting the notion that they suffer from a "mental" illness.

I don't see it as an illness. To me, it seems like part of myself that evolved, part of my personality. And, I mean, it sounds crazy, but it is almost like a dual personality, the happy side of me and the sad side of me. And I mean, that's how I referred to it a lot when I was growing up. I mean biologically, I would have to say, "Yeah, I have a permanent illness or whatever." But I don't like to look at that. I would prefer not to think of it that way. I mean, if there was another word, I wouldn't use illness. I guess, disorder. (pause) I'm comfortable with mental disorder. [female nanny, aged 22]

You said [on the phone], "I've been dealing with this for 20 years and I'm writing a book about this illness." See, I don't like to think about having an illness that's going to be with me for my life. I just feel that like once things are going better in my life I'm just going to be happier. . . . I just want to believe that I'm having a natural reaction to adverse events in my life and that through counseling and through the medication and through improving things in my life that I can just reach a happy sustainable state. [male law student, aged 32]

Well, do you have an illness? what do you have?

I tend to think of it as a condition. I don't think of it so much as
an illness, although it feels like an illness sometimes. I think it's
an unintegrated dimension of myself that's taken [on] kind of a
life of its own, that has its own power. And I think of it, in some
ways, as a very human condition. I think it does have meaning in
some way, I just haven't really finished figuring it out yet (laughter). I don't want to think of it in sort of a pathological way, that
it's part of myself that went bad somehow. I think of it as a part
of myself that's very valid in terms of understanding what life
means or something like that. [unemployed female, aged 35]

If you say illness, that means there's something wrong with
you . . . especially a psychiatric label. That means I'm defective. If you told me I was diabetic I wouldn't think of it as bad.
That would be acceptable and I would do whatever I have to to
live with that. But to tell me I had a mental illness, that made
me feel defective. [female nurse, aged 37]

Adopting the view that one is victimized by a biochemically
sick self constitutes a comfortable "account" for a history of difficulties and failures and absolves one of responsibility. On the
negative side, however, acceptance of a victim role, while diminishing a sense of personal responsibility, is also enfeebling. To be
a victim of biochemical forces beyond one's control gives force to
others' definition of oneself as a helpless, passive object of injury.
James Holstein and Gale Miller comment that "victimization . . .
provides an interpretive framework and a discourse that relieves
victims of responsibility for their fates, but at a cost. The cost involves the myriad ways that the victim image debilitates those to
whom it is applied."[21] The interpretive dilemma for respondents

was to navigate between rhetorics of biochemical determinism and a sense of personal efficacy.

> There was a sense of relief when I started finding out that the medication was helpful, because then I could say it was a chemical problem and that I'm not looney tunes and that, you know, it's not a mental illness which sounds real bad to me. . . . So, in a sense it was very comforting to be able to use the word chemical imbalance as opposed to mental illness. [male salesman, aged 30]

> The illness thing I suppose I finesse to a certain degree. . . . I mean, when a depression becomes profound enough to require hospitalization, I'd say I'm in the category of the ill or the emotionally ill, but I don't think of myself as an ill person generally. I think of myself as a pretty high functioning person who has some experiences like this along the way. [male professor, part-time, aged 48]

Respondents generally fall into two broad categories regarding their hopes that they can put depression behind them. First are those who view having depression as a life condition that they will never fully defeat and second are those who believe that either they are now past the depression forever or that they can attain such a status. As might be expected, the two categories are generally formed by those who have experienced depression as an ongoing chronic thing, on the one hand, in contrast to those who have had periods of depression punctuated by wellness. The role of medications is interesting in establishing for some the idea that depression is something they can leave behind. Among the words that reappeared in comments about drugs was "miracle." Although, as noted, most of those interviewed at first took medication reluctantly, several reported that often for the first time in their lives they felt okay after a drug "kicked in." Generally, subjects were split between those who felt that while there was always the possibility of a reoccurrence, they essentially could get past depression and those who have surrendered to its inevitability and chronicity in their lives. The following comments summarize the two positions:

> I've stopped thinking, "OK I'm going to get over this depression. I'm going to finally, like, do this primal scream thing, or whatever. . . ." [At one point] I did buy into [the idea] of the pursuit of happiness and the pursuit of fulfillment. I hate that word. And the mental health equivalent to finding fulfillment is to fill up the gaps inside of you and everything grows green. And that's what [psychiatry] is really striving for . . . and that's the standard life should be lived on. . . . But then I finally realized that well, maybe I'm in a desert. Maybe your landscape is green, but, you know, I'm in the Sahara and I've stopped trying to get out. . . . I'd rather cure it if I had my choice, but I don't think that is going to happen. My choice is to integrate it into my life. So, no, I don't see it going away. I just see myself becoming, you know, better able to cope with it, more graceful about it. [female mental health worker, aged 27]

> I would say that this particular period of my life is a period where I don't have the fear or feeling [that depression will reoccur]. That's why, for me at least, I'm more inclined now to take the depression as an aberration and to take me in my more expansive, expressive state as the norm. For me, maybe I'm deluding myself, the way I feel now, and it's been three years since the hospitalization and I take no medications of any kind, [is] that I may be out of the woods, so to speak. . . . At the moment

I don't have a fear of reoccurrence, but I do remember having it.
[male professor, part-time, aged 48]

Unfortunately, the norm is for people to have repeated bouts with depression. In this regard, the process described here has a feedback-loop quality to it. Individuals move through a crisis with all its attendant identity-altering features, come to grips with the meaning of their experience by constructing theories about causation, and then sometimes reach the point where they feel they have gone beyond the depression experience. A new episode of depression, of course, casts doubt on all the previous interpretive work and requires people to once again move through a process of sense-making and identity construction. In this way, depression is like a virus that keeps mutating since each reliving of an experience, as the philosopher Edmund Husserl tells us, is a new experience. Chronically depressed people are constantly in the throes of an illness that is tragically familiar, but always new. As such, depression often involves a life centered on a nearly continuous process of construction, destruction, and reconstruction of identities in the face of repeated problems.

CONCLUSION

This chapter proceeded from the assumption that in order to understand people's thoughts, feelings, and actions we need to inquire into how they arrive at definitions of the situations in their lives. Chronic emotional illness poses especially difficult problems of sense-making because the source of the problem is unclear and its course uncertain. The interview material presented illustrates that peoples' experience with clinical depression is an exercise in negotiating ambiguity and involves the evolution of an illness consciousness often extending over many years. The effort to describe how those living with depression interpret and respond to their problem over time complements the large volume of survey research studies on depression that neglect the processes through which illness realities are socially constructed.

Conceptually, the chapter's analysis focused on the intersection of the ideas of career and identity. Following the lead of sociologists who have demonstrated the value of the career concept for framing a range of human processes, this chapter was organized around four generic stages through which all respondents moved as they tried to comprehend their puzzling life condition. Everyone initially felt discomfort and emotional pain which they could not name as depression. This was followed by the recognition that something was "really" wrong with them. In turn, people experienced a crisis that thrust them into a therapeutic world of mental health professionals. Finally, the crisis precipitated a stage of coming to grips with a mental illness diagnosis. Each stage corresponds to ongoing identity shifts as individuals come to view themselves as damaged and in need of repair by psychiatric experts. These identity transformations hinge, for example, on the way individuals reinterpret their pasts in the face of the depression diagnosis, deal with information control about their problem, experience hospitalization, understand the meaning of taking medication, and evaluate the validity of the illness metaphor.

An essential filter for inclusion in my study was that individuals had at some point been diagnosed and treated for depression by doctors. For that reason there is a built in bias in the sample toward acceptance of a medical definition of depression's cause and the proper response to it. In contrast, there is no way to know how many people are troubled by bad feelings that never acquire a name or receive medical treatment. I suspect that, if we could somehow count them, the greatest numbers of such individuals would be found at the lower levels of America's class structure. After all, the poorest and most disenfranchised members of the society have least access to the medical system and typically have real life situations that appear to explain their pain. For example, why would we expect a parent, without secure work, struggling to support a family while living in a dangerous housing project, to define his or her distressing feelings as illness? Such people have good reasons to feel terrible, none of them apparently connected to having a disease.

There are probably millions of people who inhabit a "parallel world"[22] to mainstream America who never define their difficulty as something requiring medical treatment. Physicians would likely say that such people suffer from "masked depression," a kind of veil of medical false consciousness that could be lifted if only they talked to the right person. These individuals, furthermore, probably experience emotional crises every bit as powerful as those described by the respondents in this study. However, instead of going to doctors, they might instead seek solace in religion, for example. They too could be described as following a career path prompted by suffering, but it would be bounded by symbols and stages wholly different from the ones analyzed here. Like their counterparts in this study who eventually come to acquire an identity as a depressed person with a biochemical disorder, they no doubt construct explanations about the source of their misery and adopt identities consistent with their definition of the situation. They simply are not illness identities. I am suggesting, in other words, that there is nothing intrinsic to the feelings experienced by people in this book that necessarily and inevitably lead to a definition of the pain as disease.

Among those whose emotional problems are eventually defined by doctors as a disease called depression, virtually everyone is told to take medications. The significance of taking antidepressant medications has thus far only lurked around the edges of my conversation. Chapter 4, however, is devoted exclusively to the meanings of taking medication since the role of drugs is central to the way every person interviewed eventually became more thoroughly socialized to a medical version of what was wrong with them. In this way, my thinking about medications extends the analysis of how individuals come to accept the legitimacy of medical definitions of their problem as primarily biological. The moment individuals first take a drug for depression surely begins a process of biochemical revision. More profoundly significant, however, taking pills hastens the revision of self already begun by the time individuals find their way to a doctor's office.

Chapter 4

The Meanings of Medication

All I can tell you is, "Oh my God, you know when you're on the right medication." It was the most incredible thing. And I would say that I had a spiritual experience.

Female graduate student, aged 24

I will never take another fucking pill in my life. And I'm not generalizing this to other people, but for me, I had gotten so fucked up with this stuff that I will never do it again.

Male professor, part-time, aged 48

One noontime I sat with a group of economists in the faculty dining room at Boston College and listened with amusement as someone complained about a colleague who "strangled his data until they confessed." Although there is considerable debate about the possibility, or even the desirability, of objectivity in the social sciences, most sociologists would likely say that we should not give up on objectivity. My own position is that no one can escape the biases that emerge out of their particular biographies and life circumstances and it is foolish to claim that researchers can leave their life experience behind when they embark on a study. Researchers, like everyone else, necessarily see the world from a particular vantage point that influences each part of the research process—the way they formulate problems, the methodologies they feel an affinity with, the observations they make or the questions asked of respondents, the kind of data they see as relevant to understand something, their choices for emphasis as analysis proceeds, and, finally, the way they render their "findings."

Since pure objectivity is impossible, researchers ought to be up front about their biases and assumptions so that readers can at least know where they are "coming from." While I see researchers' occasional claims to total objectivity as silly, I tell my students in research methods classes that to wholly give up on objectivity is to invite intellectual chaos. I understand objectivity as a goal to be pursued by honestly responding to collected data so that the analysis truly emerges from what people have said. Such an attitude also involves going out of one's way specifically to look for data that might contravene emerging theories. In short, researchers ought to adopt whatever safeguards they can to avoid so thoroughly falling in love with their theories that giving them up becomes impossible.

Of all the chapters in this book, this one on drugs might be the most potentially compromised by the intensity of my own feelings. In the spirit of my methodological injunction to students, I want to briefly preface this chapter's data and analysis with some elaboration on my personal attitudes about medications. In Chapter 1, I indicated that I continue to take medications, but with great ambivalence. In fact, I have not been free of antidepressants for many years, although I shift from time to time to a new one hoping that it might finally "do the trick" for me. I reluctantly stick with medications because I am afraid that things could become much worse if I were to stop and I don't want to chance that. Along with an antidepressant, I also have "permission" to use, "as needed," an anti-anxiety drug called Klonopin for sleeping. I try to restrain my use of this drug because, unlike the antidepressant I take, Klonopin can be physiologically addicting. I'd like to cut it out altogether, but the withdrawal symptoms (irritability and the awful sleeplessness for which I take the drug in the first place) are hard to deal with and the drug's promise of an occasional good night's sleep is extremely seductive. Through the years my attitude toward drugs has remained steady—a mixture of hostility and dependence.

When I try to examine the hostility part of my response to medication, I realize how deeply my feelings about drugs are tied up with my views about psychiatry and its prevailing definition of depression as a biological disease. I respect what I take to be the sincere impulse of medical scientists to help people, but I also wonder whether psychiatrists' willingness to so thoroughly embrace the use of drugs might be related to their own relatively suspect status within medicine. It certainly would affirm psychiatry as a "medical" specialty if it could be demonstrated that affective disorders have as clearly an organic source as diabetes, epilepsy, or heart disease. However, a plainly organic etiology has never been established in the case of uni-polar depression. That people sometimes feel better after taking antidepressant medications is hardly definitive evidence that depression is caused by an underlying physical pathology. Such logic would require us to say that the individual who feels better after a glass or two of wine with dinner was de facto suffering from some biological impairment corrected by the alcohol.

My own view—rooted in personal experience, listening to others, a lifetime of reading social science, and what seems commonsensically true—is that depression arises out of an enormously complicated, constantly shifting, elusive concatenation of social circumstance, individual temperament, and biochemistry. As such, I would never flatly declare that medications that revise body chemistries should be avoided. Too many people have been dramatically helped by medication to take such a position. At the same time, I strongly resist an approach that systematically minimizes the role of social experience in shaping emotions, good ones and bad ones. To resort primarily to pills because other approaches for treating depression have not worked nearly as well may make sense as a practical strategy. That pills sometimes greatly help people, however, does not warrant the prevailing medical judgment that depression has, first and foremost, an organic basis.

Connected with my professional and personal resistance to wholly biological explanations for any human behavior, I have misgivings about the current practice of psychiatry on political grounds. Whether the proposed psychiatric cure for emotional problems has been talk, as in the past, or medication, as is presently the case, the solutions have neglected the larger structural bases for emotional distress. For example, if, as studies routinely show, women suffer from depression twice as often as men, it strains credibility to believe that such a finding can be accounted for by biological differences alone. To me, there is an obvious validity to the assumption that something about the patterned social situations of women accounts for the statistical gender difference in all the studies. If this is so, a medical treatment focused exclusively on changing patients (either changing the person's self through talk or their biochemistry with pills) leaves wholly unattended the structural sources of human pain. As such, most psychiatric treatment is inherently conservative by implicitly supporting the systemic status quo. Medicine nearly always interprets illness as a reflection of individual physical pathology and rarely as *a normal response to pathological social structures*. Following this line of thinking, I find the current medical rhetoric that hypes medication as the cure for depression to be both scientifically arrogant and politically retrograde.

Along with the millions of people who now take pills for depression, I honestly hope that their current promise doesn't become tomorrow's problem. However, using history as a guide, we should not be sanguine about any category of pills hailed as "wonder" drugs. Instead, we should wonder about the claims. Let's remember that beginning in the 1950s such psychotropic drugs as Valium and Librium were claimed to provide revolutionary cures for a range of anxieties that were disrupting people's lives, especially women. In a short period of time, millions of people were poppin' pills to get through their days less painfully. By the 1970s medical and social scientists[1] were coming to see the incredibly widespread use of these minor tranquilizers as an emerging social problem. In retrospect, the early medical claims for the efficacy of tranquilizers seem grossly overblown and plainly dangerous.

As promised in Chapter 1, the last chapter will specify the broad cultural arrangements in America that might illuminate why increasing numbers of people are feeling sick with depression. I hope that the more extended cultural analysis there will be provocative and persuasive. At this historical moment, though, I fully expect American medicine to increasingly endorse the view that medication is the best way to deal with depression. The chemical revolution, fostered by an extremely powerful medical establishment and by Americans' readiness to look for quick scientific fixes, has an extraordinary cultural momentum. Right now, in fact, one drug, Prozac, which has been around only since 1986, is being used by an estimated 6 million people in the United States. Initially meant for treating depression, Prozac is now being prescribed for, among other things, obsessive compulsive disorder, weight loss, and excessive shyness. In his controversial book, *Listening to*

Prozac, Peter Kramer raises troubling questions about the likely future practice of a "cosmetic psychopharmacology" made possible by a drug that seems to alter human temperament and to make some people feel "better than well."[2]

My comments thus far suggest some of my deep reservations about the overuse of antidepressant medications. Perhaps, like many sociologists who write about medicine, I feel a strong concern about one group of people—physicians—being in such an authoritative position to shape a whole society's thinking about the character of illness and what needs to be done about it. Recognition of medicine's great achievements does not prevent me from holding the view that science is itself a belief system with great potential for error and for the misuse of power to control people.

This chapter is most fundamentally about how people with depression come almost invariably to accept the medical version of what is wrong with them and what to do about it. Right now, the prevailing cultural view is that a healthy revision of self is best accomplished through a revision of one's biochemistry. Despite the growing "faith" in medication as the preferred way to combat depression, the analysis throughout this chapter will show that the decision to embark on a course of drug taking is not a simple matter of unthinkingly following a doctor's orders. In fact, a patient's willingness to begin a drug regimen and stick with it involves an extensive interpretive process that includes consideration of such issues as the connection between drug use and illness self-definitions, the meanings of drug side effects, attitudes toward physicians, evaluations of professional expertise, and ambiguity about the causes of one's problem.

I have been particularly anxious to begin this chapter with disclosure of my own sentiments about medication. It is probably a combination of these personal impressions and my sociological impulse to question the legitimacy of medicine's preeminent status relative to other belief systems that shapes the framework of my analysis here. You may, therefore, find me somewhat irreverent when I later equate respondents' increasing commitment to a medical version of reality with published descriptions of the recruitment, conversion, and deconversion of individuals to a variety of religious groups.

Respondents' stories that center on feelings of desperation, lack of perceived meaning in life, and then sometimes a "born again" drug miracle bear an instructive resemblance to accounts of involvement with a range of religious groups. Like religious conversion, capitulation to a biomedical version of depression's causes and proper treatment is accomplished through a socialization process that entails a radical transformation of identity, a "process of changing a sense of root reality."[3] I believe that this way of looking at things comes out of an honest reading of the data rather than from my subjective discomfort with the growing dominance of biochemical explanations for depression. Of one thing I'm sure—I am not alone in my confusions about the role of medication in the treatment of depression. Let me tell you about the drug experiences of a 30-year-old salesman whom I'll call Randall.

At about 6'4", with broad shoulders, weight in proportion to height, wavy red hair, and a strikingly handsome face, Randall is quite an imposing figure. It was not altogether surprising that throughout his years at a Catholic high school and later in college, he had been a standout basketball player. Like many superior athletes he was known and valued primarily for his athletic skills. These skills ensured his acceptance to a first-rate college despite his relatively poor grades in high school. As he put it, "Grades-wise I didn't do real well . . . but it didn't matter because I played basketball well. So that [grades] just wasn't an issue. Just keep playing and that's what everybody pushed me to do. I don't even know if I liked to play basketball. I was good at it and I enjoyed being good at it." On the basketball court Randall continued to perform at a high level. However, this was misleading because, he reported, "by the time I was a senior in high school, depression was pretty much a constant thing. I was always depressed. Depressed was my natural state."

Like nearly everyone interviewed, Randall was aware of unusually bad feelings for a long time without knowing what to call them. He said, "The thing was, I knew all the feelings, but I never associated them as 'I'm depressed.'" He found naming his emotions especially difficult because talk about feelings was absolutely taboo in his family. Were I to identify a single theme in Randall's interview aside from his troubled dealings with medications, it would be his distress about having to "stuff his feelings" throughout all his growing up years. Particularly traumatic was the death of a younger brother when Randall was 12. He described the family's response to the death this way:

> I can remember, I was about 12, in 1973. That summer, I had my first depression. I didn't know what it was. And nobody else knew what it was. My family didn't know what it was, and basically they just ignored me as far as, you know, [saying] "it will go away." I had a brother who died that April, and basically nobody did [anything] as far as dealing with feelings. I can remember . . . I have five brothers and sisters, and he died in April and we came up to [names a college] for my father's 20th college reunion. We stayed over in one of the dorms. Like, that was our big outing together as a family, to just kind of relax. And that was the only thing [we did] really.
>
> Basically they didn't have a funeral. They had a Mass of the Angels, and then from there, you know, a party afterwards.

People came over, and said, "Oh, I'm sorry." You know, all that. But basically there was no grieving. This kid was real sick anyway, so it was a blessing. That's what they said, "It was a blessing." And basically, feelings were not felt at all. That was the beginning. That was the first time I can remember [depression]. I can remember being suicidal after that.... That was the beginning of . . . stuffing feelings and not feeling feelings. I do believe that depression for me is rooted in not feeling feelings. Not being able to express anything. And they [feelings] just grew. Not long after, probably a year or so after that, I started to drink. And from then on, I was not a happy person ever.

There may not have been much family discussion about feelings, but Randall could remember voluble arguments between his parents and a lot of acting out among the children. As he saw it, the relationships between his parents and himself, as well as with his siblings, were not exactly abusive, but they were certainly disturbed and disturbing. As a result, he "hid out" whenever possible. Through all this, he said, "I wasn't supposed to be angry. You're not supposed to be angry. So I wasn't angry. So I walked around smiling, like, you know, false. And basically I hid all these things. I had all these things to hide that nobody could know about.... There was a lot of guilt and shame. That's what I carried around. [But] at the time I probably couldn't have told you what I was feeling."

Randall initially medicated himself with street drugs and alcohol. He told me, "I drank from 14 to 21. I was stoned constantly.... I got stoned probably on weekends till I was 15 and then pretty much whenever I could. ... The drinking wasn't a conservative thing. I said, 'Well, I'm going to drink because I don't like the way I feel.' You know, drinking made me feel good." At a point it became apparent to his basketball coach that something was truly amiss. At the coach's insistence Randall saw a counselor for a short time, but the meetings were perfunctory and made no difference in the course of his drinking. "I was just unhappy. . . . I continued to drink and the more I drank the better I felt. By the end of my high school [years] I would drink every day. I got high at 7 A.M. [and then I would] go out to lunch and drink some more." Once in college the substance abuse pattern deepened and he "drank like there was no tomorrow." He remembered, "I was physically addicted at this point. If I couldn't drink, I couldn't sleep. So I drank pretty much all the time and I used a lot of drugs. I didn't know what the hell was wrong with me, but I was suicidal."

Any denial about depression ended abruptly in 1983 when things got so bad that Randall needed to be hospitalized. His condition became clear to him after "they gave me a blood test and said, 'You're depressed.' And I believed them." What followed was a string of hospitalizations—"in for a month, out for a month." It was also the beginning of his licit drug therapy. No one consulted Randall about whether he ought to take medication. He was simply told that it was necessary to begin a course of treatment. At the time, Xanax, a tranquilizer in the same family of drugs as Valium and Librium, was prescribed. Unfortunately, no one seemed to understand just how habituating Xanax could be. Eventually it became plain, at least in Randall's case, that a highly addictive medication was being prescribed, in large dosages, to a person with an "addictive personality." As he recounted the doctors' immediate reliance on medications ("the doctors were going to cure me with drugs and they got me hooked.") Randall became agitated and the tone of the interview became angry.

During the next 20 minutes or so of our conversation Randall described his ongoing involvement with a range of psychotropic medications. His thoughts illustrate the profound confusion depressed people often feel about the biochemical genesis of their difficulty and the value of medications. However much he has thought about his drug encounters over the years, Randall has not been able to develop a consistent attitude about their worth. One moment he describes himself as having a chemical disorder that requires the use of medication. Later, he diminishes the value of pills in staving off his episodes of depression, although believing that they help him emerge from depression. He feels dependent on antidepressants and therefore on the physicians who prescribe them. At the same time, there is a clear edge of anger in his feelings about psychiatrists. After all of this, he denies having a disease and instead offers the view that his problem is more primarily spiritual than medical. At best he is ambivalent, uncertain, and inconsistent in his feelings about doctors, their pills, and medicine's version of the depression reality. Such expressions of confusion are common. Randall is not a muddled thinker. He is in a muddled situation.

Here, in abbreviated and edited form, are excerpts from our conversation about medications. It centers on two apparently contradictory thoughts: a belief in the biochemical origins of depression and anger at psychiatrists' reliance on medications.

You can get to a certain point in treatment of depression [with] drugs and therapy and stuff like that, but you can only get to a certain point. My own belief is that the depression is an inability to cope with the feelings that I come across every day. And depression is, I think, its own entity within me. I mean it's chemical. . . . I was hospitalized for most of '83, about six or eight months, on and off. And, you know, the doctors were going to cure me with drugs. [But] they got me hooked on one drug. It was supposed to be a cure-all.

This was an antidepressant?

No. Well, it was called Xanax and it was being used as an antidepressant. . . . I mean, I learned how to be depressed in a psychiatric hospital. I watched people. I learned the words. . . . How to get drugs, how to manipulate [psychiatrists]. But the problem was that on the drugs, like Xanax, I didn't feel anything. I was taking one milligram every three hours, or whatever. I didn't feel anything. I couldn't express anything. I mean it was just like each hour I'd take another Xanax, and that's the way it was.

You don't appear to think too highly of psychiatrists.

I don't think very highly of psychiatrists. You can tell. I tolerate them because I have to take this medicine. [But] everything can be cured with a drug, everything. They've got a drug for everything. . . . They like to tinker with the body through these drugs rather than trying to have people express what they're feeling. They just took one look at me and pronounced me depressed and put me on a battery of antidepressants. . . . They're not very human. They don't look at the humanistic side. You know, where I was coming from . . . I thought I had a case to sue them . . . for medical malpractice.

The people at the hospital where you were?

Yeah, mainly around the Xanax. I overdosed on it on the end of November of 1983, and the whole time they just kept telling me, "Randall, just keep taking the Xanax, you'll be fine." I was an admitted addict when I got there. But the hospital, through my psychologist's own admission, pushed the tranquilizers. . . . They just pushed the Xanax. They just pushed it any time that I got angry.

So you've had some real bad experiences with medication.

Yeah. But, I mean, it can bring me out [of depression]. But it can't keep me from going in. . . . I believe there is something different in my brain, physiologically different. But I don't know how it happened. Nobody in my family ever had anything like this. I kind of believe that there is something physically there and I can use medicine, but it's not a cure-all. I don't know whether to call it a disease. I don't like to think of it that way. I don't go around thinking my disease is acting up. I don't really think about it like that. I kind of think it's something I have to live with and just make the best of. And that's where the spirituality enters. I mean, doctors and medicine can only do so much, but if you've got somebody with a broken spirit [there isn't much that medicine can do].

My conversation with Randall covered other terrible difficulties involving medications, including a serious suicide attempt in which antidepressants were "the lethal part of the cocktail." On the lighter side, we talked about the rituals associated with drug taking. For instance, we had a mutual laugh about air travel and always packing our medications in carry-on luggage. We agreed that having airlines lose our clothing might be a considerable inconvenience, but having our drugs lost would really be a catastrophe. We also shared information about such things as noncompliance with "doctor's orders," about personally constructed experiments with timing and dosage of medications. However, the common denominator linking Randall's with the others' experiences is their shared commitment, despite sometimes dreadful experiences and a continuing range of difficult side effects, to stick with drug treatments. Most of those interviewed have moved through a socialization process that imbues them with the belief that medications are the way to go. For the remainder of this chapter I want to consider how and why this happens.

INTERPRETING THE DRUG EXPERIENCE

The perspective taken in this chapter fits with a general literature in social psychology arguing that the subjective experience of taking drugs emerges from individual and collective interpretations about the drug taken. Among the classic studies on the subject are Alfred Lindesmith's[4] analysis of heroin addiction and Howard Becker's[5] study of marihuana smokers. These studies attest to the validity of the symbolic interactionist notion that the meaning of all experiences, including drug-induced physiological experiences, requires labeling and interpretation. Becker, for example, illustrates that one must "learn" how to smoke marihuana. Aside from adopting the correct techniques for ingesting the drug, one must learn to perceive its effects as pleasurable. The effects of marihuana are not intrinsically pleasurable and in order to continue using the drug people must rely on a subculture of fellow users who help to provide positive interpretations of the drug's physiological effects. These studies rest on the notion that taking drugs is not an event, but an ongoing process of meaning-making during the period of their use.[6] Once we conceive of taking psychotropic medications in processual terms, it makes sense to adopt, as I did in the last chapter, a "career" model for ordering the data.

In Chapter 3, I identified clear stages in the evolution of an illness consciousness among depressed persons. Certain events in the course of an illness become critical identity markers that reflect a profound shift in how people see themselves. You may recall that Anselm Strauss[7] refers to these moments as "turning points" in identity. At such junctures individuals are transformed in a way that requires a redefinition of who they were, are, and might be. The following data illustrate that the eventual decision to take medications was a major benchmark in the way my respondents came to see themselves, the nature of their problem, and their images of the future. The consequent decisions to continue and then eventually to stop a drug regimen are complicated and sometimes the product of years of confusion, evaluation, and experimentation.

Although it would do an injustice to the complexity of people's responses to drug treatment to say that everyone moved through absolutely determined stages of interpretation, the stories I heard suggest clear regularities. These "moments" in the way respondents simultaneously tried to make sense out of drugs and their illness include an initial *resistance* stage during which they were unwilling to take antidepressant medications. However, despite their ideological and psychological opposition, those interviewed eventually became desperate enough to try medication and thus capitulated to the advice of medical experts. During a second period of *trial commitment*, individuals express a willingness to experiment with drugs only for a short period of time. Having made the decision to try medications, they begin to accept biochemical definitions of depression's cause and persistence. Such a redefinition is critical in becoming committed to a medical treatment model. For several, taking the drugs has a marginal or even negative impact on their problem. However, by now even these individuals have become *converted* to a belief in biochemical explanations of depression and begin a search to find the "right" drug. Finally, even among those who experienced a "miracle" and felt "saved" by medication, several eventually have other episodes of depression and become *disenchanted* with drugs. They feel a need to get off the drugs "to see what happens," to see whether they can "go it alone."

Resistance

On rare occasions persons I spoke with sought out physicians explicitly to obtain antidepressant medications. Perhaps this will increasingly be the case as both psychiatry and pharmaceutical companies "educate" the public about the nature of depression and as drugs like Prozac are touted in the media as revolutionary cures for depression. Normally, however, the idea to take medication is first raised by a therapist or doctor, a suggestion that is met with considerable resistance. Typically, respondents offered a number of reasons for initially saying no to drugs. Some described themselves nearly identically by saying, "I'm the kind of person who doesn't even believe in taking aspirin for a headache." Others were appropriately concerned about the unknown and possibly long-term effects of powerful medications. It is interesting that even respondents who had earlier in their lives experimented with all kinds of drugs (e.g., marihuana, cocaine, and LSD) were opposed to taking psychiatric medications. Without denying their stated reasons, there appears to be a central underlying dynamic to their resistance. Taking an antidepressant medication would require a dramatic redefinition of self; it would be a clear affirmation that they were a person with a stigmatized emotional disorder. In this respect, a willingness to begin a regimen of psychiatric medications is far more than a simple medical decision. It is a decisive juncture in one's self redefinition as an emotionally ill rather than merely troubled person.

I didn't want to be told that I had something that was going to affect the rest of my life, and that could only be solved by taking pills. It was sort of definitive. I had a label and it was a label that I thought was pejorative. I didn't want to be this quietly depressed person, that there was something wrong with me. And it was sort of a rebellion in that [I said] "No, I'm not like that. I don't need you and your pills." [female nurse, aged 37]

My internist said, "You're depressed. You need an antidepressant." I mean, I didn't understand the word exactly. She sent me to [names a psychiatrist] for antidepressants. I went to [names psychiatrist] and said, "I don't need antidepressants, but I do need somebody to talk to." Drugs. I was against drugs. I didn't understand them either. But if he would talk to me, maybe we could work our way out of it. [female college professor, aged 49]

I'd get depressed and I'd stop eating. So now I knew I was really depressed. They wanted to put me on antidepressants and I said I wouldn't. And they said, "You have to." [But] I didn't want anything manipulating me. From an early age having had asthma and having had this sense that there's always some drug trying to fix me. Fix my asthma. Fix this. Fix that. I didn't like that. And I felt . . . there were times when I blamed the drugs for some of my depression and problems. I felt like any more drugs would have control over me. [female travel agent, aged 41]

I have to tell you, there was a battle on this (taking drugs) because I am the type of person, if I have a headache I'm stoic about it. I won't take any kind of a pill. And so all of this was against my better instincts. [unemployed male waiter, aged 33]

I tried Prozac . . . briefly. It gave my hands the shakes and I said, "Forget this. . . . Let me fix up all the problems in my life first." I was edgy about it [medication]. I didn't really want to play around with my body chemistry. At that time I did not think that there was a chemical component to my depression. I knew I was unhappy. But, I had successfully resolved so many issues before . . . [and] I felt that I could resolve this. And I also know about chemicals that they all have side effects. . . . [So] there were reasons that I was opposed to medication for me. I was not opposed to it for anyone else. [female software quality control manager, aged 31]

It was awfully depressing to me, if you don't mind my using the word, to reduce a human being to a series of chemical reactions. Why bother? Why be conscious, you know? [unemployed female, aged 35]

For several respondents the first clear communication that they needed medications followed a crisis that pushed them into a psychiatrist's office or, sometimes, into a hospital. New patients often perceived doctors as unwilling to pay significant attention to their feelings and were, as they saw it, altogether too quick to prescribe medications. Especially in hospitals, respondents sometimes acutely experienced the paradox that psychiatrists didn't want to spend much time hearing about their feelings even though it was their bad feelings that forced them into the hospital. As individuals often saw it, their souls were wounded. Such a perspective on the causes of their misery did not seem to square with the assessment that they had a disease in the form of unbalanced brain chemicals and should be treated with medication.

While people suffering from depression often express anger toward those they view as implicated in the creation of their problem, I was surprised throughout these interviews by the virulence of the animosity expressed toward psychiatrists. Eventually, many of those interviewed found psychiatrists whom they trusted and from whom they benefited. However, early in their treatment, individuals saw psychiatrists as oppressively evangelistic "true believers" in biochemical causes of depression, a view that they did not then hold. Their initial negative evaluation of psychiatry and psychiatrists is caught in the frequency and regularity with which respondents angrily labeled their doctors as "pill pushers."

> This particular doctor was such an asshole. He sounded like a used car salesman for antidepressants. He was just like so gung-ho. "Oh yuh, you're the typical depressed [person], here's the drug that will cure you. Let me know if you go home and just want to kill yourself or something. We'll try something different for you." And I hated him. I just really hated him. [unemployed female, aged 22]

> So I ended up going to a private hospital. . . . It was a nightmare. I wouldn't take my meds consistently. They ended up taking me to court . . . to force me to take my meds. They showed that I wasn't capable of making my own decisions. . . . They told me, "You need this medication" and I thought they were poisoning me. I was all paranoid. I was so scared. I thought that they were trying to kill me. That was basically the bottom line for the first month. I must have taken at least 20 different medications. . . . Antidepressants was the main thing. [unemployed female, aged 23]

> You never see a doctor in a hospital. I mean, you see mental health workers and, you know, the doctor sort of, you know, walks in once a week and dispenses pills and then walks back out. You know, he's a very regal kind of figure who is untouchable. [female mental health worker, aged 27]

By the time patients arrive for treatment in doctors' offices or hospitals they have already moved through a number of changes in self-definition. When asked about the unfolding of the recognition that they were depressed, individuals ordinarily describe an early time of inchoate feelings of distress, followed by the feeling that "something is really wrong with me," and then to some variant of "I can't continue to live like this." Even after a crisis severe enough to precipitate hospitalization, individuals are, as we have seen, still resistant to taking medications. Resisting medication is a way of resisting categorization as a mentally ill person. However, the depth and persistence of their misery proves great enough that, under the proddings of physicians and sometimes other patients and family members, individuals begin to waver in their resolve not to take medication. Several persons described themselves as eventually "coming around" to the decision to take drugs because they became willing to try anything to diminish their suffering. Over and again respondents portrayed their capitulation to medications as a consequence of the desperation they felt.

> But I also didn't want to do it [take drugs] because I felt such shame. I felt like, "Well I'm not depressed, someone else is depressed." Like I couldn't believe it was me. It was like some wonder drug or something. And I was thinking, "No way, I don't want to jump on this bandwagon." I was so scared of it. I felt like five years from now they'd find out that it gave me cancer or something. I just didn't want to take medication at all. But then at the same time I wanted so desperately for something to fix me. So I was just willing to try anything. He just said, "Give it a week, think about it." [unemployed female, aged 22]

> I knew this was something real different from what it had been. I wasn't really able to function, particularly because I got so tired, and I wasn't eating, and just, you know, more panic, and just [being] exhausted. So, I started on the medication and

I remember I felt really uncomfortable about taking it. It felt like it was [now] at a whole different level. If I couldn't sort of cure myself. . . . If I needed medication I thought, "This is really serious." [female physical therapist, aged 42]

I was very leery of it [taking medications]. I mean I was concerned about what the effects might be and I didn't like the idea of putting myself on some sort of medication, but at a certain point it just seemed to me that I had to try it and the problem was so great that I really wanted to do anything that would alleviate it. [male professor, aged 48]

The big Prozac controversy . . . scared my parents and scares my girlfriend. It kind of scares me, if you read about this stuff. But by that time I am so convinced that "Shit, anything if you're depressed is better than being depressed." I knew I had to do something. [unemployed male waiter, aged 33]

And in fact, I never wanted to take the drug. I mean I took the drug because I believed it would keep me alive. [female free-lance writer, aged 41]

In an especially evocative comment, a respondent equated taking the medication with "swallowing her will."

I have a hard time taking medication. . . . I don't like taking pills. I didn't like taking aspirin. I mean, I've generally been very conservative at that, so I kind of swallowed, you know, my will and that's when I took Prozac. [female baker, aged 41]

The moment individuals decide to try medications is decisive in beginning a reorientation in their thinking about the nature of their difficulty and of their "selves." Social psychologists have long understood that embarking on a new life direction, especially one that departs from earlier held views of reality, requires the construction of a new "vocabulary of motives"[8] and new "accounts"[9] for behavior. Labeling theorists,[10] for example, argue that eventual commitment to a new subculture involves successive redefinitions of self made in response to others' labeling and to one's own changed behaviors. Instead of understanding behaviors as always being propelled by clear motives, we know that behavioral changes often precede motive productions. Taking the medication is the beginning of a process of a commitment to biochemical explanations of affective disorders.

Trial Commitment

In his well-known paper entitled "Notes on the Concept of Commitment," Howard Becker shows that commitments to new ways of life do not happen suddenly, all at once.[11] Commitments are built up slowly, gradually, and often imperceptibly through a series of "side bets" or personal decisions, each of which, at the time, seems of little consequence. People, for example, may become committed to work organizations through a series of side bets such as paying into a pension plan, accepting a promotion and new responsibilities, buying a home based on current income, and so on. As Becker explains, each of these apparently independent decisions is like putting individual bricks into a wall until one day it suddenly becomes clear that the wall has grown to such a height that one cannot climb over it—a commitment has been made that is not easily reversed.

The decision to take a medication is sometimes preceded by a *negotiation* with doctors about how long one is willing to try it. Here the analogy to involvement with religious groups may be profitably drawn. In their paper on modes of conversion to religious groups, Lofland and Skonovd describe five different "conversion motifs" that vary in terms of such factors as the degree of pressure involved in the conversion, the length of time involved, and the degree of emotional arousal during the process.[12] Along with intellectual, mystical, affectional, and revivalist motifs, the authors describe an "experimental" conversion motif that corresponds to this juncture in the drug-taking process. In experimental conversions, there is "a relatively low degree of social pressure" as "the recruit takes on a 'try it out' posture."[13] Negotiations reflect patients' ambivalence about psychotropic drugs and signal both to physicians and themselves that they have not yet accepted doctors' definitions of them as having a biochemically based illness.

And so then I started taking this Prozac. And the only reason I would take it is that he promised I would only be on it for three months. I ended up being on it for nine months, probably longer, nine or ten months. If I had known that, I don't think I'd ever have gone on it because I just didn't want to put any kind of substance in my body. [unemployed female, aged 22]

The psychiatrist . . . said, "Look, I just think you should stay on it through the end of the year, you know, and then you can go off it." So I decided. . . . I wasn't thinking of it quite so blatantly, but I was sort of thinking, "All right, I'll just take this eight months and see what happens." [female mental health worker, aged 27]

Negotiations aside, taking medications coincides with a growing acceptance of official medical versions about the causes of depression. Everyone who suffers from depression feels obliged to construct theories of causation in order to impose some coherence onto an especially hazy, ambiguous life circumstance and to evaluate the extent to which they are responsible for their condition. Although it is impossible to ever fully resolve whether nature or nurture, or some combination, is responsible for depression, every person I interviewed eventually accepted in greater or lesser degree a biochemical explanation of depression.

> I figure it comes from . . . a combination. In some people it may be triggered by one particular thing . . . but I think in most [people] it's probably a combination of genetics and bad chemistry and the stresses of life. . . . But mine, I think, is pretty heavily biochemical and genetic. My father apparently had it. We didn't find that out until after his death. [unemployed male, aged 58]

> I think it is biological. No matter how hard I've tried to shake the depression at times, it still seems to pop up when I don't want it to. That's what's annoying. I found that from talking to a lot of people you can try and try and try, but just when you think things are okay and maybe you've got it under control, then there comes a day when, "Why am I crying? Why am I depressed? Why do I hate life today?" There's nothing to hate. It just happens. [female nanny, aged 22]

> I think there was a certain point when the chemical thing just took off on its own. I think before that I had a chance to impact on it. It was much more interactive. Once it took off on its own I needed medication. There wasn't anything else that was going to get me out of that. [male therapist, aged 45]

> Got a cold? Take Vitamin C! Got depression? Take the damn antidepressants! [female baker, aged 41]

Conversion: *Muddle or Miracle*

Once patients have accepted and internalized a rhetoric of biochemical causation they become committed to a process of finding the "right" medication. Such a discovery often proves elusive as people enter upon a protracted process of trial and error with multiple drugs. This process is often extremely confusing as they deal with a variety of side effects ranging from such relatively benign problems as dry mouth, constipation, and weight gain to more dramatic experiences like fainting in public places. In several interviews drug "horror stories" were a prominent theme, as in the case of a hospitalized woman whose therapy, along with drugs, consisted of physical exercise.

> I was on every drug under the sun. Just everything [said with exasperation]. It was like a cocktail. I mean I was really out of control. . . . I'll never forget this little vignette where they would drug me and say, "Well, you've got to get out there and be more active. . . . I'll never forget tennis. . . . I was so drugged up I could barely see my fingers and this therapist took us out to the tennis courts. He was hitting balls and I couldn't even see the ball. This asshole, I couldn't even see and he's worried about my backhand. It's stupid. You know, at the time I don't think I thought it was too funny. I thought, "What's wrong with me." So things went from bad to worse. [female social worker, aged 38]

Another young woman told of dealing with drug side effects.

> I was on this medication that made me thirsty all the time, so I had to carry around like a six-pack of soda (laughs). It was Elavil and it made me tired all the time, and it made me gain weight. I mean, I was a zombie at that point. It made my mood

brighter, but I hated all the side effects. I felt like a lab experiment. [female nanny, aged 22]

Sometimes individuals stayed on a medication for months that had no discernible positive effect or which they perceived only modestly influenced their condition. The search for the "right" drug seems analogous to a process of serial monogamy in which individuals move through a series of unsatisfying, bad, or even destructive relationships, always with the hope that the right person will eventually be found. Just as individuals internalize the notion of romantic love with its attendant ideology that one's perfect mate is somewhere in the world, respondents maintained their faith, in spite of a series of disappointments, that they would find the right medication.

Anyway, I think I continued on the Imipramine, but they gave me other drugs. Out of all the drugs that I had I can't say that any one really made me feel better. You know and I can only say that when you find the right drug you really know. "Oh, this is what it means to be better." But I do remember it wasn't Imipramine. [female graduate student, aged 24]

It's [names drug] been effective and I haven't felt the need for anything else. But I also have the feeling, "I wonder if there is something better that I could take a lower dose of that would be effective." Or, "Isn't there something else now that might be better." I always feel that way (laughs). [male professor, aged 48]

I'm feeling very hopeless [right now]. I'm still taking the Trazadone. I'm also taking an anti-anxiety drug once in a while and I feel like I'm treading water. I'm waking up at five o'clock in the morning even with the Trazadone. I wake up in horror that, you know, I'll be a bag lady, that I'm not going to be able to get through my work day today. Every once in a while I wonder "Have I tried enough stuff. Is there something that would work better?" [female college professor, aged 49]

The first thing that they tried was the Prozac. They didn't tell me about some of the side effects. Unfortunately, it reduces your sex drive, but my sex drive wasn't that high anyway because I was depressed. And also, I think I just have a normal low sex drive. So it makes it even more non-existent, which they don't tell people. I'm not the only one in my woman's group [who has discovered this]. A lot of people kind of discover it. And then it does a number on my appetite. But I can live with the side effects because that's a lot better than living with the depression. [unemployed disabled female, aged 39]

Many of those interviewed never find a drug that significantly influences things for the better. These people continue to take the medications, but remain only partial believers in biochemical explanations. However, some describe the "miracle" of medication. It is among these people that the metaphor to religious conversion is most apt. For them, the drug truly provides a "revelation" because it makes them feel "normal," often for the first time in their lives. In these instances, any trace of uncertainty about the biochemical basis for their problem disappears. Finding the right medication is, in fact, described as a spiritual awakening, as an ecstatic experience.

All I can tell you is, "Oh my God, you know when you're on the right medication." It was the most incredible thing. And I would say that I had a spiritual experience. [female graduate student, aged 24]

So I started taking this Trazadone. It may have been a week or two. I had never experienced such a magical effect in my whole life. Thoughts that I had been having . . . I had been having these horrible, tortured depressed thoughts and the only thing I can say is that they just stopped being in my head and it was like they had run around in my blood and I just didn't think that way any more. And I started thinking better thoughts, happier thoughts. It was very clear to me that it wasn't the same as being high. Astonishing. It was wonderful. . . . After two weeks . . . I mean, it was just magical. My life began to change profoundly at that point. [female college professor, aged 49]

And then I start seeing this therapist last September twice a week and he recommends going to see a psychiatrist. I go to him and he recommends Doxepin and I start taking that. And then at the end of November it just kind of kicked in. It was a miracle. It really was. Quite extraordinary. [male therapist, aged 45]

Well, I'd had a headache for four months and they treated that with Amitriptyline. And then I changed doctors. I went to the [names a university] health plan. Anyway, I saw a psychiatrist and had been seeing her for a while and I guess probably giving all the classic symptoms that I didn't know existed. And finally she said, "Well, you know, I think one of the problems here is that you're depressed and I'm putting you on Imipramine and see if that's going to work." And when it started working it was like a miracle. It was just like "wow." I know specifically of other times I was very depressed and then when I got out of it I would describe to people "I feel like I've come out of a tunnel." [female librarian, aged 43]

I noticed that the medication seemed to melt away like this physical pressure inside my head. I felt like more clear-headed.

And I noticed within about two weeks that I stopped having the thoughts about escaping by being dead. I thought more [like] "Well I'm alive and I have these problems and what can I do to deal with the problems?" [This was] instead of just wishing that I were dead. And so I think it [the drug] has dramatically affected [me]. [male law student, aged 32]

Although it is more fully within the province of Chapter 5, "Coping and Adapting," to discuss the "positive" features of depression, I want to mention here the claim of several respondents that the agony of depression has been instrumental in their spiritual growth. One unanticipated aspect of depression revealed in the interviews is the connection between depression and spiritual life. Several people in my sample have seriously experimented with Buddhist teaching which, they claim, more satisfactorily than Western religions understands the place of human pain and suffering. Others connect their depression with creativity and insight. The following woman, quoted at length, although working as a mental health aide, has aspirations as a writer. Her comments illuminate the breathtaking impact of feeling normal after years of nonstop pain, the religious-like dimensions of the drug conversion experience, and the uncertainty attached to giving up any long-held identity, even one that has been deeply troublesome.

How would you describe the experience of Prozac?

I went on Prozac. I was like cracking up a couple of years ago, and sort of got back to the mental hospital—time number five. And I think the psychiatrist I was seeing, she didn't know what to do with me, so she sent me to this . . . psychopharmacologist, and he prescribed Prozac for me, and within five days, it was very, very strange. . . . I mean, it was hard to explain, but, I was just incredibly fearful and anxious, and I really at that point was going to kill myself, because I just was like, "Forget it." You know, "I've worked too hard and tried to conquer this thing too much, and I can't do it." And there was a tremendous amount of anger. But within five days of going on the Prozac it was like the obsessions reduced, and it was a very weird feeling. What was strange about it was that it took away the feeling of depression that I've had in my stomach for years, ever since I was a little girl. It was gone. And I remember not wanting to tell anybody about it, because I thought, this is really strange.

Not wanting to tell anybody because?

Like, "I think this is working." I was kind of like, "Jesus Christ, what's going on here." Because I'd been on medications that never had done anything for me, and this was so dramatic. . . . It was also very dramatic because I was on the brink of really cracking up, and then within five days I wasn't anywhere near cracking up. And actually, it's interesting, because I loved it, but I also wanted to go off of it, because I was sure it was going to take away my creativity.

So, it's back to the pain/creativity link.

Oh, because I couldn't write. I was used to being in an anxious state all of the time, and suddenly I didn't care as much about my writing any more. That was what the weird thing was. It [writing] didn't mean as much to me. Nothing meant as much to me. In a way that was incredibly freeing. And at the same time, I built my whole identity around being a person who was, you know, driven, intense, and I tried sort of whipping myself up into an intense state, you know, and it didn't work.

You mean, something that you had no trouble with before . . .

It (the intensity) wasn't there and as much as I hated it before, I also felt like it was who I was, and the Prozac took it away, and I remember thinking, "This is very nice. I should take this when I go on vacation, you know, and [otherwise] get me off of this stuff, because this is going to make a moron out of me."

So what's the end of the story? Still taking it?

Well, I remained on it, but the course is kind of rocky because then I was a convert to Prozac, and I was like, "This stuff is incredible." I was thinking, "This stuff is just the greatest stuff I've ever taken in the world." I mean, "this is a miracle." And I would think, "This is a miracle." And it was a miracle, it really was a miracle to me. For that one year, I was so happy. . . . And at this point the Prozac has become so intertwined with the millions of meanings that I've given it. Even a God [meaning] for a while. [female mental health worker, aged 27]

As Max Weber pointed out years ago, even charisma becomes routinized.[14] People's commitment and conversion to drugs is completed when those drugs become a routine part of their daily life. The process of adopting the medical version of depression's proper treatment is accomplished when the respondent's initial resistance to drugs completely vanishes. What normally started out as a tentative and ambivalent experiment with medications typically becomes a taken-for-granted way of life. In effect, the people interviewed have undergone a socialization process that has transformed the meanings to them of medication. The negotiated experiment begun with trepidation has become institutionalized, habitualized, and ritualized. To use the vocabulary offered by

Peter Berger and Thomas Luckmann, a once alternative and alien "symbolic universe" has become an accepted and seemingly immutable reality.[15] That is, taking medications now appears as an absolutely unquestioned feature of daily reality. Consider the casualness with which those initially opposed to drugs sometimes come to regard them.

> What's interesting to me about the drug now, or at least my attitude toward it, is that I regard it almost as a food supplement. It's just something I eat that's going to have a certain effect. So I don't quite see it as unnatural the way I used to. [male professor, aged 48]

> I'm convinced maybe I have to take it for the rest of my life. I'd certainly rather feel like this than feel like that, and if it's two little pills I've got to put in my mouth every day that makes me stay this way, then so be it. [unemployed male waiter, aged 33]

Disenchantment and Deconversion

Those who study conversions must include in their analyses the factors that sometimes account for the disenchantment, defection, and deconversion of large numbers of people from their respective groups or belief systems. Some, of course, retain their commitments to alternative realities over the long term. Equally, though, are those who come to question the utility and correctness of the explanatory schemas they had experimented with and then fully embraced. Of course, even converts stand at different places on a continuum of commitment. Some are never fully convinced of the value of new behaviors and beliefs, are easily disenchanted with new problem-solving perspectives, and return relatively quickly to old perspectives and identities. A few among those studied stayed on drugs for only a short time, deciding that they were not sufficiently effective to put up with noxious side effects. After experimenting with medications, these people were easily able to return to the view that their problems were environmentally based and that drugs would not be their salvation. The failure of a belief system is much more devastating, of course, when people have embraced it unreservedly. This was certainly the case for those who had experienced a drug miracle, but subsequently suffered a relapse. The young woman quoted at length earlier described her response to the eventual failure of the drug after her ecstatic revelatory experience.

> Then I decided I was going to go away to [names a southern state] for two months and do an internship in interviewing women down there. And then again I thought, this is the kind of thing I can do, because now I'm on Prozac and I won't freak out, whereas before that kind of change would have freaked me out. And I went, and I freaked out, and that's when I completely like, relapsed. . . . Now I have a somewhat more balanced view of the Prozac in that I can become obsessive, anxious, depressed on it, even very obsessive and anxious and depressed. It's not a miracle drug. It hasn't saved me. And it's been a long time coming to terms with that. It helps somewhat, sometimes, and that's where it's at. And, I did for a while think, "I am going to be cured." It was the ultimate disappointment. You know, it was connected with an intense sense of loss and a sense of redemption, and I do not overstate [things]. It really was that. [female mental health worker, aged 27]

The complexity of stopping medications is evident in that even when they do not appear to fundamentally alter depressive feelings, respondents sometimes become psychologically dependent on them. Once having experimented with the drugs and having accepted biochemical definitions of their condition, they feel uncertain about stopping. Whatever their current problems, several individuals were afraid that things might deteriorate if they ceased the medications.

Can you see yourself getting off this medication?

I really don't want to because I'm afraid. I don't really have any side effects other than the upset stomach, the appetite fluctuation, and the sexual dysfunction which I can live with. [Recently] I said [to my psychiatrist], "Well, I can't tell the difference [between] being on it or not being on it. And she said, "Well if you stopped taking it . . . you would notice it because you would fall back into the depression." That's how you'd know that it was working. So I said, "Well I don't want that because there's nothing worse than not being able to sleep, not being able to eat, and not being able to function." [unemployed disabled female, aged 39]

I'm afraid to not take it, but it really hasn't done much of anything. [female college professor, aged 49]

I mean, it's almost to the point now where I take it sometimes but like I really don't feel like I have the need for it. But I'm sort of afraid not to take it. . . . I'm on such a low dosage [now]. He's [doctor] got me on one pill a night. And it's taken, you know, ten years [to get to that point]. [male administrator, aged 54]

If I had listened to myself I would have just said, "Screw the medication." But also I think I was probably afraid, afraid that if I went off them completely that I would get worse, and I guess there is some evidence for that. [male professor, part-time, aged 48]

Ultimately, the respondents in this study, like the epilepsy patients interviewed by Peter Conrad, become, at the least, ambivalent about the role of medications in dealing with their difficulty.[16] They may feel dependent on the drugs and worry about the consequences of stopping, but they also begin to question the wisdom of staying on the medications. Just as Conrad's epilepsy patients eventually discover that the medications are not the "ticket to normality," it soon becomes apparent to most sufferers of depression that a medical cure is not forthcoming. In both instances, patients become disenchanted with drug side effects, begin to question their efficacy, experiment with dosage levels, and sometimes decide even to stop taking them. Conrad describes a number of noncompliance responses of epilepsy patients that reflect efforts to regain control over their illness. He notes that "[self] regulating medication represents an attempt to assert some degree of control over a condition that appears at times to be completely out of control."[17] His findings certainly seem generalizable to the case of depression, as the following comments illustrate.

I guess I myself was curious to see what would happen if I were to stop taking it. Partly my wife didn't like the idea that I was on a drug. She's concerned about long range effects and I guess I was a little concerned about that too. [male professor, aged 48]

I think the medication was more of a hindrance than a help. The Zoloft started making me have crying spells. . . . He wanted me to try Buspar, but I finally told him, "Look I want the business with the meds stopped." [female telemarketer, aged 23]

I just decided I wasn't going to go the route of something that could possibly give me brain damage. And I just decided that

I would suffer through whatever happens. And I just quit. [male professor, aged 66]

I had gained a lot of weight on the pills. I was always a very thin person and here I was carrying forty more pounds. My sense of physical identity was damaged and I wanted out. [female social worker, aged 38]

In other cases individuals finally rebel against taking medications as a way of reclaiming selves that they believe have been lost because of their involvement with antidepressant medications. These persons who vow never to go on the drugs again have plainly had a deconversion experience.

Now, in between the new and the old [medications] there would be a period when they would take me off the thing. And my friends during that stretch without fail would say "You seem like yourself again." And if I had listened closely I would have said, "Gee, the implication of this is that these pills are fucking me up." [Finally] I would go in and say "Can I get off it? Can I get off it?" And he would say, "Try it longer." Finally I thought "I'm not going to ask this son of a bitch any longer. I'm just going to take myself off it." And I did and he either forgot about it or didn't raise it. I just took myself off. . . . [And] I will never take another fucking pill in my life. And I'm not generalizing to other people. . . . But for me, I had gotten so fucked up with this stuff that I will never do it again. [male professor, part-time, aged 48]

I mean, I put my foot down about the Trazadone. I was at the point where I could say, "I'm just going to stop." [female librarian, aged 43]

CONCLUSION

Although the people you heard speak may stand at different points in their drug-taking careers, most commonly move through a socialization process that involves overcoming initial resistance to drug taking, negotiating the terms of their treatment, adopting new rhetorics about the cause of depression, experiencing a conversion to medical realities, and eventually becoming disenchanted with the value of medications for solving their problems. This process bears a strong similarity to descriptions of religious conversion and deconversion. That is, one's willingness to begin, sustain, and sometimes stop a doctor-prescribed regimen of antidepressant medications must be understood in the broader context of adopting a new, identity-altering view of reality; namely, that one suffers from a biochemically based emotional illness. For this reason, the experience of taking antidepressant medications involves a complex and emotionally charged interpretive process in which nothing less than one's view of self is at stake.

The process described in this chapter helps in thinking about some of the social psychological dynamics that are part of the "medicalization"[18] of society more broadly. Implicitly, my analysis refers to an ongoing struggle between professional and lay definitions of illness, reality, and self. As several observers have noted,[19] the behaviors of persons in today's "postindustrial" society are dominated by "experts." Experts advise us on virtually every aspect of our lives. And dominant among these experts are physicians who tell us when our bodies and selves need repair and the proper procedures for doing it.

The data presented illustrate the power of the "medical model" in defining the appropriate response to emotional problems. The medical model is used to support the political reality created by a coalition of physicians, teachers, judges, and other health professionals. Peter Berger and Thomas Luckmann[20] refer to this coalition as "universe maintenance specialists." These specialists from different disciplines set the norms defining proper and improper behavior, deviant and conforming behavior, normal and pathological behavior, sick and healthy behavior. Thus, therapy "entails the application of conceptual machinery to ensure that actual or potential deviants stay within the institutionalized definitions of reality. . . . This requires a body of knowledge that includes a theory of deviance, a diagnostic apparatus and a conceptual system for the 'cure of souls.' "[21]

Nowhere, of course, is the struggle over definitions of illness reality and, literally, the mind of the patient more apparent than in psychiatry. The materials presented earlier illustrate that acceptance of medical versions of reality is not automatic. Psychiatric patients are initially resistant to illness definitions of their problem and "come around" to prescribed medical treatments only with great difficulty. Although everyone I spoke with eventually capitulated to medical versions of reality, conversion was often incomplete as individuals lost faith in the efficacy of drug treatment and sometimes rebelled against it altogether. It seems reasonable to speculate that as part of a general and increasing "democratization" of professional/client relationships, resistance to medical authority will become more intense. Moreover, the terrain of this struggle over reality is most likely to be in the psychiatric arena where the legitimacy of a purely medical model is most suspect.

The people interviewed eventually realize that doctors, despite their best efforts, will not clear away their confusions about depression. The socialization process described earlier involves hope that medication will provide the solution to their problem.

In most cases, however, this optimistic attitude was replaced with disillusionment and sometimes anger. The failure of medical treatments for depression supplies fertile soil for the emergence of self-help groups that offer the view of affective disorders as troubles that must ultimately be remedied by the individuals who suffer from them.[22] Such a definition suggests an anti-psychiatry ideology that demands, at the very least, a greater democracy between doctor and patient in efforts to treat the problem. The data and analysis in this chapter point to some areas of conversation that are likely to become central in the working out of the "identity politics"[23] inevitably a part of depression's treatment.

Chapter 5

Coping and Adapting

If I didn't do my work and I didn't focus on the work, then all there is is pain. The work takes me away from the pain. If I didn't work then I'd have to think about how miserable I was and how I didn't have any friends and how no one loved me. It was awful.

Female graduate student, aged 24

I believe that depression is actually a gift. That if we can befriend it, if we can travel with it, that it is showing us things. Somewhere along the line we've got to integrate it into our lives. All of us are depressed some way, somewhere at some time. If we don't allow it in, it can be destructive. If we allow it in, it is a teacher. I'm saying embrace it. Be in it.

Female freelance writer, aged 41

An emphasis on *process* has been an underlying motif throughout. In particular, I used the notion of "career" in Chapter 3 to play out how an individual's identity as a depressed person comes into being, and Chapter 4 describes a socialization process that normally eventuates in acceptance of a biomedical version of depression's cause. This chapter on coping and adaptation[1] parallels and extends these earlier themes since bad feelings insistently require that something be done about them. As Kathy Charmaz shows in

her powerfully written book *Good Days, Bad Days*,[2] chronic illnesses can utterly dominate people's lives. Those with severe and
debilitating diseases are enveloped by and immersed in them.
Often, their whole lives are necessarily organized around the contingencies of their medical problems. Although Charmaz restricts
her conversation to such illnesses as multiple sclerosis, depression
no less than unremitting physical diseases dominates the lives of
sufferers and calls forth continual efforts at adaptation.

In an autobiographical memoir of her emergence from nearly
two years of "madness" and life in an asylum, Susanna Kaysen observed that one of the great pleasures of mental health is that she
needs to spend far less time thinking about herself.[3] To be sure,
a subjective sense of wellness most fundamentally means being
able to move through life without constantly worrying about one's
readiness to meet everyday obligations and challenges. Well people
enjoy the taken-for-granted assumption that their bodies and
minds will not interfere with the requirements of everyday life. As
discussed in Chapter 2, however, those with depression may find
even the simplest tasks and rituals of daily life impossible. Even in
its more benign forms, depression shapes how a person plans for
and moves through each day. In the longer term, depression nearly
always influences how people think about critical choices related
to careers, friendship, and family.

Kaysen's observation about the inability of mentally ill people
to forget themselves strongly resonates with my own experience.
When depression/anxiety dominates my life I can think of little
else than my(self). If I am fortunate enough to get any sleep in the
midst of my worst nights, my first thoughts upon waking center
on just how bad the day is likely to be and how well I'll be able
to meet its demands. Depressed people become experts on the
smallest nuances of their psychic states and the physical feelings

they produce. Sometimes a day might turn out better or more miserable than anticipated by this initial scan of my body and mind, but always the intrusive negative feelings require an assessment of how things are likely to go. My waking hours are then characterized by a nearly continuous monitoring of how well or badly I am doing. On very bad days, as much as I might want to focus on things outside of myself, I can't. For instance, since I am unable to muster enough concentration to read a newspaper with any comprehension, attention to local, national, or international events is impossible. In fact, the strain of the effort to forget myself as the day proceeds only affirms the power of depressive feelings over my will to transcend them.

On many occasions I have told people close to me that the difference between my good and bad days seems like the difference between being dead and alive—the contrast is that sharp. On the cherished good days I am able to glide through things, attending to the same tasks and projects with ease, clarity, and pleasure that 24 hours previously might have seemed tortuous. I never stop being amazed by the fluctuations in the state of my mind from day to day, week to week, month to month, and, most extraordinarily, sometimes from hour to hour. For this reason, I listened with interest to a TV interview in which the author Michael Crichton compared his own bouts with depression to changes in the weather. One day the weather is bright and sunny in the morning, but by mid-afternoon a gloomy cold front might descend. There might be several pleasant days in a row, followed by a month-long cloudy spell with some really stormy periods. And there have been years when the weather was pretty lousy most of the time. I mean to say that when the depression weather is most bleak, forging ahead unselfconsciously simply cannot happen. An injured, hurting, pained self dominates thought, perception, and action. Depression makes it impossible to "lose" one's self in the flow of life activities. To the contrary, sufferers become swamped by their selves and then lost in them.

It is not surprising that people with depression are often accused by those close to them as being thoroughly self-absorbed and insufficiently attentive to anyone's needs but their own. In their less charitable moments, family and friends of depressed people view them as selfish, as rarely thinking about anything or anybody but themselves. As you will see in Chapter 6, intimates eventually and wisely realize the need to distance themselves from a depressed friend or family member in order not to become sick by association. Eventually they realize that efforts to pull another out of depression are destined to fail and, ironically, will only catch them in the vortex that is already enveloping their child, sibling, friend, or mate.

The idea that the sick person is not doing enough to help him or herself is implied in the self-absorption criticism. One of the strongest norms surrounding illness experience is the expectation that the sick person "work" diligently at living as normal a life as possible. Even people who are literally dying from chronic diseases are expected to minimize the extent to which they are a burden on others and do whatever they can to normalize their circumstance. For example, in her wonderfully detailed treatment of the history of tuberculosis, Sheila Rothman uses the illness narratives found in letters and diaries to show how "invalids" suffering from "consumption" were expected to devote themselves— indeed, devote their whole lives—to getting better.[4] However difficult or deadly one's illness, sick people have only so many "sympathy credits"[5] they can use to legitimate total immersion in the sick role.[6] At a point, the failure of sick people to do something for themselves generates anger among family and friends who come to believe they are being unfairly manipulated in the name of illness.

It is important to mention another feature of depression in this context. Over and again, interviewees contrasted depression to visible physical problems, such as broken bones, complaining that the invisibility of their disease and the lack of any physical manifestations of its presence was a critical factor in diminishing empathy for them and their condition. In this regard, depressed people share much in common with those who suffer from chronic physical pain that has no demonstrable source. A nearly universal response to chronic pain sufferers, especially when medical tests show "nothing wrong," is a gradual belief that complaints about the pain are exaggerated.[7] We might suspect that of all claims about suffering, psychic pain has the least credibility because it possesses no clear locus and medicine is unable to produce the functional equivalent of an X ray to affirm that it has a material cause. One woman who cut her face and arms during difficult depressions told me she did it for two reasons: the physical pain momentarily blunted the far more difficult mental pain, and the effects of the self-mutilation were available to others as an undeniable and palpable sign of pain they couldn't otherwise see. Jim, a part-time teacher, conveyed the substance of these ideas with his comment that

> I must say that I think there is quite a bias in our society about people who suffer from emotional illnesses. I mean, if you break a leg or something, it is a discrete event. You get sympathy, people sign your cast, you get cards. . . . Depression or any other emotional illness is much harder to handle. . . . People, even your closest friends seem very uncomfortable. They don't know what to say. Some friends kind of evaporate. [male professor, part-time, aged 48]

Organizing the 24 hours of everyday life in the face of depression poses the most immediate and most continuous problems of adaptation. However, depression, like any serious chronic illness, forces decisions that shape the overall contours of one's life. Those who have had extended hospitalizations or are subject to disabling episodes of major depression find their life choices and chances greatly foreshortened. The numbers in my sample speak for themselves. Most of those interviewed have somehow gotten through college and their words surely demonstrate their insight and intelligence. Yet many are unable to hold *any* job and others find that their chronic illness keeps them chronically underemployed. Even when they develop resume writing strategies to conceal long periods of unemployment and then lie on job applications about their history of mental illness, many have learned they must radically revise downward their occupational aspirations. Similarly, most in my sample have had difficulty in establishing long-term personal relationships because of their depression and, like the person who concluded, "I'm beginning to think that I'm not very marriageable material," they realize that a conventional family life will not be possible for them. Thereby, depression renders problematic a range of decisions, from those as immediate as accepting a dinner party invitation to choices about attending school, embarking on a particular occupational path, or planning a family life.

Depression, like many illnesses, requires ongoing answers to a series of related questions: What is wrong with me? What should I be doing about it? Is this something that can be fixed if I try hard enough? What do other people expect me to do about this? What, if anything, can I learn from this difficult experience of mine? As a result, my interviews are, from beginning to end, stories of adaptation. The first open-ended question in each interview asks

"Whether or not you could attach the word depression to your situation, when was the first moment you realized that something was wrong with you?" As they fill in the natural history of their experience with depression, individuals comment, without prompting, on the things they have done to get rid of it and then eventually to live with it. In this chapter I want to look at the regularities that emerge over the course of time in the way individuals adapt to and cope with depression. I suspect these regularities apply to a range of chronic illnesses, both mental and physical.

The particular contents of people's stories, of course, vary quite widely, but their overall form shows remarkable consistency. Initially, respondents describe a series of strategies to deny, run away from, or outrun their intrusive and prolonged bad feelings. Somewhere along the line depression grabs them from behind and it becomes plain that no diversionary tactics, however intensively engaged in, will allow them to distance themselves from their problem. With this recognition, their consciousness turns to what is necessary to "fix" their difficulty. The analogy here is to a piece of broken machinery. The presumption is that just as one might fix a watch by opening it and setting right the mechanical defect, the same can be done with their emotions. Thus, ill people are transformed into patients who rely on psychiatrists, society's designated experts on fixing troublesome emotions. I was not prepared for the frequency and intensity of anger expressed toward psychiatrists as respondents spoke about their search for the "right" one. This anger, I now believe, comes partly from patients' eventual recognition that, in most cases, doctors cannot fix them and somehow they must learn to live with the depression. Once this truth is absorbed, people often respond to pain in a more spiritual fashion, trying to find ways, if not to embrace it, at least to incorporate depressive illness into their lives. Thus, the process of adaptation moves full circle. It starts with diversion and ends with incorporation.[8]

DIVERSION

As Karl Marx argued in a very different context, action typically follows consciousness.[9] If the intention of Chapter 3, "Illness and Identity," was to document how people come to perceive and label their problem as depression, the attention here shifts to behavior in the face of the pain eventually labeled as depression. In other words, the contrast between this and earlier discussion is between *perception* and *action*, between recognition of what the problem is and what to do about it. Each of the stages described in Chapter 3—inchoate distress, the sense that "something is wrong with me," crisis, recognition of depression as one's illness, and perception of the condition's permanence—has clear behavioral analogs. Each of these identity turning points is associated with responses designed to mitigate the problem, to cope with and adapt to the condition *as one understands it at that moment*. Since ideas about what depression is and what it means for one's life seep slowly into consciousness over time, decisions about appropriate responses to feeling dilemmas also have an emergent character. Definitions of what is wrong and decisions about remediation are the two central interpretive axes involved in the social construction of any illness reality.[10]

As discussed in Chapter 3, respondents initially have no idea about the sources of their uncomfortable feelings or even that there is something "wrong" with them. What they do know is that certain activities, at least initially, take the edge off their melancholy or dull their particular variant of anxiety. In fact, during the earliest stages of the depression career it would probably be wrong to say that respondents were strategically choosing behaviors to feel better. Strategy implies a level of recognition, intentionality, planning, and assessment of cause that likely does not exist early on. They were simply drifting toward activities that made them feel happier, more secure, and more content. A 22-year-old woman, unemployed at the time we spoke, described her life during the summer following college graduation this way:

> I think I spent that whole summer really partying a lot. I would go from therapy to play softball for a bar I used to hang out in with friends. Just totally blot out anything that was going on. I spent the whole next day—I was doing a social work internship in the Bronx—and I would like try to focus on everybody but myself. Like that went on for months. [unemployed female, aged 22]

Others described similar behaviors, all of which involved throwing themselves into things as a way of diverting attention from the depression. Here, as at many points during interviews, I could strongly relate to the stories I was hearing. I currently weigh about 180 pounds, but in the late 1970s my weight was down to 160 pounds because I was playing basketball three hours a day with students at Boston College. At the time, I thought of myself as just participating in the new fitness consciousness that was sweeping America. Like everybody else I was getting into shape. In retrospect, I feel certain that I was literally running as hard as I could from the discomfort of depression. Pick-up basketball games required an intensity of effort (especially for a "thirties-something" person guarding an 18-year-old) that for a time allowed me to forget myself. In hindsight, I can understand how the extent of my involvement in the game seemed strange to those around me, but at the time I just knew it made me feel better. As described in the interviews, any of a variety of involvements worked as long as they were sufficiently engaging.

I did things to ignore depression. My big thing was like just ignore it. Get busy. Do things. Don't feel. That was my thing. Don't feel. And it's easy to do. I mean, I could write a book about how I didn't feel. You know, things that I did. Fifteen magazine subscriptions, you know? Anything not to feel. I spent a lot of time after I got out [of school] trying just to only feel good. Only be happy. 'Cause after all, I didn't want to be depressed, you know? [male salesman, aged 30]

I just knew I felt better doing drugs. [male law student, aged 32]

On weekends I used to go to church. So I got really into religion and into you know, going to CCD (Confraternity of Christian Doctrine) class. And then I was on the board that runs the church. I was on that for a couple of years. And I sang in the choir. So I just did a lot of diversionary things. [unemployed disabled female, aged 39]

During the number of years actually prior to the Trazadone and stuff I was a shopaholic. I mean, I never got myself in trouble with it, but I bought stuff I didn't need. Shopping was my form of meditation or escape or whatever. I paid cash for everything, but it really was a tremendous waste of money. Recently I've been going to movies. The shopping is long since gone. And the movies are a mixed blessing. If it is a compelling enough movie, it will take me away from the terror. [female college professor, aged 49]

Well, you know, [I was] keeping myself up by my studies. It
helped me forget the intensity of the depression. . . . And I was
beginning to develop political interests and so that also helped
me in a different way to get over the depression. . . . I realized
later on in my life that [without the political involvement]
I simply would have gone out of my mind. I realized later that
that must have done me a great deal of good. I managed to keep
myself occupied in the single-minded pursuit of an object. . . .
In my late teens I began to develop great interest in sports and
that was one factor which relieved my depression at that time.
I was really mad about sports. [unemployed male bookkeeper,
aged 51]

At the point where it becomes impossible for individuals to sustain the definition of their pain as normal, as pain without pathology,
they also realize that they needed and used activities to blot it out.
It is sometimes said that anxiety lies behind productivity, that a certain amount of anxiety is valuable to provide the motivation for hard
work. Among those in my sample, many were high-achieving persons. Several did outstandingly well in school, for example. It might
then reasonably be asked, "If they were suffering so, how could they
possibly work so hard?" The question points to still another paradox
of depression. Before it completely flattens them and makes work
impossible, working at a furious pace gives some people respite from
the pain. Sometimes individuals plainly knew that work was their
diversion from very difficult feelings. One of my former students
who was in graduate school when I interviewed her recalled

Well, take this depression that I had three weeks ago. After two
years of not being depressed, to have that come back. Terrifying.
I had all those papers to write and I was so glad because having

work, having school is a diversion from the depression. There's something to sink my teeth into. . . . I'm just thinking about that year when I went to you and how suicidal I was and how depressed I was. I did damn well that semester. I got my work done.

That's amazing.

To tell you the truth, I think the depression helped it, meaning I can't write when I'm not depressed. I go off and do things and daydream. The work saves me. I mean look at all this stuff (points to previously written notebooks and journals). . . . Two years of not writing anything on my own. And this semester . . . this is the first year that I've been in school that I haven't been depressed. I completely blew off the semester. I went out with friends. I did all these social things that I didn't do for ten years [while I was depressed]. Work. Forget it. And then [names a professor] says to me, "How could you not do any of your work?" I said, "For 16 years I was a good little girl. I did everything I was supposed to do. I did real well."

It sounds like in some curious way the depression focused you.

Because if I didn't do my work and I didn't focus on the work, then all there is is pain. The work would take me away from the pain. If I didn't work then I'd have to think about how miserable I was and how I didn't have any friends and how no one loved me. It was awful. [female graduate student, aged 24]

A 49-year-old female college professor believed she would be dead without her work.

I think that teaching was one of the first major antidepressants that I discovered. It was reliable. I still do have a little withdrawal when I'm not teaching. I mean I'll have withdrawal when I don't teach for six weeks. So it's not really a drug. It's like they talk about healthy addictions.

It's a focus and an involvement.

Right. It's not fair for me to call it an antidepressant even. I don't know, I think I get more out of teaching than other people do. I really feel real and alive [when I'm teaching] and [it helps me] through some really difficult stuff. . . . It's worked for me even when I've been profoundly depressed. . . . Recently I have been extraordinarily depressed and am right now. And the fellow I occasionally see, the psychiatrist for meds, he's learned, but he'll say, "Can you go to work?" And I'll laugh. And I say, "Look, the day I can't go to work I'll be dead." [female college professor, aged 49]

And a 27-year-old mental health worker said:

You see, the thing that was hard to explain is that I was depressed inside of me all the time. [There was] this feeling of emptiness; a feeling like lead. That's what it feels like to me in my stomach, [something] that I can never [get rid of]. . . . And the way I learned to make it go away . . . was to write. . . . It worked to relieve the depression. It was like the heaviness would go away. And then I would get praised for it, and I would feel . . . I mean, I wouldn't feel depressed. [female mental health worker, aged 27]

Special mention should be made of children's coping strategies. Children, of course, have absolutely no way of defining their bad feelings as depression, but as any psychology text will affirm, they plainly know when things are not right in their families. Several

respondents in this study described the kinds of abuse, both physical and sexual, that has only in recent years been grabbing the attention of the media and social scientists. Only now are we coming
to understand the extent of the violence in American homes at all
points along the class structure[11] and the long-term effects of that
trauma on the mental life of its victims.[12] From among those who
described their childhoods as taking place within a dysfunctional
family, some version of "I hid out" was used to describe efforts to
escape a situation that seemed terrifying and which they intuitively knew was wrong.

> I could close that door downstairs and when I was very young
> I would go to my grandparents for the weekend because I would
> tell my parents I need some peace and quiet. And I think this is
> one of the ways I coped then. You know, I needed to shut down
> a little bit. [female librarian, aged 43]

> The only really tough part was well, school. At school I went on
> autopilot. School. I don't know how I went through it, because
> I think I just sort of shut down whatever emotions there were
> and acted like nothing was going on. And at night, I would just
> lock myself in my room, except my sister shared it with me. Or
> I would go downstairs and put the stereo on, and sit there and
> do my homework, and have the music blast out whatever the
> yelling was. And so I did that. I was trying to sort of drown it
> out. [female nurse, aged 37]

TRYING TO FIX IT

As my own biography and the materials in Chapter 3 illustrate,
once it becomes undeniable that something is really wrong, that

one's difficulties are too extreme to be pushed aside as either temporary or reasonable, efforts begin in earnest to solve the problem. Now, choices to relieve pain are made with a conscious and urgent deliberation. The shift in thinking often occurs when the presumed cause of pain is removed, but the difficulty persists. Tenure is received, you finally get out of an oppressive home environment, a destructive relationship is finally ended, and so on, but the depression persists. Such events destroy theories about the immediate situational sources of depression and force the unwelcome interpretation that the problem might be permanent and have an internal locus. One has to consider that it might be a problem of the self rather than the situation. Such a turn in thinking generates its own confusions since now the problem requires a name. Is it a "condition," an "illness," an "imbalance," or a "disease," and are words like "mental" or "emotional" appropriate?[13] Although the cause of the deeply unsettling feelings remains obscure, there is perfect clarity that something has to be done to make things better.

Initially, respondents had the idea that if they just thought enough about things or did some experiments to see what made them feel better, they could solve the problem by themselves. Like physician-phobic people who try to solve a persistent and debilitating cough by searching through the drugstore for a more effective medication, many individuals first preferred to seek a solution on their own rather than see any sort of therapist. This reluctance to visit a therapist sometimes came from Puritan upbringings that taught them to be self-reliant, to be stoic, and to solve their problems without complaint or help. For people like Jack, an unemployed waiter, who had been taught that "anybody who saw a psychiatrist was weird," the idea, at least initially, of getting professional help was out of the question. Instead, they elected to try solving their problem as though it were a giant jigsaw puzzle. If they could identify all the relevant pieces to their emotional puzzle and array them for inspection, it would eventually be possible, they thought, to put their life picture together and move ahead comfortably. So, they tried in a variety of ways to fix themselves.

I decided to do junior year abroad. So that was going to fix me. [unemployed female, aged 22]

I threw myself into books, [into] my stacks of romance novels. Not the kind of books I would normally read often. Because I didn't have the concentration for science. But, just enormous stacks of novels that I would just chew my way through. And then there comes a point where distraction is just not practical. And then you say, "Okay, I've got to do something." And you do as much as you can. It's not so much that you say, "I've tried to fix it and failed," as that you do all the things that are possible. You try the medication. If you haven't resolved issues you talk issues. [female software quality control manager, aged 31]

I guess I didn't want to see myself as sick or in need of some major kind of therapy, some major intervention. I wanted to see if there were some methods that I could follow that would help me to be more effective. [male college professor, aged 48]

[I was] thinking all the time, trying to figure out what was wrong and what I would have to do to make things better. [female college professor, aged 49]

I'm such an analytical person that I tried to figure out what was going on. I tried to analyze it, which made me even more miserable because I couldn't figure it out. [female house cleaner, aged 23]

> I wanted help. I was desperate for help. I just wanted somebody
> to fix this or tell me what the hell I needed to do. . . . I always
> tried like hell to find some key to it. [unemployed male, aged 58]

Eventually, everyone who tried to figure things out on their own had to conclude that their mechanistic assumptions about feelings were wrong. It took a while, though, before they could fully accept that a logical approach and hard work would not set them straight. Often they were misled by some diminution of their depression. Since depression tends to vary in intensity over time and periodically disappears, individuals sometimes presumed a cause-and-effect relationship between their interventions and an improvement in mood. When depression returned, they still might have faith that by fine-tuning the tools they had earlier established for feeling better, the problem would be solved once and for all. Of course, each time depression returned it diminished their faith that they could handle it themselves. Several shared the experience of one woman who told me, "I thought that I would pass through it, that I would figure it out, and it would be okay. And in a sense that was true. It did lift and things got better, but then it's happened again. The first couple of times it happened, I was so sure that it would never happen again, that I would never feel that way again. . . . [Thinking that way] I made it harder on myself."

Each interview has a distinctive tone and flavor. My interview with Keith, himself a therapist, centered, in fact, on coping and adaptation. Keith described a life devoted to psychological development that he believed would insulate him from a recurrence of an earlier depression he had attributed to a long-term physical problem with his back. His tone was upbeat and after describing how awful the earlier period had been, Keith depicted his progress in developing strategies to ensure that he would not suffer another depression. He described the earlier depression, the failure of spirituality to help him, and then the new, more effective strategies he had put into place to avoid depression. Here is part of our conversation on these themes:

> I think what I realize now, and it is somewhat painful and a rebuilding process for me, is that [I thought] spirituality was one of several things that actually were kind of a defense for me against the kind of emptiness that the depression kind of dropped me into. So spirituality really didn't help me. Spirituality as I understood it didn't help me. That's a great sadness for me. . . . I used to feel that I'd done a lot of spiritual work. I put a lot of time into it and therefore I would be protected. And there is a certain amount of ego in that. And it didn't work. That had a tremendous impact on me. I don't have anything to put in its place. . . . I couldn't meditate when I was depressed. I just couldn't.

> *So where are you now?*

> I feel good. I feel like a lot of what's happened for me is I've changed some of the fundamental structures of my life. [At this point, he talks about significant changes in his work situation]. I'm processing things in a different way. I've kind of moved myself out of that [bad work situation] a lot. . . . It feels like my life has changed. Some of the fundamental kinds of underlying things that were responsible for the depression [have been taken care of]. The choices that I wasn't making or the choices I didn't experience as choice, [but] . . . they are choices. You can't see that they're choices because they have been made so long ago. They seem so fixed into place that they seem like fact. But it's not. To realize that is transformative, very empowering.

And I think for me [that] is mainly responsible for the lack of depression. [male therapist, aged 45]

I had become friends with Keith before this interview. We first met at a support group for people with depression and had been in fairly close contact over several months before I got his thoughts on tape. For that reason I was not surprised to get a call from him about two weeks after our interview. I assumed he was interested in getting together for the kinds of casual conversation we had been having periodically. I was saddened to learn that the purpose of the call was to tell me that he had fallen into a depression even worse than his first. Well aware that our talk just two weeks earlier had been so upbeat, he told me that the failure of all his therapeutic work—his "insurance policy" against depression—was making the current pain that much more unbearable. Like nearly all 50 persons interviewed, Keith realized that he could not fix himself and eventually saw a psychiatrist. Sometimes individuals voluntarily visited a doctor at a point of desperation, when nothing they did seemed to help. In other cases, crisis and hospitalization required a doctor's attention.

Chapter 4 was devoted exclusively to the process through which patients come to take antidepressant medications and the way they interpret the meanings of those drugs. Implicitly that discussion was also about coping and adaptation. Drug taking was a big enough piece of the depression experience to warrant a separate chapter. In that discussion and at other points along the way, both my analysis and the comments of interviewees deal with attitudes toward physicians. By the time I talked with them, most of the people interviewed had years of experience with psychiatrists. While some of those you have already heard speak had nothing but positive experiences with psychiatrists, most were, at the least, ambivalent about psychiatry, and several were downright angry and hostile toward all therapy and therapists. The depth of their feeling toward therapeutic experts who tried to fix them when they couldn't fix themselves calls for description and comment now.

LOOKING FOR DR. RIGHT

Nearly everyone interviewed for this study has seen several psychiatrists over the years. In some cases, it required extraordinary attention to follow a person's complicated history with as many as a dozen different doctors. Sometimes, the number of doctors mentioned was a result of a person's having been treated in different areas of the country and in different hospitals, but far more often individuals gave up on doctors whom they believed simply did not understand them, were not humane enough, or, they felt, were incompetent. Generally, respondents were ambivalent about therapists of all sorts. Some, however, were decidedly unambivalent when they variously described someone who had treated them along the way as arrogant, elitist, insulting, ineffective, crazy, rigid, distant, cold, cynical, and without empathy. Others angrily described one or more of their doctors as "a fuck-up," "a real pig," a "supercilious prick," a "quack," a "really sick bastard," as "really weird," "an absolutely hopeless jerk," or "brutal to me."

There is no doubt that psychiatry has been "taking it on the chin" in recent years. Celebrated cases such as the suicide of Paul Lozano, a promising medical student and recipient of "unorthodox" treatments for depression by a Harvard psychiatrist, Margaret Bean-Bayog, make daily news stories for weeks at a time. The allegations in that particular case were that the psychiatrist had made Lozano completely dependent on her through a controversial therapy and that she was herself sexually obsessed with him. Stories about therapists having sexual relationships with dependent patients have become common in the print media and on TV talk shows. Together, these accounts have fostered vigorous discussion about professional ethics within the therapeutic community and a more general public debate about the worth of therapies of all sorts. However, even in the context of such unflattering publicity, the sheer volume of angry and negative comments I heard is striking. Why would patients routinely become so disenchanted with doctors whom, I assume, were honestly trying to help them?

Perhaps the relationship between extremely distressed, vulnerable patients and powerful psychiatrists intrinsically generates friction, discomfort, and anger. The gap between the expectations that patients bring to psychiatric professionals and what their doctors can actually deliver may be so great that disillusionment is inevitable. In fact, close inspection of respondents' words persuades me that the instability of the patient/therapist relationship may stem from profoundly different definitions of what the relationship is all about and what it ought to yield. The therapeutic encounter seems full of possibilities for mutual misunderstanding. Jessie Bernard observed years ago that couples do not see their marriage the same way; that there is a "his" marriage and a "her" marriage.[14] Might patient and doctor also have very different versions of therapy's "reality?" Doctors may hold one set of assumptions about therapeutic relationships and patients quite another.[15] Patients want understanding, warmth, even love. Instead they find detached professionals who often do not even inquire about their feelings, only their symptoms. A tip-off to the possibility of mutual misunderstanding is found in the way that patients talk about searching for the "right" doctor.

It is really hard with depression. It's like you've got to get to the right doctor who's going to understand it. [unemployed female, aged 22]

I heard that the [names a therapy institute] would take people on. I signed up for five years of psychoanalysis and that was destructive to me. The woman who became my analyst completely misunderstood the problems. She kept criticizing me. I mean, it turns out that [it] was just wrong. She wasn't right for me anyway. She wasn't very good. And the analysis really hurt me. [female college professor, aged 49]

I think in '81 . . . I started to feel a lot of stressing out. . . . I was seeing one therapist for a while, and that didn't work out, and I started seeing another one. . . . I think he's the best doctor I've ever had. He just knows what the hell I'm talking about. He's empathetic but he's not, you know, coddling. He knows what's going on. You know, we're on the same wave length. We're sort of the same age [and have] the same [aged] kids. [male administrator, aged 54]

In these and other descriptions respondents repeat the theme of finding a therapist who is "right for you." As I re-read stories about relationships with therapists "gone bad," I could not help thinking that were the words and contexts of the accounts changed slightly, they might be stories about soured romances. The accounts parallel comments often heard in everyday conversation and popular music about falling in and out of love.[16] People's relations with a series of therapists might be understood as similar to a pattern of "serial monogamy": finding someone you believe is right for you, becoming dependent on that person for meeting certain needs, making a commitment, eventually realizing that you may have made the wrong choice, leaving the relationship, and searching once more for the person who is *really* right for you. Taking liberty with the title of a pop music hit from a few years ago, depressed patients may be "lookin' for love" in at least *one* of the wrong places. To see plainly the parallel with troubled romances or marriages, here is a description of a difficult "breakup" after 12 years. At the expense of taking things somewhat out of context, I want to highlight phrases in the following comment that could easily be used in a description of a failed love relationship.

> *There began to be no surprises.* His reactions to what I would bring in didn't help me to reframe the issue or to look at it in a different way, whereas in the early years [he could help me to see things differently]. And I also began to think, "Am I replicating the actual situation that brought me to his office?" because he was the blank screen unemotional type and it *began to remind me a lot of my mother.* There were another seven or eight months when I continued going to him. And I had cut the meetings down. At my suggestion I cut it to every other week. . . . Remember, this is a guy I had been going to off and on for 12 years. *I certainly have some positive feelings about him, but increasingly negative.*
>
> One particular day I go to the office and . . . he didn't show. I found out later that his car had broken down on the turnpike, but his not showing was enough . . . That was a key thing [because] he was in a position of having to call to set up the next appointment. . . . [When] he called me on the phone *I was about to leave town and I said, "I can't talk to you right now, I'll call you when I get back."* Then he sent me a few notes and I ignored the notes. It really felt liberating. . . . I'm a very loyal person and sometimes to the point of being against my self-interest. Very loyal in the sense that I allowed myself to be administered all these drugs against my better judgment and it takes an awful

long time for me to lose my faith in someone. And he had been helpful over some stretches. And all I'm saying is that *the break in the continuity gave me enough reflection time* ... I was [also] talking to a friend of mine who had gone to him, and in recent years we had quite a few reservations. All of that kind of gelled.

[Then there was] a dispute over the bill which really sent me up the wall to such a degree that I went to the bank and came back the same day and thrust the bill at him. *That's when I cut myself loose. I was a bit afraid* ... *to cut loose completely from him* because I thought in the back of my mind there could be a recurrence. But then as month after month passed by with no pills and only minimal support from him ... *I seemed to be functioning pretty well and everything. The need seemed to be less and less until finally I made the break.* [part-time male teacher, aged 48]

If intimacy presumes equality, the hierarchical nature of professional/client relationships virtually ensures some degree of disaffection on the part of patients. Moreover, inequalities of power occur in the context of extraordinary vulnerability for the patient. Hurt and bewildered, patients are expected to share deeply private feelings, emotions, and experiences. Patients expecting emotional reciprocity from their physician healers will be disappointed. A professional demeanor—clinical, objective, and detached—is more likely what they will find.

That patients seem not to be getting what they want from physicians is reflected in their openness to "alternative" treatments. A survey[17] conducted by researchers at Boston's Beth Israel Hospital found that more than a third of 1,539 people sampled had made use of "unconventional practitioners" such as acupuncturists, herbalists, and chiropractors. The same study estimates that Americans spend $10.3 billion yearly on unconventional healers, nearly as much as they pay in out-of-pocket hospital bills. Of particular relevance here are the ailments for which alternative help is sought. Anxiety and depression were, in that order, the top two problems (back pain was a very close third) for which alternative help was sought. My guess is that the professional bias toward detachment pushes patients both to frequently change doctors and to seek "alternative" help. Predictably, the most profound expressions of anger toward psychiatrists that I heard were reserved for those who exercised complete control over respondents in hospitals when they had little choice about their treatment.

I remember I saw this doctor who looked like a frog. I hated him. No. He looked like a pig. I didn't like his personality and he kept asking me questions about sex and stuff. It made me uncomfortable and I just didn't like him as a person. He was a shrink. And then comes that whole power thing. Psychiatrists and mental health workers, but particularly psychiatrists, have the power to decide when you are going to leave, if you are going to leave, if you can go out on a pass, when you can go out on a pass, if you're good, if you're not good, that sort of thing. And I wanted to get out of the hospital, you know, especially after two or three months and I was feeling much better. But he wanted me to open up. I remember that. I needed to open up. You have to play by the games to get out. You have to do what they say. By the fourth hospitalization, third or fourth, I knew how to play the game so well. So anyway I would tell him what he needed to know. I would talk to him because if I didn't talk to him then I couldn't leave. And I remember this pig, whatever. He had me sit in this swivel chair and [for] the first four weeks, maybe, I would not even look at him. I didn't want to talk to him. [female graduate student, aged 24]

This guy was just a supercilious, superior, arrogant prick. . . . I had the feeling that he was just looking down on me as a semi-vegetable, and did me absolutely no good at all. He was a resident, and what does he know? That was the feeling I had. . . . He was a tall, red-headed guy with a mustache and this arrogant manner, because he was this great resident from Cornell, you know, and I didn't know shit. And he didn't either. And I was really angry at this guy, because he wasn't helpful. . . . So I was for a while having to put up with that. [male administrator, aged 54]

My feeling about psychiatry is really that psychiatrists can generate a lot of anger in patients. I felt as a patient that when I was at my most vulnerable many people did not treat me well and hurt me. . . . And I was a teenager on top of that and nobody likes teenagers. So, I think you make a choice if you are going to survive as a patient. The choice unfortunately . . . It's like a commitment. You have to learn the rules and choose whether you are going to play by them or not. It takes learning the rules. [female social worker, aged 38]

The doctor I had [in the hospital] was an idiot. Excuse me (laughter). . . . I hadn't liked doctors up until then. I've hated them. I haven't gotten along with them. I've looked at them very negatively. They're all rich Yangos.

Y-a-n-g-o? Is that your word? Or should we look it up in the dictionary? (laughter)

I don't think you'd find Yango. (laughter)

What would it say in the dictionary if it were there?

"A doctor-type guy (laughter)." The doctors I've had, I've had some really bad experiences with them. . . . They didn't help me. This doctor [in the hospital] . . . did experiments on me. I felt like a guinea pig. It was very experimental. He didn't know what to do with me. He had no idea. None. He was just clueless. . . . So my doctor was a Yango. . . . He was like in his seventies and he lost his hearing aid. . . . He just didn't know what he was doing. He didn't understand anything I was saying. . . . I didn't believe he was a real doctor at first. I asked him for his license and if it had said "Yango" I would have believed it (laughter). [unemployed female, aged 23]

Another feature of the relationship between psychiatrist and patient that defeats illusions about intimacy is that patients, in effect, pay for any expressions of sympathy they might get. A therapist might appear as a concerned friend, but the credibility of the gesture is necessarily suspect since it would not be offered without a fee. Although the comparison might be unkind, the patient who believes absolutely in the honesty of a therapist's expression of concern could be as misled as the "John" who believes a prostitute's praise for his sexual performance. Of course, both communications could be heartfelt, but the economic context of their occurrence raises doubt about their motivational purity.

Jim, whose breakup with a therapist I recounted earlier, was delighted when this person visited him twice during a hospitalization. Thinking that the visits were a demonstration of genuine concern for his well-being, you can imagine Jim's chagrin when the therapist later asked, "Can you find a way for me to get paid for those two visits? Can you inquire at [names hospital] for me to be reimbursed?" Jim's response as he told of the incident? "I thought he wanted to visit *me* (Jim's emphasis), Doctor G to Jim; that it was a compassionate thing. And then he wants to get paid."

The German social theorist Georg Simmel eloquently touches on these issues in his discussion of the emergence of a money economy in nineteenth century, industrial Europe.[18] As he saw it, the honest warmth and freely given emotions of persons in agrarian societies stood in contrast to the rational and artificial relations among urban dwellers in Europe's developing capitalist economy. "Money," Simmel wrote, "with all its colorlessness and indifference becomes the common denominator of all values; irreparably it hollows out the core of things, their individuality, their specific value, and their incomparability." Although no one thinks that doctors should provide their help for free, the following two people would no doubt agree that human relationships built on asymmetries of power, one-sided sharing of intimate information, professional detachment, and money can feel wholly alienating.

One hundred and twenty-five bucks a shot. In the medical world, I just can't understand. People with a straight face just charge you that much and they don't even tell you how much time they're going to give you. You know, I had asked a few times and they would say like, "Oh he sees you 20 minutes." It'd be 15. And they would think nothing of charging you the full fee and there is nowhere else I know of where that happens. . . . It's a rip-off. It makes me furious. It's a rip-off of really dependent people. [unemployed male waiter, aged 33]

Tell me a little more about your feelings about psychiatric experts.

Oh, psychiatric experts . . . Without going into particulars I found few that I feel are competent, that can really empathize with someone. . . . The one that had me committed . . . I would see him once a week [after I left the hospital] and my wife would also see him. He would never take notes, never write things down. And I always thought to myself, the man must be brilliant if he can keep track of everything that's going on. And when I was committed to the hospital, the first thing he said to my wife after he talked to her on the phone, he said, "Don't forget to bring the insurance form." [male file clerk, aged 38]

In trying to fathom the extent of anger expressed toward psychiatrists I have emphasized some of the structural elements of the doctor/patient relationship that make it inherently unsteady. I have been arguing that doctors do not easily meet some patients' expectations for empathy and intimacy. In the end, though, the biggest disappointment for patients may be the eventual realization that doctors can't easily fix them. These days depressed people are likely to have strong expectations that physicians should solve their problem. After all, TV spots lament the fact that so few persons with the symptoms of depression are diagnosed since it is such a treatable disease. I have heard some commercials boldly claim that 80 percent of those with depression are responsive to treatment. In addition, it is hard to get through a day in America without reading and hearing about the magic of Prozac and other drugs that are part of the newest generation of antidepressants. The words "treatable" and "responsive" are absolutely true. Medicine helps those with depression to feel measurably better. The problem is that the words treatable and responsive, used as they are in a context of unbounded optimism, are probably often heard as a promise of "cure."[19]

Among the 50 people in this study are a few who say that as a result of medical treatment (primarily drug treatment), their depression has vanished. For the others, as you have heard, the depression comes and goes, the medicines only modestly alleviate their problems, or seem to do nothing at all. Data from 50 people chosen in a nonrandom way hardly allow definitive statements about the efficacy of medicine to deal with depression. Yet the continuing problems of so many in this sample, myself included, make me ask why this would be so if depression is so easily dealt with. Then, when I periodically go to a self-help group for depressed people, I have to wonder why so many are there. I have never met a person in this group who was not being treated by a doctor and few who were not taking drugs. Still, as individuals introduce themselves in discussion groups and say a few words about their continuing and substantial problems, it is plain that medicine has a long way to go before it can claim to have eradicated the suffering associated with depression.

One of the most well-documented relationships in all social psychology is the link between frustration and aggression.[20] Frustration breeds aggression. Such a simple, nearly commonsensical association makes the anger expressed toward psychiatrists understandable. Depression itself and then the treatment for it can be hugely frustrating. Belief that this treatment, this new therapist, this new form of therapy, or this drug that you haven't yet tried might be the thing to finally cure you generates for many a frustrating cycle of high hope followed by varying degrees of disillusionment. When patients realize that their doctors can't cure them, faith in their expertise fades and may be replaced by animosity.[21] Despite their physicians' best efforts, most of those I have talked with come to realize that their therapists will not clear away their confusions about depression. In a more fundamentally existential way, many conclude that their depression is likely never to be fixed once and for all. Such a consciousness, in turn, requires a shift in thinking about coping with depression. The new thinking is typically less mechanistic and more spiritual in nature. As the reality of pain's permanence sinks in, the goal shifts from eradicating depression to living with it.

INCORPORATION

One of the tricky things about formulating an analysis that focuses on change and process is that each respondent is to some degree "in a different place" regarding their interpretation of depression. One of my interviews was with Alex, a recently graduated 32-year-old law student, who called after seeing my newspaper advertisement. When I described the study, he explained that although he now understood himself to have been depressed for much of his life, he had only recently been diagnosed and was, at the moment, first experimenting with medications. He seemed eager to talk with me, in part I suspect, as a potentially useful exercise for making sense of things. He was concerned that I would not be interested in talking to him because he was "probably just a novice" compared to most of the people I was speaking with. I assured him that I would likely find his conversation valuable precisely because he was at an early stage in sorting things out. When we met, much of our discussion did, in fact, center on his current dedication to fixing the depression and getting rid of it.

During interviews, respondents often wanted to know what I had thus far learned about one or another aspect of depression. Alex wanted to know how successful others had been in curing themselves. I told him that, at least among those I interviewed, most people eventually realize that their depression is unlikely ever to be fully fixed. He was, naturally, unhappy to hear this assessment and throughout the interview persisted with the view that if he tried hard enough he was sure he could get over his problem. He was not alone in thinking that assembling the right tools would insulate him from depression. Others, like a young woman whose trouble had finally been named as depression just before we spoke, had this to say.

Given the tools that I've learned . . . this overwhelming shadow is not over me, day after day after day. I have learned things that work, just like a drug would work. But I don't think I ever could have learned them if I hadn't been healthy for a while. Like I do stuff with plants, crafts, go for walks, hang out with friends, do fun stuff, not just go to meetings (AA meetings) all the time, not just worry about my family relations. But [I] write or take courses I'm interested in, art work, and read . . . Just be freaking social. [unemployed female, aged 22]

As I often did during interviews, I used my own experience to ask a question or generate a response. For example, when individuals first expressed the feeling that they were stuck with the depression, I offered that for me depression is akin to being tied to a chair with restraints on my wrists. I explained that it took me a long time to see that I only magnified my torment by jerking at the restraints; that my pain diminished only when I gave up escaping from it. This analogy made sense to many who then recounted how they too arrived at the recognition that no set of tools, however skillfully applied, would let them completely defeat depression. They might learn how to substantially mitigate its effects, but most came to accept that even when they were feeling well the depression was always lurking somewhere in their mind or body, likely to return despite their best efforts to stay well. One of my conversations on this point went as follows.

I have a feeling of unpredictability and lack of control over something that has a life of its own [and] that contradicts my feeling of mastery. And I know that now. I've had this experience for so long that I'm going to be up and that I'm going to be down and I suppose it makes it a little bit easier. I mean, I know that it's going to happen. It is out of my control and therefore

I shouldn't feel so dreadful when it does happen because it's just part of the rhythm of my life I suppose. And that's the way I sort of look on it now as opposed to the way I used to look on it, with a kind of terrible dread. Is it going to be a good day or is it going to be a bad day?

What you seem to be saying is, "OK, this is a part of my life."

Well, I can say that. Sometimes I can even implement it, but not always.

Implement it?

Well, act on it. Act on it in the sense of take it in my stride, try to make the best of it without feeling the need to be angry and struggle against it and really be under the thumb of these feelings. But then there are times when I just can't do that and I'm so miserable that it gets the better of me. It's at those times that I feel I want to withdraw and that there's nothing I can do about this.

Does all this add up to a kind of fatalism? "This is the way it's going to be for the rest of my life."

I think I've reached the point of seeing it that way. I find it hard to imagine any radical, permanent change forever leaving this experience behind me. [male college professor, aged 48]

And others expressed a similar outlook with words like these.

I believe that people hobble along, and you can learn to limp gracefully and nobly, or you know, you can scream about it. . . . I've had the same image [as yours] of my wrists being, not tied to a chair, but being tied, and wanting to get out, and realizing that you can't get out, and that to me is like a tragic realization. That you can't get out. And that's the way the cookie crumbles, as they say. Why you and not someone else, I don't know. And that leaves me with a feeling of real sadness and disappointment in life. And that's what I tried to make sense of. . . . I don't believe that, you know, I'll ever be a happy person. And, when I stopped believing that is when I started to get better. [female mental health worker, aged 27]

Depression is unfortunately a really significant part of my experience of life. You know, I'm screwed up in ways that other people aren't. . . . And I would hope [to learn] coping strategies; maybe like a way of looking at it that's really therapeutic, that helps to cut it or deflate the power of it. Like I say, "The kingdom of God is within me." I mean, statements like that, I really focus on. That's really significant to me in relation to my depression, because it means that there is good in me and that basically the answer is within me. So, I'm sort of moving in the direction of accepting it. [female physical therapist, aged 42]

I'm sure that the psychiatrist I see would cringe at this, but, to me, I will always be a depressed person at some level. . . . On some days I'm sort of hopeful and other days I'm, you know, everything is hopeless. But basically I am a depressed person. I mean, there just are ups and downs, and whatever. So, it's sort of like a wild animal that I have to tame. And there is this sort of battle with the psychiatrist that I'm seeing now. Basically what he's saying is that "You don't have to be this depressed. Your life doesn't have to be that way." And I think, "That's why you're (the psychiatrist) here talking to me." And I'll say, "But that's who I am. That's my way of looking at the world." I accept the fact that I will always look at life this way. And whereas he is saying, I can just sort of throw this all off, I'm saying, "This is the way my life is, you know, and I can't change that." [female nurse, aged 37]

AA says you have to admit that you're an alcoholic, otherwise it won't work. That means that I had to admit that I can't overcome this thing. I'm still not able to say that but I'm getting closer and closer and closer to admitting that it's a permanent condition in my life. It's been a change in that direction. . . . I still have not accepted my depression totally. . . . I'm coming to acceptance. [male professor, aged 66]

I remember when I went into therapy. I said, "Okay, this time I'm not going to drop out like all the other times. I'm going to make a two-year commitment. Well, now it's been five years. . . . And Prozac isn't the miracle thing, and I don't feel like going from drug to drug to drug. . . . So I'm starting to think, "Okay, it's not going to be fixed." [female graduate student, aged 32]

The recognition that the pain of depression is unlikely to disappear eventually provokes a redefinition of its meaning, a reordering of its place in one's life. As I contemplated writing this section of the book and re-read passages of the sort in the preceding, I considered the appropriate words to characterize respondents' new ways of thinking and acting about depression. At first, the tone of their comments seemed "fatalistic," but this did not perfectly capture their perspective since fatalism connotes a kind of helpless capitulation. I considered the word "surrender," but this also seemed too passive and defeatist. When the writer quoted at the outset of this chapter said, "I believe that depression is actually a gift. . . . If we don't allow it in, it can be destructive. If we allow it in, it is a teacher. I'm saying embrace it, be in it," I considered "embrace" as a possibility. But this word didn't quite fit either. In the end, since respondents' "post fix-it orientation" seemed to contain elements of both acceptance and resistance, the words "integration" and "incorporation" seemed most appropriate. Their new approach involves fighting against depression as best they can while constructing a life premised on its continuing presence. Such a reorientation, I discovered, involved a cognitive and attitudinal shift from the medical language of cure to the spiritual language of transformation.

Although questions of spirituality were not in my head when I began interviewing for this book, I was quickly sensitized to the spirituality/depression link. At the very beginning of each interview I asked a series of factual, demographic questions about age, occupation, ethnicity, marital status, education, and religion. When it came to religion, I was struck and initially somewhat puzzled by the number of people who spoke about having grown up Jewish, Catholic, or Protestant, but had since divorced themselves from these religions. Many of these same people, however, quickly added that they were nevertheless highly spiritual individuals. When I probed on this point, it often evoked lengthy descriptions of experimentation with different forms of spirituality, but especially with Eastern religious and meditative practices. Particularly, there was far more interest in Buddhism among this group of 50 Americans than chance alone could possibly explain. When I admitted my ignorance about Buddhism, several explained in nearly identical words that they found valuable its tenet that "pain is inseparable from life." Al, the custodian, explained to me that "when the Buddha had pupils he would ask them 'Are you in pain?' If they said 'yes', he would say 'What are you attached to?' In other words, our ego attachments cause us pain. To the degree we are attached to things is the degree of our pain."

In another interview spirituality was the dominant theme. Laura had been a foster child, constantly shuttled from one family to another. In some of these homes she was abused in unthinkable ways. Even as a child, she told me, "I felt like I had a mission and to do what I came here to do, I had to go through some lessons." At a later point, she explained her lifelong spiritual involvement.

My interest and my study in Buddhism? It was more practical in my life and it was something that I could use to get through things that were difficult. It was a way of understanding . . . in a larger sense, perhaps why I went through a lot of things that I went through. It was just a help. It helped me enormously. It made me feel that my own life was unique. I didn't feel that somehow it was just me. And having that stronger spiritual sense of community was really helping me see myself in a larger sense. And so, the sense that there was a large community in the spiritual work fascinated me and helped me feel that I didn't have to be sort of a victim. I didn't have to be just little ole me. [female travel agent, aged 41]

Perhaps I should have more quickly grasped the value of spirituality in the lives of many depressed people since the perspective of symbolic interaction, which directs all of my analysis in this book, is rooted in the notion that human beings confer meaning onto *everything* in their worlds. Those who moved toward a more spiritual response to depression had simply realized that they could, indeed, refashion the meaning of their pain. This insight, though, could apparently be achieved only after they had internalized the idea that the pain was not going to disappear. Correspondingly, the ideology of a 12-step program like Alcoholics Anonymous is that it can only work for those who commit themselves to a higher power and honestly admit their powerlessness over alcohol.

Much has been written about the religious features of AA and other change-oriented self-help groups.[22] In his ethnographic study of AA entitled *Becoming Alcoholic*,[23] David Rudy observes that "individuals who successfully affiliate with AA have not merely found a technique which helps them to stop drinking; they have also found a new life style and philosophy, a new perspective from which to view the world, and a new identity." In short, successful coping with alcoholism requires a symbolic transformation in the meaning of the problem. Similarly, the spiritually committed among my respondents recognize the need for a redefinition of pain's meaning. In the context of a discussion on spirituality I asked one person, "How do you distinguish pain that is a normal part of human existence from abnormal pain?" I got this reply.

> I think that when you try to make that distinction, you get into trouble because what you're basically saying is that there is some kind of pain that is of alien form to us, and should not be, and I've come to see it for myself that there is no pain that should not be, that pain is not a bad thing, it is not sickness. It can be very uncomfortable, but it's not evil, and that's the difference. I think people almost see pain as like theologically evil. It's something that came from the Devil and we have to get rid of it if we want to live in God's graces. I mean, pain is as much a part of this world as anything else sent down. It's from something outside of us, and there is some kind of reason for it, and I think that it's possible even for pain to be integrated into a culture in a way that's celebratory, [but], I don't think we do it. . . . I remember once reading this description that Margaret Mead had written. I can't remember where it was, but it always stayed with me. [It was about] this idiot boy . . . maybe it was [in] Samoa, but they were having this dance, and the whole community was participating in the dance, and what they did, was they dressed him up as a steer. They put antlers

on his head, and he became very much a part of the dance. And he was driven into a frenzy over this, and there was a place for his craziness, and it was an integral part of the community. It wasn't something that was outside of it. [female mental health worker, aged 27]

This last quote suggests that there can be a social value to mental illness. There is an association between the development of the kind of spiritual sensibilities I have been describing and the pain of depressive illness. Sometimes respondents initially displayed incomprehension when I asked, "Is there anything good about having depression?" They would ask in return, "What do you mean?" "Of course, there is nothing good about depression," they must have been thinking. Even after I explained, as an example, that a substantial body of literature[24] relates mental illness to creativity; that perhaps it was the madness of Van Gogh that generated his brilliant vision or the vicious pain described by Sylvia Plath that made her poetry possible, some individuals flatly denied any benefits to depression. They were, however, a minority. Most people were not stumped by my question and had a ready answer.

Sometimes the answers bordered on elitism. Several felt that they had a deeper and more accurate picture of human nature and social life than happy people. They subscribed to a kind of "bliss means ignorance" view and sometimes expressed disdain toward family and friends whose happiness they saw as built on a distortion of what the world is "really" like. Others viewed depression as the price paid for insights that were inaccessible to others. A woman whose first depression "hit" when she was an adolescent told me: "Somehow I felt that my depression made me better, that I was deeper. You know, sort of the tortured artist type of thing. I wrote poetry while everyone was hanging out and playing."

Another woman who got depressed at about the same age agreed that depression "meant I was a deeper person, that I was somehow special." A 48-year-old professor of English who analyzes poetry for a living answered my question by saying, "Well, I would use it as a justification almost. 'I have to accept this pain because of my insight. This is the price you pay for seeing more deeply into reality,' or something like that."

The claim that depressed people sometimes see reality more accurately than others could have empirical merit.[25] The source is now long gone from my memory, but some years ago I read about a laboratory experiment that impressed me. Two groups of subjects were used in the study. Those in one group had a history of diagnosed clinical depression and those in the second had, by all appearances, a healthy mental life. The individuals in each group were placed before a machine showing lights blinking in an apparently random fashion. In front of the light board was a series of buttons and the subjects were told to experiment with them to see if they could learn how to control the pattern of the blinking lights.

Like many laboratory experiments, this one was based on deception. Pushing the buttons could have no effect whatsoever on the lights. There was nevertheless a revealing difference in the reports of those in each group. The depressed subjects claimed that nothing they did had any effect on the pattern of the lights. The clinically "normal" subjects, on the other hand, claimed that they had been able to exercise control over the pattern. While we should vigorously question the generalizability of such artificially created situations, at least in this case, depressed individuals had a more accurate perception of reality than healthy people. One respondent tried to make the same point with her comment that "What other people call depression I don't see as hopeless thinking. I think it's looking at things the way they really are." Were she right, it would be an extraordinary irony since mental illness is conventionally defined by a person's presumed inability to perceive reality correctly.

While a relatively few among those interviewed claimed greater intellectual prowess because of depression, there was widespread agreement that it had two clear benefits: It deepened one's capacity for empathy and provided an important learning experience. The word "sensitivity" came up most frequently when the values of depression were cited. From among the many who believed depression had given them a more profound appreciation for others' difficulties, these statements were typical: "I think part of depression is an intensified humanity, a real sensitivity to what goes on in the human world." "What's good about it is at least it's made me sensitive about different things." "There is no question about it, just humanity. It can make you more humane." As for depression's lessons, these comments were typical: "Maybe this is pie in the sky, but with each one [episode of depression] there has been a progressive move upward for me in terms of learning." "Pain is very focusing. It makes you recognize what's at stake in life." "I really feel that I'm here on earth, that this is school, and there are things for me to learn. And whatever has happened has happened for a reason. It's part of my learning plan." All these ideas are well summarized by the following respondents.

I think depression has made me a stronger person somehow. I mean in learning to handle this kind of thing. I think that I've had to develop skills and abilities that I wouldn't otherwise. And sensitivities too. I think it's made me more compassionate. I think, because of it, I know what it's like to go through something like that and I'm more curious about other people and what they're going through. [I'm also] more intent in trying to make some meaning out of the whole thing [life], which is getting back to the spirituality thing. I try to make some meaning out of my life, and not just sort of go from spot to spot. You know, sometimes it seems the general culture doesn't provide very much in the way of the meaning for your life. And so in a way this (depression) is part of the meaning of my life. (heavy sigh) It's something that at times I would have loved to be rid of, but I'm afraid that if [it were] excised, there's something important about me that would be excised with it. [unemployed female aged 35]

You know, people say, would you like to have had a different life. I say absolutely not. I'd live it all over again. But I think it takes awhile to get there. To see some of [the pain] as a real gift. . . . I wouldn't give up one minute of it, not one minute of the pain. As horrible as it was, I don't see how I could be what I am without it. So, in a Buddhist sense I embrace it when it comes to this stuff. The dark side, all the awful stuff has to be just as much part of my life [as the good stuff]. The yin and the yang can't exist without each other. [female travel agent, aged 41]

CONCLUSION

There is a parable about human troubles that has every person's most powerful sufferings hanging from a tree. Each leaf, we might imagine, tells of an individual's life travails. The pains and injuries that all others have endured over the course of their lives are plainly documented. Every person is then given the choice of a second life from all those displayed, to be lived with exactly the difficulties advertised. The parable has it that in the end everyone chooses their own life over all others. We might speculate from my recent discussion of spirituality that the individuals who have spoken, despite the horrors of their depression experiences, would likely choose their lives over again. With all its difficulty, it is *their* life and they see suffering as inseparable from who they are and the sensibilities they value in themselves.

From time to time as I have been writing this book, I have felt uneasy about the negative and somewhat pessimistic tone to my descriptions and analyses. While others are writing upbeat books whose themes involve "overcoming" and "conquering" depression,[26] the message in this book has been about the enormous complexity of depression and my great uncertainty about the prospects for beating it. For that reason, it has been heartening for me to report on the ways people find value even in life's most difficult trials. Indeed, the materials in this chapter on coping and adapting affirm the theoretical view that because we are symbolic animals, we have the potential to create social worlds consistent with our needs. Although it sometimes seems so, human beings are ultimately never completely victims of their environments, social or biological. Ward Abbott's account of how some artists transcend their immediate lived-worlds[27] illustrates the power of symbols in transforming the experience of even the most oppressive circumstances.

The artist is doubly subversive in that only a bullet can stop him. He feeds on changes as others shy away from them. Joseph Brodsky, exiled in Siberia, infuriated officials by *enjoying his life there.* Unlike a banker, the artist carries his work in his mind. To express it, he needs only a stub of a pencil and a scrap of paper, or charcoal and any surface. One of the last acts of Gaudier-Brzeska in the trenches of World War I, surrounded by death and desolation, was to carve, out of a bit of blown-up rifle butt, a splendidly Brzeskian sculpture.

There are, of course, limits to our capacity for determining the nature of our environments. However much the artists Brodsky and Gaudier-Brzeska were able to redefine their lives in Siberia and World War I trenches, they still had to cope with both the physical features of their wartime surroundings and the socially constructed decisions made by powerful people who put them in those situations in the first place. Likewise, the consciousness dictated by the historical period into which we are born, the normative demands of our cultures, the requirements of our particular location within a social structure, and the frailties of our bodies and minds are genuine constraints. However, the optimistic message suggested by much of the data in this chapter and throughout the book is that human beings have extraordinary capacity for adaptation because of their unique ability to define the meaning of their life constraints and to determine how they will respond to them.

Every chapter in this enterprise is predicated on the idea that human beings make meaning. However, they don't do it alone. Another key assumption of symbolic interaction theory is that the meanings we create are jointly produced in the sense that they arise out of the process of interaction with others.[28] No meanings exist apart from social context and communication. Sometimes to convey this idea I ask students to imagine being alone on the moon, with amnesia about the values of their culture. Then I ask, "Under these conditions could you commit an evil act?" After some conversation the students come around to the idea that the meanings given to their own behaviors, attitudes, and feelings are contingent on the presence of an audience. Our sense of self, in fact, is created and sustained by seeing ourselves from the standpoint of others, putting ourselves in their place, imagining how they are evaluating us, and anticipating how they are going to react to us. We, in turn, are audiences or mirrors in which others see and evaluate their social reflections.[29]

In the next chapter, I turn my attention to the problems of meaning-making for those who are close to and care about a person with depression. After all, mates, lovers, friends, parents, and siblings are deeply affected by the depression of someone important in their lives. If all meanings are jointly produced, it is a simple conceptual extension that depressive illness is socially contagious. Family and friends must themselves cope with the depressed person close to them. In turn, how depressed people experience their own illness is related to the responses of these "significant others." Thus, a complete analysis of depression requires that we try to see it from the standpoint of family and friends. Their stories form the substance of chapter 6.

Chapter 6

Family and Friends

The thing about depression is that it is so overwhelming and anyone who takes it on is going to lose. As a family and friend— anyone who is close—it's too overwhelming. And the only way to deal with someone else's depression is to maintain your own life and to understand that person and empathize and be there as you can be. But to recognize that fundamentally it's their experience and you're not going to shift it. All you can do as a friend is to allow it [to happen] and to be there again and again and again.

Male therapist, aged 45

This chapter is chiefly about the limits to sympathetic involvement with a depressed person. My main question is "How do family and friends go about establishing clear sympathy boundaries in order to avoid becoming engulfed by another's depression?" As with every issue raised in this book, my own experience provides an initial guide for analysis. By now, my wife and I share a whole inventory of verbal and gestural signals about the state of my mind. She pretty well knows by my demeanor, facial expression, and general responsiveness to things how good or bad I feel. Normally each day still begins with her question, "How did you sleep last night?" I think she continues to ask the question out of honest concern, but also because my answer helps her to gauge how we will relate that day.

Years ago, when we were both new to the consequences of depression, Darleen was very solicitous of my feelings and unfailingly tried her best to pull me out of black moods. When she attempted to cheer me up by pointing out how good my life really was, I alternated between appreciation for her concern and upset at her incomprehension. It took years before she realized that nothing she could say or do would make much of a difference; even worse, that efforts to comfort me might only invite more negativity.

Although I too have concluded that she can't turn things around for me, I continue to complain about my pain. Often, in the midst of a difficult period, I resolve to keep quiet, to be stoic, to bear the discomfort alone. Nearly always, though, my pain spills into complaint. As soon as the complaints are issued, I feel badly about being a complainer. However, I need to complain because (1) I hurt, (2) I hope that somehow the intensity of my words will finally convey the depth of my suffering, and (3) the complaints function to signal my unavailability as a husband, father, and household member. After many years, my retreats to the bedroom are no longer alarming. The whole family has worked out an accommodation of sorts. Dad goes off by himself and everyone else carries on without too much inquiry about his well-being. Even though I understand that I can expect far less sympathy after so many years, I still feel isolated and often angry that my distress is sometimes only barely acknowledged.

The potential problems in managing relationships with sick people can be truly daunting. The illness of someone close demands ongoing negotiations[1] about the degree of help, concern, and sympathy one should offer. In a beautifully written book, based on her experience with "chronic fatigue syndrome," Kat Duff wisely advises that "not only is it better for the sick to be left alone at times, it is also better for the well to leave them at times. Healthy people can be contaminated by the gloom and depression of the ailing if they come too close or have too much sympathy."[2] However, as the accounts in this chapter will show, sustaining an appropriate level of involvement with a depressed person who is a friend or family member can sometimes be extraordinarily difficult.

In the only systematic study I know on the etiquette of giving and receiving sympathy, Candace Clark describes the social flow of sympathy as part of an "emotional economy."[3] The partners in any relationship share a mutual "sympathy biography" and the "margin" of sympathy available to each person is determined by how much each has given and received in the past. Moreover, the way all of us manage the exchange of sympathies is dictated by cultural norms that apply to everyone. For example, requests for sympathy will not be honored if individuals ask for more than their difficulty warrants, have made illegitimate sympathy requests in the past, or have not abided by the expectation of distributive justice that demands reciprocity in sympathy exchanges. As a general rule, each of us expects to get approximately what we give and an individual who makes great sympathy demands without repayment may run out of credit altogether. Should a person become "bankrupt" in a particular relationship, he or she will have to draw on sympathy accounts that remain "open" in other relationships.

Based on a range of data sources (interviews, greeting cards, observation) Clark documents a number of other somewhat less obvious features of sympathy economies. For instance, to receive their "fair share" of sympathy, individuals must ask for it with great enough frequency. Ironically, when a person rarely asks for sympathy, he or she is less likely to receive it than another who more routinely makes sympathy requests. Those who infrequently ask for sympathy come to be defined as "strong" and self-sufficient; consequently, their requests are taken less seriously ("Oh, you'll be OK.

You always manage things well."). Relevant to the circumstance of chronic illness, Clark notes a curvilinear relationship between the time span of problems and the amount of sympathy offered. Less sympathy is given to short- and long-term problems than to those with a "middle-range" time frame.

From among the several of Clark's important observations, I found most relevant to my immediate concerns the connection between individuals' social statuses and the "width" of their respective sympathy margins. Spouses, for example, are expected to honor sympathy requests for problems that would seem too trivial in another relationship. Husbands and wives can complain to each other at length about a bad day at work, for example, and feel wronged if their partner does not pay close attention and extend considerable sympathy. The relationships between parents and children are bounded by quite different rules. In this case, the margins are asymmetrical since parents are expected to freely extend far more sympathy to their children (especially, of course, young children) than they can legitimately expect in return. In similar fashion, the extent of sympathy persons can expect from "close" friends, acquaintances, or strangers in a public place will be enormously variable.

Clark's analysis allows the presumption that individuals will negotiate the boundaries of involvement with a depressed person differently depending on their respective social statuses. The complexities of establishing a comfortable level of involvement will vary for the spouse, parent, child, friend, or sibling of a depressed individual. I might also speculate that gender, race, ethnicity, social class, and age will importantly affect the construction of sympathy boundaries. Thus, as Clark clearly acknowledges, we ought not make too rigid an analogy between emotional and market economies. Unlike market economies where everyone is subject to essentially the same rules of credit, supply and demand,

and equity, there are a multiplicity of emotional economies established along different status lines, each of which is bounded by distinctive expectations and obligations.

For most of the remainder of this chapter I will report on the experiences of individuals who want to honor commitments to a depressed friend or family member, but also want to avoid being devoured by their illness. Because it would be imprudent to make bold generalizations from only 10 interviews with family and friends, I have chosen a different mode of data presentation here than in earlier chapters. Although I have provided modestly detailed descriptions of particular individuals in other chapters, most of my earlier analyses depend on the comments of many respondents. For the remainder of this chapter, in contrast, I will tell four stories about caring and commitment. You will hear from Rachel whose husband suffers from severe depression that began after contracting viral encephalitis, from Anne who has dealt alone with the depression of her two children after a divorce, from Marco who, at age 14, became the primary caregiver to his depressed mother, and from John who tries to help several friends in trouble. While I cannot claim them to be representative, these "case studies" should at least sensitize you to the different demands depression makes on mates, parents, children, and friends.[4]

IN SICKNESS AND IN HEALTH, TILL DEATH DO US PART

Several of Rachel's friends thought she was crazy for going ahead and marrying Ted. During the three years they lived together before getting married, Ted sometimes drank too heavily and occasionally was mildly depressed, but the real trouble started with what first seemed only a bad flu. It all happened "like the drop of a hat," Rachel told me. She had become somewhat concerned when Ted's flu, with its high fever and sweats, went on for several days since he rarely remained sick for more than a day or two. Despite feeling awful, he went back to work on Monday and seemed to get through the early part of the week. The Thursday of that week was Thanksgiving and since she had to return on Friday to the insurance company where she was "a kind of employee-at-large, doing some selling and customer service," they took separate cars to Ted's brother's home in Rhode Island for the holiday. When she arrived home on Friday evening, Ted wasn't there as they had planned. He was in a Rhode Island hospital, having suffered a seizure. After the call from Ted's brother, she "got in the car and rushed down to the Rhode Island hospital," and that, she told me, "was the beginning of the whirlwind." A day later he was released from the hospital, came home, shortly thereafter had another bad seizure, entered the Massachusetts General Hospital in Boston, and then fell into a coma from what was subsequently diagnosed as viral encephalitis.

For more than a week no one knew whether Ted would emerge from the coma at all and, if he did, his prognosis "could be anywhere from complete zombie to full recovery." Fortunately, Ted gradually got better although "there were a lot of mental problems to begin with . . . [and] it was a long road back." After several months of recuperation at his parent's home in the Midwest, Ted returned to Massachusetts and Rachel began to learn firsthand that the neurologists were correct with their prediction that he would continue to have *grand mal* seizures. They were at home the first time Rachel witnessed a seizure and she recalls, "I went screaming from the bedroom, and called somebody else to come help because I had never seen anything like that." As time went by Rachel became something of an expert, even calmly instructing nurses what to do when Ted had a seizure during one of his hospitalizations.

During a several-month period of experimentation with numerous epilepsy medications, they went to a movie and dinner one evening. Ted had a seizure in the restaurant and, as Rachel recalls, this setback "just triggered something in Ted and slowly he went into a depression." She went on to explain that he wasn't working and stayed home all day. "He was isolated," she said, "because we lived in [names town] which is in the middle of nowhere. He couldn't get anywhere. We had one car at the time and I was working all day. And that's when I started to notice that he wasn't getting out of bed in the morning. He was still in his pajamas when I got home at night. He's a neat freak [but] he hadn't cleaned any dishes if he'd eaten. That's when I started to notice the depression."

Such turmoil was new to Rachel since she had always enjoyed good physical and mental health. When I asked, "What was your life like prior to all this," she said, "It was smooth. It was up. It was great, happy-go-lucky, carefree. [I] never had a problem." She continued, "I didn't have a clue. I had no idea what I was in for and it's a good thing nobody told me (laughs)." Ted's illness began in November 1986 after they had been living together for two years and despite its critical implications for their joint future, they decided to marry. When I asked the obvious question, "Did you consider bailing out of the relationship," she told me, "It was going to go one way or the other. . . . I mean, several of his sisters had said to me, 'Don't feel you have to stick around because you feel sorry for him'. . . . But it never occurred to me. . . . It just always felt right to stay with him. . . . We were planning to get engaged before he got sick anyway. . . . I mean, many people told me to feel free to leave, to walk away . . . but I always wanted to stay." Part of committing to the relationship was the feeling that she ought to "help him through it." She said, "I always believed he could get through it, though there were some times when I was right in the middle of it [when] I thought, 'My God.'"

At a point it became clear that the depression was a far larger problem than the epilepsy. The latter was eventually controlled with drugs, but Ted's slide into depression continued. As part of her decision to see Ted through the problem, Rachel took it as her responsibility to monitor his moods and behaviors with the idea of intervening before the depression thoroughly captured her husband. Making sense of Ted's depression was a completely new thing for her because in her family only an uncle she barely knew had been depressed. He lived a distance away and so, she said, "I never saw [it] day to day. I never understood it. It was always like, 'Yuh, uncle Joe's depressed,' but it didn't affect me."

Now, with Ted, it was decidedly a continuous day-to-day thing. When I asked her, "What did you make of it at the beginning?" she replied, "We did a lot of crying together as I was trying to understand. . . . I panicked [at this early point] because I didn't know what to do. . . . I lived close to where I worked, so I could come home at lunch times. I would come home at lunch and force him to get up. I would try calling him a lot of times during the day. I was trying to force him to [come around]." She also learned to recognize the signs of a deepening depression. When earlier she described Ted's seizures, she told me that they were always preceded by an "aura" that allowed him to warn her before it began. As she told it, she began to recognize the "aura of depression." When I asked her to explain, she told me, "Oh yeah [there's an aura to depression]. If he comes home and he's very quiet, and he'll just sort of look at the floor or stare. He's not talking. He's not active. That's the start."

As hard as she tried to set him on a positive course, things only got worse and then completely fell apart after a drinking binge with a friend. Here's what happened: "We lived on a river and a friend of Ted's had come over and they had taken the canoe out on the river and they were fishing. And Ted had gotten drunk. When they came to shore Ted fell out of the boat. He didn't even make it to the land. I came home and got him undressed because he was soaking wet. I got him in the shower, and then after that, I mean he was just crying and crying. You know, 'Why me? What's happened? I don't understand. I just want to end it all.'" The next morning she took him to the hospital. "You know, I pretty much forced him to go. He wasn't happy about it." You can imagine Rachel's surprise when, after their arrival, Ted persuaded the attending physician that the problem was *Rachel's*, not his. "He convinced them that I was the one who had the problem; that I was the one who was overreacting and being silly, and that it was me (laughs). . . . And so the woman then called me into the room and was saying, 'Well, maybe you're overreacting.' And I was like, 'Hold it.' And so we left. I don't even remember what happened. Maybe they set up an appointment for him to come back. I don't remember what transpired."

Although Ted continued to deny his depression for a time, Rachel finally persuaded him to see a psychiatrist. "It took a while to find a good one," she told me, and by the time of our interview they had "been through a slew of 'em." Although the psychiatrist they finally settled on provided antidepressant medications, Rachel's private view was that Ted's depression was linked to his occupational instability since, she told me, "I had seen it. If he was working it was okay. So the goal was to get him into a job he could handle." Still, job or not, the first three years of their marriage were tumultuous. There were cycles of exhilaration and depression. "Well," Rachel explained, "every time things were [down] something good would happen, so we'd get up again. You know, he'd get a job. [And then] Oh my God, he got fired [and] what am I going to do now? Okay, so [then] he gets this rehabilitation thing. That was really exciting. We're on the edge of our seats. Is he going to get in? Is the insurance company going to cover it? So there were highs and lows."

I found one of the episodes in this developing joint history with depression especially enlightening because it reveals how the behaviors of sick and well people are deeply and synergistically related. At this point Rachel was no longer shocked or surprised by an approaching depression. What made the following incident different, however, is that it led to *Rachel's* momentary breakdown. As you will see, her inability to hold things together became a turning point in the way this husband and wife saw and understood each other. At the time, Ted was working and had just finished the week. By Friday night, Rachel began to see the aura of a new and serious plunge into depression. Ted had been having difficulty at work and she saw his drift toward catastrophic thinking. She said, "I watched and by Saturday morning . . . he was building things up in his mind. He was making so much more of this situation at work than it needed. And it was snowballing." Our conversation on how it all unraveled went this way.

So you see this happening?

Oh yeah, well I could watch it. We didn't do much around the house in the morning. He said, "I'm not going to let it bother me," but then he took a nap for six hours during the day. Then he woke up. He was trying to convince me he was [physically] sick. But yet he wasn't getting sick. By Saturday I recognized it [depression]. So we talked for a little while and I said [to myself], "Okay its four o'clock in the afternoon, I'm like making an agenda for him. Get up, take a shower. I want you to vacuum. I need you to do this, this, and this." And he was okay then, because he had something to do.

So you did this on purpose to keep him going.

Oh yeah, to get him up and get him going.

So when you see that aura of depression you sort of get into a game plan of what to do?

Yes. Yes. So he was okay Saturday night. Sunday, he slept a lot, but I kinda made it a fun day. It was the Super Bowl. It was a really cold day, and there was golf on TV, so I said let's pull the sofa out in the living room. Let's cuddle up on the sofa with all kinds of blankets, and the dog can come play with us, and we had fun. And we had dinner, and I said to him, "I'm gonna go take the dog for a walk, do you mind doing the dishes?" [He said] "No, no problem." Well I came back. I'd been out with the dog for maybe 20, 25 minutes, I came back and there was no dish done. And I walked up and said "Ted, Ted," and I couldn't find him. He was in the bedroom sobbing. Just sobbing. Again, it was that overwhelming feeling. And you know, I recognized it, I wasn't shocked.

This was like other times?

Oh yeah. Yeah. And it's a recognized behavior. . . . That was the Sunday night he was crying [and] I talked him out of it. He was okay. We talked for awhile, he seemed okay. Monday morning he woke up and he was having a panic attack. It's the only way

I can describe it. He was shaking. He couldn't move. He was terribly frightened of going to work because he had made so much out of it.

So he had been obsessing about this work thing all weekend?

Yes, all weekend. And it got worse and worse. I said, "Come on, take the dog for a walk." I get to work [on Monday] and I'm thinking to myself, "Nobody at work needs to know what's going on, you'll be fine." I called the psychologist. Left a message on his answering machine: "We need to see you, please call tonight." So I felt a little relief that I had done that. I was like, "I'll be fine, no big deal." And something happened at work that just triggered something in me, and I burst out crying. And I'm sobbing and sobbing. And my boss, she didn't know what to do. But she knows [my] whole situation, so I told her what was happening. She said, "Go home. You need to take the day for yourself. Just go home." So I wasn't going to argue, because I couldn't concentrate on work. So I went home, and as soon as I got home I called Ted. I said "Ted, I'm home." And he said, "Are you okay?" And I said, "Well, to be honest with you I completely lost it at work today." And I told him what had happened. I said, "Now I understand that feeling you must have had last week when you were fighting off tears and your frustration."

So this was a revelation for you actually?

It was a revelation for me, but more than anything it was a revelation for Ted. He was so excited that I broke down. He said to me, "I'm sorry you broke down and I'm glad you're okay, but God I feel so much better." He said, "I'm not the only one that burst out crying at work because something strange happened." I said, "Oh no, I understand."

At that moment you really did have a deeper appreciation . . . ?

Oh, because I sat there trying to fight these tears off for awhile. And Ted had described to me the week before how he was trying to fight off tears.

And all I could think of was, "This must be what Ted's going through. . . ." So he was so happy (she laughs) that I reacted this way. And that caused him to rally. And he came back and he was fine.

In a curious way, your own misery sort of energized him. I mean, your own misery is an antidote to his misery.

It is, because I tend to be strong when I need to be strong. And when he's doing okay then I collapse. But this is the first time I collapsed while he had collapsed.

However profound Rachel's new level of empathy, it was irrelevant for keeping Ted well and she knew it. As time went by and he continued to be depressed she felt less able to do much about it. She knew, in fact, that during one of these periods he would try suicide. She explained, "I literally was preparing to come home every day from work and find him dead. I was so prepared for it that the day it (a suicide attempt) happened, I knew exactly what to do." To be absolutely certain I understood, I asked, "You saw this coming, like a train on the tracks?" and she answered, "Oh, big time, big time . . . [and] there was nothing I could do. I tried everything. I tried taking him to the psychiatrist. I was constantly setting up appointments with different people and it just wasn't working and I couldn't do anything about it." This 1991 suicide attempt (his second) was precipitated by a job loss. Prior to it, "He had pulled away from everybody. He wouldn't see anybody. . . . There was nothing I could do. And I just prepared myself every day when I came home from work. . . . It was awful."

In earlier chapters I described the feelings of isolation that accompany depression. My interviews with family and friends persuade me that their isolation can be equally great. In a way, their experience parallels that of the person close to them because they too have the feeling that no one can understand them. Rachel explained, "There were people at work who knew, but by the same token they couldn't help me. They could just listen." When I expressed the thought that her pain might very well equal Ted's she agreed with the simple comment, "It was horrible." Despite her constant efforts to get Ted to talk, Rachel finally realized that they would never really comprehend each other's perspective. She made the point by telling me, "His perspective of it was 'I'm such a burden to her why don't I just kill myself . . . and that will free her from having to put up with this.' That's how he thought . . . but yet he couldn't understand what I was going through, from my perspective of it."

By the time we spoke, Rachel had come to the somewhat grim, but realistic conclusion that she could not be Ted's savior, however hard she tried. This is the way she put it: "Whatever I was communicating to him he was receiving completely differently. So every time I thought I was helping, it was making matters worse. So I guess I must have at some point sat back and said, 'I'm doing all I can and if something else happens, I know I've done my best.'" Later in the interview she made the same point, but even more forcefully, when she said, "I guess it got to the point where if he can't help himself, I can't help him. I can't do it for him. It's got to come from him. I can't get him out of depression. He's got to get himself out of that depression."

Ted survived his 1991 suicide attempt and despite the kinds of personal trials his illness has brought to their marriage, Rachel remains committed to him. She has, though, abandoned the idea that her heroic efforts will make him well. As the interview moved toward its conclusion, I asked Rachel how she saw the future. Her focus immediately shifted to her wish for children and her fears that Ted's illness would make that impossible. She said, "I'm actually going to be 36 next month. For so long I had said to myself, 'I'm not even going to worry about kids. I'm not even 35 yet.'" "But now," she continued, "I find we're five years behind all our friends." However, each time Ted becomes depressed Rachel realizes how difficult the decision to have children will be. She recounted recent thoughts on the issue by saying, "When Ted went through this depression a couple of weeks ago, I thought to myself, 'My God, what would happen if I had a child?' All this energy for years I've put into Ted . . . I'm not going to have it anymore. So that's a big case scenario [because] everything I do I have to think about how [it's] going to affect Ted."

Having already interviewed Ted, it was easier to appreciate Rachel's version of events. Nevertheless, anything I write on these pages misses much of the interview's energy and emotion. If you could actually hear the determination in her speech, you would likely share my view that despite the overwhelming difficulties imposed on their marriage, Ted and Rachel will stay together. Partly, I make this prediction because Rachel seems so resolute a person and plainly loves Ted. Strength and love, though, are probably not enough to sustain a relationship troubled by depression. In the end, those who care for a sick spouse must learn flexibility in dealing with the other's tragic difficulty. Storms are, after all, far more likely to destroy the unbending than the pliable tree. I might even speculate that the survival of a marriage in which someone is depressed requires the eventual recognition that one cannot solve a partner's depression and must gain distance from it. The therapist whose words begin this chapter no doubt had it right when he said, "All you can do . . . is to allow it [to happen] and to be there again and again and again."

WHAT'S A MOTHER TO DO?

I first met Anne at a meeting of a self-help group for people with depression or manic depression. I knew that each week a family and friends contingent gathered and I had arranged with the president of the organization to describe my study and to ask for volunteers. After a very brief presentation, Anne was the first to approach me. She was, in fact, attending the meeting with her son Jay, whom she told me had been diagnosed with bi-polar depression. As she saw it, Jay suffers primarily from depression. Within a few days we had made plans to meet at her apartment in Boston's exclusive Back Bay area.

At 59, Anne is a tall, exceedingly handsome gray-haired woman whose demeanor and speech convey refinement and dignity. We sat in the dining area of the small, two bedroom apartment she shares with 26-year-old Jay, who only months before had returned home after his third extended hospitalization since high school graduation. I thought the interview would be primarily about her relationship with Jay, but it shortly became plain that I would hear a great deal about two other people: her daughter Linda, now 28, who also has been hospitalized multiple times with depression, and her ex-husband whose erratic behavior she now attributes to alcoholism and mental illness. Only her oldest child, a son finishing law school, has "never had any evidence of mental illness."

Although Anne is a nurse, nothing in her professional training could prepare her for the strain and sadness of caring for two children who have been in and out of hospitals since 1980. During the approximately three hours we spoke, Anne returned often to the theme of responsibility as when she said, "As far as my sense of responsibility, I still have it. . . . It has been so ingrained in me that it [has been] a very difficult concept for me to give up." She told me, "The frustration of being the responsible person has left me very angry, very tense and angry." At the time of our interview, consequently, Anne was struggling to find a better balance between her felt obligations as a mother and her wish to make a life for herself. She has been regularly attending the support group where we met for more than six months, drawn by the repeated message among the family and friends members that "I didn't cause it and I can't cure it." Although she finds solace in "seeing [others] who have been through it [and are] still surviving," she is having trouble acting on the group's collectively held view that caretakers of depressed people need to maintain a healthy distance from those they care for and about.

It is not hard to understand why Anne would have such difficulty with making a life of her own, independent of her sick children. Approaching 60, she stands at the tail end of a generation of women who were socialized to believe that child raising and fostering their husbands' careers were their primary life obligations.[5] Although Anne remained employed throughout the course of her 23-year marriage, she served a "second shift"[6] at home, never questioning that her family's well-being was really her number one job. Like other women her age, Anne was likely influenced by the philosophy of child rearing articulated in Dr. Benjamin Spock's famous book *Baby and Child Care*.[7] Earlier generations of women felt they had done their job well if their children were well disciplined and prepared to conform to society's institutions. Beyond this, however, Spock proposed that mothers were literally responsible for molding their children's personalities. "Deep in their hearts most middle-class, Spock-taught mothers believed that if they did their job well enough, all their children would be creative, intelligent, kind, generous, happy, brave, spontaneous, and good—each, of course, in his or her own special way."[8] You might imagine the guilt generated for such mothers when their children were unable to function socially because of an illness characterized by desperate unhappiness.

Anne's family problems started to overwhelm her in 1980. Her mother was dying of cancer at the same time that Linda's mental health began to deteriorate. Then a ninth grader, Linda "had a bad year. . . . [Her father] was not particularly involved or responsible [and] the guidance counselor was calling me at work if Linda wasn't at school. And Linda was so depressed that I really was afraid that she might kill herself. You know, I didn't know when I got those calls if I would find her alive when I got home. . . . I mean, it was [all] just numbing." A psychiatrist at a local hospital claimed that Linda was just going through an expected period of adolescent adjustment. When Anne protested that the problems were greater than that, the psychiatrist dismissed her concerns. She told me, "I felt like I was in the third grade being put down by a teacher . . . and I figured, 'Well, these are the experts.'" Anne's diagnosis proved correct when some months later Linda had a full-blown episode of manic psychosis.

This began a series of meetings with mental health professionals. The upshot of these sessions, as Anne perceived it, was "that certainly the family was the cause of Linda's trouble. . . . It's not like they said, 'Now if you had been a better parent,' but it was [implied]." These communications actually affirmed Anne's own belief that Linda's breakdown was her fault. She told me, "I assigned myself the role of taking care of everyone and, therefore, it was my fault. . . . When things weren't okay then it was my job to get everything as close to normal as possible." When I asked where this idea came from, she replied, "I know it [the role] so well, it's like breathing. [Maybe] it's something that I inherited as a genetic thing." She seemed eager to continue this line of thought and told me, "As [for] my children, I had to be sure that they were well taken care of. . . . I don't know that I did that good a job, but I had that sense that it was my responsibility . . . and it never occurred to me that I couldn't meet my expectations." With such a perspective her response to Linda's illness is understandable. "I felt that if I worked hard enough [and] fast enough that I could make her better. Anything [the doctors] suggested I jumped on with great enthusiasm." Later, she added, "The fact that I cannot take care of everything . . . is very difficult for me to accept."

At home Anne was also dealing with a very successful professional husband whom "a number of social acquaintances referred to as my fourth   and my most difficult child. . . . He was totally unpredictable. He could be very loving and very supporting. Or he could be very angry and you never knew what was going to happen." Despite feeling great anger toward her husband, she decided, with the help of a therapist, to "save the marriage and keep the family intact." It is interesting to note that Anne reported feeling closest to her husband during his own periodic depressions. She explained, "At least three times that I know of, he had a three-month episode of not feeling well . . . and he would sit with blankets by the fire. And he would play Pink Floyd and cry. Cry about the loss of his father. Cry about the tragedies of his childhood. Cry, cry, cry. And I would sit and rock and hold him and feel like the person he needed. To that extent, his depressive reactions made me feel more a partner in his life. . . . I can remember feeling closer to him during his depressive times than any other times."

Through all this Anne persisted in efforts to make a happy home. Although "the family wasn't chaotic in a wild sense," it was clear that "the kids didn't particularly want to bring friends home." Anne found her own refuge in the domestic roles of cleaning and cooking. These involvements served both to divert her attention from family problems and to make things that were emblematic of a happy household. The importance Anne attached to her roles as mother and housekeeper is evident in this comment: "We tried having a housekeeping group come in and the house looked a lot better. Anyway, we stopped having the housecleaning service come in [because] I think I needed [to do the cleaning]. That was one of my diversions. I [also] cooked a lot because nobody came into the kitchen and I had the place to myself and I was busy." In response, I asked, "So you were doing therapy by keeping busy?" and Anne replied, "Oh yes, definitely. And I had a product when the meal was on the table. I had accomplished something good. There was that sense of satisfaction. We had desserts every night. Everybody's favorite was served at least once a week." However, even as she tried mightily to create normal appearances, Anne knew it was only an illusion.

We spoke for more than an hour before Anne mentioned Jay. He was in the background of the narrative because, until his senior year in high school, he had been in the background of the family. Although a star athlete in high school, he had been an unusually quiet child. "He was always the quietest child in the room in any class that he was in." "He was," Anne continued, "just quiet." "And people like my brother would say, 'Don't worry about Jay, because he's going to be okay.' And [so] I interpreted his solitary activities as a strong thing. He didn't have to please people." This interpretation proved wholly wrong when Jay was hospitalized for major depression just prior to his high school graduation.

Anne remembered, "He missed his high school graduation. And this is one of the first times I've been able to say that without bursting into tears. He was in the hospital on the day of his high school graduation and both of us wept. I felt like he could have gone through the ceremony and been okay, but [the doctors] said 'absolutely not!'"

Jay passed through this episode, but suffered another only a few months later during his freshmen year in college. At this point, the family fell apart altogether. "Jay was out of control . . . [and] never got back on track. . . . My daughter came home from [names college] . . . and she was ripe for hospitalization. [And] my husband was becoming more and more strange . . . and that March went into an alcohol rehab center. . . . So I had three family members in the hospital." Among Anne's few potential family resources was her father who "always felt that depression was a matter of will power and [if you were sick] somebody wasn't trying." During all this she was working around the clock to pay the bills, propelled by an energy generated from "a profound sense of desperation." These events occurred in 1987. Since that time, Anne's husband has left her and remarried. She recalled with some bitterness that, despite his own emotional troubles, "He was very angry at the children's illness and felt that it was their own fault; that certainly it was not anything he had done. [As he saw it] he had paid the bills . . . and gave them a good life and here they were failing him."

At the time of his father's wedding, Jay was in a halfway house that allowed him to come and go as he pleased. After returning from the ceremony, he swallowed a package of Benadryl, a common antihistamine bought over the counter. He was discovered in a groggy state and brought to a local hospital. When Anne arrived, she found him in a unit "one step down from intensive care." "He was sitting there wired to the EKG machine because his heart did have some arrhythmia." When Jay saw his mother, "he burst into tears . . . and so it was easy to interpret that he didn't want to die. . . . He just didn't like the way he was living." Whatever insights Anne had about her son's feelings and motives, she had little control over what physicians did to him. She expressed deep resentment about not being involved in his treatment plan. She knew Jay had agreed to it, but when she got the call at work that he had received the first in a series of twelve ECT (electro-convulsive shock) treatments she "just became weak in the knees," explaining that "I couldn't stand the thoughts of it."

By this point in the interview I was feeling astonished at Anne's ability to continue in the face of such overwhelming, ongoing trauma. I remembered her comment about feeling closest to her ex-husband during his weakest moments, and I asked, "Do you feel that all this extraordinary turmoil has deepened your relationships with your kids?" This question provoked the most emotion during the interview. Anne became teary and choked with emotion as she tried to answer. I will give you her response in detail because it suggests the intensity of love that makes it so difficult for parents like Anne to distance themselves from their children's troubles.

> It opens up a dimension of love. You know, I'm trying to think of how I can compare it. Jay was a track star when he was in high school. I was an obnoxious mother. I loved those meets. I would come in with gallons of Gatorade and iced tea. The whole track team was hydrated through my efforts week after week. I yelled longer and louder and harder than anyone. I guess it was an embarrassment to Jay. And you know, we've talked about that now, [and] I think he would have been just as happy if I had stayed home. But he was a marvelous runner.

And it was a special moment. I loved those moments. And I loved that it was my son.

We rarely touched. Jay still doesn't like being touched. And I thought I loved him [but] when I saw him at the [names hospital], with those EKG leads, the tears just burst forth and it was a different love. It was just overwhelming. You feel the affection, but it goes into a depth that you may never have known you are capable of. That's what I found. I thought I knew I loved my kids, but at that moment when they were so sadly afflicted, the depth was just . . . There was a purity. The sadness was a dimension, but there was [also] a feeling of love. You have the love that you felt [before] but it just expands to fill a space that you never even knew existed. . . . It's [a love] closer to truth. . . . I wouldn't want to have this [the tragedy of depression] visited on people, but I believe that I've had some special moments that other people don't have. . . . There's probably a better word than beauty. . . . I knew that truth was a factor in it [but there is also] a certain honesty. It was a very unguarded emotion. . . . I grew up in a household with a lot of mixed messages and never was able to trust my own emotions. But this one came without any [difficulty]. . . . To truly feel my own capacity to love, which I had not felt before, is liberating.

About a month after interviewing Anne, I spoke with Jay. I found the first hour or so of the interview difficult because he was so tentative, answering most of my questions with one-liners. Eventually, he loosened up and offered more voluble answers as he tried to articulate how difficult he finds his life. Along the way, Jay acknowledged that his mother deserves greater freedom and he certainly feels awkward continuing to live with her. In an effort to become more autonomous, he has pieced together enough coursework to receive a college degree. However, he is still too sick to work full-time and does not feel nearly strong enough to leave home.

For her part, Anne has begun to take some preliminary steps in "trying to recreate [her] life." In 1990 she went to a two-session waltzing class where, she told me, "I met a man about my age and impulsively gave him my telephone number." She became close with Paul, but by last fall they concluded that theirs "was not going to be a permanent relationship." She half joked about a fantasy that "[She] will meet somebody that has similar problems and we'll go off into the sunset, solving our problems and the children's problems all at the same time." Instead of hoping for a magic resolution to her family's problems, Anne is better served by acting on the advice of those in her Wednesday night support group who tell her, "There's no way that you can live your child's life and you're going to have to relinquish a lot of your responsibility." Putting such an injunction into practice will be difficult for a woman whose life has been constructed around an especially demanding version of motherhood. I hope she finds a way to redefine her obligations to her children since both her own and their future well-being may significantly depend on it.

WHAT DO YOU OWE YOUR PARENTS?

Marco contacted me because he wished to be interviewed about his own depressions that have twice forced him into hospitals, in each instance for several months. By the time he called, however, I had completed my 50 interviews and explained that I was now more interested in talking to the family and friends of depressed people. As I began to thank him for calling anyway, Marco volunteered that when he was 14 his mother became severely depressed for nearly three years after a pregnancy ended with a stillbirth. He described briefly that neither his father, his younger brother, nor a much younger sister were emotionally equipped to deal with the trauma of his mother's illness. Marco, consequently, both took over the household and became his mother's primary caregiver. His dual career as a depressed person and as a caregiving child intrigued me and we arranged to meet. For nearly three hours we spoke of the obligations of a first-born Italian son to a sick mother and the powerful bond of kinship forged by the lifelong efforts of two family members with the same devastating illness to care for each other. At age 43, Marco still feels very much "like my mother's son." "I'm sensitive," he explained, "and have all these psychological characteristics . . . that I see in her."

In many ways, Marco's description of his home life fits Hollywood's stereotyped image of working-class Italian families. Marco himself did not leave home until age 29 and his 36-year-old unmarried sister continues to live with their parents. During his early years, the family lived in a section of Boston called the North End that today is still the city's "Little Italy." His father was a "real go-getter" who worked full-time as a mechanic for a large company while doing a number of part-time jobs as well. He described his father as "somewhat authoritarian,"[9] but "not the way most authoritarian fathers are [who] keep long distances from their children. He wasn't like that. He would take the family out [on] Sundays and go for rides . . . but he did have a very stubborn streak."

Prior to the regular Sunday outings, the whole family attended church. "The other Italian Catholic and Sicilian cultural thing I would have to throw in here," Marco added, "is that you don't have sex before you get married at all, especially the daughters in the family." When I remarked that his description somewhat reminded me of the portrayal of the Italian family in a number of movies, Marco agreed by saying, "If you look at *Moonstruck* and Cher in that movie, even though she's not Italian, she played the role of an Italian daughter very well. She looks like my sister. My sister could fit the role of that woman in the movie."

Any comparisons with family portrayals in movies like *Moonstruck* ended as Marco began to describe the extent to which his family was *depression-struck*. His mother had married at 20 to escape an abusive household in which she was the youngest of 12 children. When Marco asked about the grandfather he never met, his mother confided that "the day her father died she had no feelings whatsoever, that it was probably the happiest day of her life." While Marco's sister and father appear to have escaped serious problems with depression, his brother, Marco believes, "suffers from depression and low self-esteem, even though he doesn't want to admit it. He never finished high school, is working part time jobs [and] he drinks a lot. I can say he's a borderline alcoholic. . . . He has had a couple of bouts with depression, [but] not nearly where I've gone with it."

When Marco's discussion turned to himself I was surprised to learn that he had been a "withdrawn, unhappy kid" who was taunted at school because of his weight. It was hard to picture the youthful, trim, athletic-looking man sitting across from me as a 240-pound adolescent. The description made better sense when he told me that his troubles as a teenager were compounded by the growing recognition of his homosexuality. As a gay adolescent growing up in a 1960s working class home, Marco told me, "I didn't feel safe with my folks because [if I told them about being gay] I felt like I was going to be abandoned and rejected."

Despite the pain of keeping his sexuality secret, Marco's remembrance of family life did not include overwhelming problems until his mother's breakdown. His father, Marco remembers, was plainly the dominant person in the home and while "they often fought about money and how they were going to support the family," he only grudgingly allowed his wife to work outside the home as a waitress. Except for these arguments, he recalled, "There was nothing wrong, absolutely nothing really wrong, until she went to the hospital [to have her child]." "She was," he went on, "really happy about the thought that she was having this kid. . . . I was 13 years old so I can remember her buying all the stuff [for the baby]. We used to go to the store and shop and we were all excited about it actually." Sadly, the baby was stillborn and "after that my mother just completely broke down."

Upon returning home Marco's mother was unable to do much of anything. Although she was never hospitalized for depression "she would have lots of crying jags." She saw a psychiatrist twice a week who put her on medications, but the problem only deepened with his father's incomprehension and anger about the situation. He explained, "My father was in a rage because it was costing him an arm and a leg. And he could not understand emotional illness. He couldn't figure out why he was dishing out 75 dollars a week to a psychiatrist. He was extremely frustrated because he didn't understand. [In turn], I couldn't understand why my father got so angry because my mother was [obviously] in a lot of pain." Marco's father who had been "sort of a workaholic" anyway, responded to the family crisis by working even harder, presumably to pay the bills, but also to retreat from a difficult situation.

Social scientists have frequently remarked on the fact that the unpaid housework of women is generally invisible and taken for granted by other family members.[10] Such work becomes very visible, however, when it is not done. As he recounted events, Marco reflected, "It just occurred to me that before my mother was sick,

I looked up to her to do this, that and the other thing." He continued, "That's what mothers do. Cook meals, set the table. Not that we weren't supposed to help, but when she was sick there was none of that at all. And what happened was that I took on that role. I needed to be strong for her at 14 years old which is kind of a weighty thing for a beginning teenager who is not sure of his sexual identity, who doesn't know what the hell that's all about, is overweight, goes to high school and has panic attacks 'cause he's afraid that kids are gonna make fun of him . . . and then he goes home to his [sick] mother."

When I asked whether there were any cultural mandates about the responsibilities of first-born sons in Italian families, Marco replied, "You know, now that you say that, there could be. . . . I think that the first-born son is expected to become the caretaker in the family if the father is not around. . . . The first-born son becomes the male figurehead." In this case, of course, Marco's father was alive, but unable to appreciate the nature or extent of his wife's illness. Moreover, he was "bent over backwards working full-time." Marco was anxious to make plain that his father did the best he could. Several times during the interview he repeated, nearly like a mantra, that "My father never abandoned his children and he never abandoned his wife." Nevertheless, it was Marco who had to take over at home and that generated strong feelings. Here's part of our conversation about his caretaking role.

Tell me more about your caretaking role.

I was going to high school. And I would come home and I would do stuff around the house.

What kind of stuff?

Clean up.

She wasn't cleaning up?

She wasn't doing a lot of the house chores. I would do laundry. And I felt that because I was part of the family and my mother was sick I had to do this. I would do a lot of the cooking. . . . I felt depressed because my mother was depressed. I felt overwhelmed because she was so sick. I felt that she had changed from the person that she was before to a person who was sort of withdrawn and not there with the family. She didn't cook meals the way she used to. She didn't do things around the house. She completely changed.

Were you resentful that your siblings weren't doing any of this?

I was pissed at my brother. My brother did shit. I couldn't understand him. He saw that my mother wasn't feeling well. And he was always like that. He never picked up after himself. He never did anything. He still doesn't do stuff like that, but I used to get pissed off. Real pissed off. My sister was, what, seven years old? I mean what the hell was she gonna do? She pitched in where she could.

I'm getting the picture of your mother as pretty much out of it most of the time.

That's right. For more than two and a half years that went on. I didn't really have any friends during high school, [but] I was very close to my mother. My relationship with my mother was much stronger at the time than my father's relationship with his wife. . . . I took on a role that he most likely should have been taking on—the sensitive, caring husband—and it really, to a degree, was a little inappropriate for me to be that close to my mother, [but] I could talk to her. [Because of my own depression] I knew what she was feeling. My father wasn't capable of doing that. So I was giving the empathy and the sympathy and the emotional caring much more so than he was doing, as well as doing some of the other stuff. I didn't know where to draw the line. There was no line. You just kept doing it. I just did it because that was what I was supposed to do. And that's the way I felt people take care of other people.

"This is my obligation?"

That's the way I felt. I still feel that way. . . . I mean, when you look at it realistically, what the hell are you supposed to do if you have a sick parent in the house . . . and you're part of the family? I don't know what other families did, but what are you supposed to do, throw them by the wayside? . . . I mean, I love my parents. . . . I did it out of love and caring and [as] a son who was, you know, the oldest.

Marco's mother eventually got better, but was never "the same person because there was something about the experience that [fundamentally] changed her." When I asked Marco if there was anything positive for him in the caretaking role, he acknowledged that "It made me feel important. It made me feel that I was more adult-like." He also spoke about the need to "push [his] own stuff aside" during that period, saying, "I don't even think I was aware how severe [my own depression] was at the time. I knew that it made me feel better to help my mother and to help the family. And I think that helped me." Apparently, the enveloping character of the caretaker role served as a diversion from Marco's own emotional troubles. Several years later, in his early twenties, he "came out" of "an extremely closeted relationship . . . that bothered me so much that I was off the walls. I was paranoid." Although his parents responded to his revelation in an accepting way, indicating that they had already guessed him to be gay,

Marco nevertheless crashed. He was hospitalized because "I had all this shit in my head with the gay thing."

During this and then another extended hospitalization four years later, it was Marco's mother who rallied to his side. The family pattern evident during his mother's illness repeated itself to the extent that his father still could not comprehend the needs of a depressed person. Thus, his mother became Marco's advocate "and she fought my father all the way about [getting] counseling. My father still didn't buy into it even when I was in my early twenties. . . . When I really got sick, the first person who understood was my mother . . . and that emotional [caretaking] bond was reversed. I got it [depression] much worse than she did, but I could see it in her eyes. She didn't even have to say anything. She was just there in a different way than my dad was because she knew what it felt like." Over the years (his mother had another significant period of depression in 1986) the shared illness of this mother and son has drawn them tightly together. Marco said, "More than anyone else I see my mother's pain and she sees it in me, and we don't even have to verbalize it."

Now that only Marco's sister lives at home with their parents, the caretaking division of labor within the family has somewhat shifted. Their mother continues to take antidepressant medications, but still suffers from periodic panic attacks and agoraphobia. These days his sister calls him when she begins to recognize the signs of a downward drift in their mother's mood, when she becomes increasingly withdrawn and anxious. What has not changed is the mutual concern mother and son feel for each other. During a recent period of trouble, Marco described how "that [caretaking] role came back and I was calling my mother [frequently] and, you know, I would just go over and talk to her. And she's constantly worried about me. Just last Sunday we were over for dinner and sitting down at the dinner table and she took my hand and she says, 'How are you doing? You know, I'm worried about you.' Because [she knows] my life hasn't been going that great."

Lessons learned in childhood have enormous durability. Toward the end of our interview the focus shifted to a recent relationship Marco has had with a man whom he met three or four years ago at an Al-Anon meeting. As easy as it is to hop on a bicycle and ride it after not having done so for years, Marco found himself naturally slipping into a caregiving role with this man. "This guy was having problems," Marco explained. "He lost his business. His mother was dying. He had a companion of 13 years [and] that was going down the drain. He was so depressed [and] that light turned on inside of me; you know, 'I've been helped by . . . doing something to help somebody else.' I got very enmeshed with this guy to the point where I was getting emotionally sick because I was attracted to him and cared about him in other ways as well. But I was looked at [primarily] as the person who was the caretaker."

The discussion of this recent relationship precipitated some thinking about Marco's difficulty in knowing how to set boundaries. I tried to push him a bit on the distinction between being a caregiver and being an "enabler." Certainly Marco understood the point that overly generous caregivers are sometimes manipulated by those cared for. He agreed that efforts to help his current friend might only have the effect of allowing him to remain sick. He also recognized an important pattern in his own life—intense involvement as a caregiver requires him to mute his own difficult feelings, with the result that he becomes sick himself.

Despite the problems overinvolvement generates, Marco sees no alternatives for himself. He tried to explain his position this way: "We're talking about setting boundaries with people that you really care about and who are emotionally sick. It cripples me, but what else am I supposed to do? It's like an all or nothing thing. . . . If we're all going to set emotional boundaries with everybody, then we're not really going to care about anybody. . . . I can't do that. I won't do that. Setting boundaries is too painful."

This last piece of conversation hits on an issue with universal significance. We all need human relationships and community involvements for the comfort and care they provide. In return, we are obliged to care for others. However, this norm of reciprocity,[11] easy to contemplate in the abstract, is a lot harder to calculate in real life. Relationships of all sorts would exist in perfect harmony if everybody's needs were exactly equivalent and we all shared a consensus about appropriate degrees of caregiving. Such is not the case, unfortunately, and that greatly complicates our decisions about involvement with others who need help.

Economists, when discussing the viability of social welfare programs, write about what they call the "free rider problem."[12] These programs are compromised or fail, they say, since so many people keep taking government money without making any meaningful efforts to help themselves or to contribute to society. Marco's comments hint at the idea that, analogously, there are "emotional free riders" who expect extensive emotional support while providing little in return. Plainly, though, Marco is no free rider. Indeed, he has paid a heavy price by giving so often to the emotionally needy even when he has few resources himself. I did not leave this interview with the same optimism I felt after speaking with Rachel and Anne. Unlike them, Marco has not moved toward a workable balance between his own and others' needs. I hope I'm wrong, but my guess is that his impulse to devote himself unreservedly to others' care while ignoring his own needs will continue to be hurtful to him. At the same time, it is impossible not to admire Marco's altruism and to see in his biography possible alternatives to a world in which people are increasingly unmoved by others' pain.

WHAT ARE FRIENDS FOR?

During the course of this research I have listened to more than 60 people detail dramatic, life-altering parts of their biographies. Often single events were absolutely pivotal in the way individuals later constructed and then understood their lives. John's story was typical in this sense. A student at Boston College, John learned of my study and volunteered to speak about his efforts to help several friends in trouble with depression and related life problems. Within the first few minutes of the interview, as though to get the record straight, John offered information that framed my understanding of everything he would tell me for the next two hours. He explained that he was raped at the age of six and only within the last six or seven years (he is now 33) has he been able to come to grips with that event and subsequent sexual abuse. He told me, "I experienced sexual abuse over many years [and] my parents were never able to understand that this is what was happening to me. They were never able to read my signals. And . . . I internalized it and became very depressed. . . . I learned to take care of myself. I somehow survived . . . [but] my parents just missed it."

I quickly realized that our conversation would extend well beyond the description of any one particular friendship. This was so because John has made it a routine part of his life to minister to the needs of many friends whom he suspects might be struggling emotionally. When I asked for the numbers he told me that he has counseled "probably a couple of dozen" friends over the last several years. John acknowledged that his desire to help others relates to everyone's earlier failure to decipher his own childhood distress signals. He seems, in fact, to have a personal mission, driven by the remembrance of his own isolation, to draw out friends who might not themselves be in touch with the nature or source of their pain. He believes, moreover, that he has refined a skill to "connect with others' pain." Added to this is John's philosophy that "To know is to be responsible." He elaborated by saying, "It's the same as with any knowledge. Once you have that knowledge, you have a certain responsibility to use it. . . . You know, I have [the] knowledge that I've gained through my pain . . . And I think that because so few people [are skilled enough] to pick up on these things . . . it kind of behooves us [who have the skill] to do something with it."

John grew up in a devout family and has always been religious. "Quite frankly," he told me, "I believe that the only way I stayed alive as an abused child was through my faith. . . . Church was a place where I felt safe. . . . I felt support [and] guidance in a way that I didn't feel it elsewhere in my life." His religiosity led him to graduate school where he earned a Master's degree in theology. However, his intention to become an Episcopal priest was never realized because the "sexual abuse stuff was starting to bubble up" and he was increasingly unable to worship. At this difficult moment he met a church-connected "spiritual advisor" who saw his desperation and "helped [him] to look at the connections between spirituality and [his own] struggles and issues." I asked, "Is your willingness to extend yourself to others related to this experience?" and John replied, "There is the element of appreciating that someone was [finally] there for me. . . . I've had friends say to me, 'Why do you give a shit? Why are you there for me? Why do you put up with me when I call you at 11 o'clock and cry for an hour?' . . . I say, 'because people were there for me and [now] it's my turn. I'm glad I can be there for you. I know what it's like. I've been there.'"

John then described a variety of strategies and techniques involved in deepening otherwise superficial friendship conversations, remarking at one point "You have to be careful in throwing out cues . . . because people may not be ready to . . . understand themselves. . . . You know, sometimes they're fishing because . . . they want to see if you're open to hearing [their problem]. Other times they're fishing because they're struggling and they don't know what [to do]. And you don't want to freak them out [by saying the wrong thing]." When I remarked that broaching intimate and troublesome life issues requires a kind of meta-language, a subtle subtext of messages during conversations, John agreed that "it is a kind of special discourse" and described his general approach this way:

> I can somehow connect with that piece [of another person] that's painful for them. I see it in their face. I see it in their body language. I hear it in . . . the way they talk. I'm usually really good at it. And . . . I send the signals that it's okay to talk about it. . . . And I start throwing out some of the things that I know are possible scenarios. . . . And sometimes people hang a coat on one of them and they say [for example], "You know, gee, it's interesting that you bring up anorexia.". . . I think that in a way what you do is empathize with people in ways that [others] don't. . . . Sometimes you're in that pit . . . [and] you need somebody to reach down and pull you out. And some of us can sense that and some of us can't. . . . Without being offensive, there are ways to say, "I'm throwing you a lifeline." And sometimes they take you up on it and sometimes they don't. . . . [In a variety of ways] I can say, "I feel for you. I appreciate your pain. And, you know, I'm here for you if you want to talk. Here's my number." Any number of things like that.

As with any sensitive form of talk, increasing levels of self-revelation require corresponding increases in trust and rapport. John provided a useful imagery when he explained, "Well, typically there's a little bit of openness because they're already starting to trust me. In most of my friendships [where the other person has a problem], they've thrown out a little stone. And I pick up the stone and say, 'Gee, this is interesting, [thereby indicating that] I understand this.' And then they throw a bigger one and it kind of builds from there. I send signals that it's okay to share that with me. It's okay to talk more. And, you know, as you listen well you leave people room to maneuver in a friendship."

As John was talking I was doing a quick calculation: "Two dozen friends counseled over six or seven years averages three or four people at any given time." Recalling Rachel's, Anne's, and Marco's incredible difficulties in managing a relationship with even one sick person, I asked, after John confirmed that he often deals simultaneously with several troubled friends, why he is not overwhelmed by their emotional demands. Using his own earlier description of the ever increasing size of the rocks passed back and forth between friends, I asked what he did when they became boulder-sized. He replied, "Some of them get too heavy to carry. I get your point. That's when my own emotional health has to come in. . . . And there comes a point when you're not doing someone any favors by letting them throw boulders at you. . . . You have to establish boundaries by withdrawing, but in a healthy way. In the context of my friendships, I've said things like, 'These are things that I really can't help you with. I hear your pain. I see where you're coming from, [but] I really encourage you to bring that up in therapy.' Or, 'I can be there for you, but I can't have calls at all hours of the night.'" Still, John admitted, "I've had to struggle with these boundaries."

The more we talked about boundaries, the clearer I became that this is the primary issue distinguishing the tasks of caregiving to family members and to friends. In her book entitled *Just Friends,*[13] Lillian Rubin explores, with her usual clarity and insight, how the obligations of kinship and friendship differ. In a fashion, her analysis explores the deeper implications of the cultural axiom that "you can choose your friends, but not your relatives." Because friends *choose* to do what family members are *obliged* to do, friendship boundaries are clearer, more flexible, and less binding that boundaries between family members. As an example, Rubin notes how personal traumas such as a divorce often envelop a range of family members, drawing them directly into another's emotional pain in ways that threaten their own identities. "For these reasons," Rubin writes, "it is easier for friends to extricate themselves from the morass than it is for kin, easier to maintain enough distance from both the painful event and their feelings about it so as not to get hooked the way family members can. Friends, therefore, can be more helpful in such moments, not requiring that we protect them from the depth and intensity of our misery."[14]

When I brought up the contrast between family and friends, John confirmed Rubin's ideas with a very personal example. It turns out that he has a brother who is terminally ill. When I asked whether it was harder to care for him than his friends, John replied, "There is this tendency for him to take advantage of me. . . . It got to the point where there was this assumption, for example, that he could just move in when he needed to have medical care and I'd take care of it. And he would tell people without even asking me, 'Oh, I'm going to be living at John's for the next month.' And I would have to say, 'Excuse me, but when did we have this conversation?'" He went on, "So there's the same limits to caring . . . but it's very hard because I'm the caregiver whether I like it or not.

I'm responsible because nobody else will [be]. There's a part of me that says, 'No, I'm not responsible,' and another part that says, 'But this is my brother and I love him.'" And later he added, "It [being my brother] makes it obligatory to struggle with it. Whereas with a friend, you're not even obliged to have to struggle with it. That's your choice. The obligations and responsibilities are different. It's maybe not so painful for a friend to say, 'Wait a minute, I'm just a friend. I'm not your mom or dad.'"

Because boundary setting is the central issue of this chapter, I pushed John to say more by asking whether he has ever had regrets about taking people on. He acknowledged that occasionally individuals have abused his friendship. In one case, "It got to the point where I couldn't answer my phone at night because I knew who it was and I knew they wouldn't take no for an answer. . . . It's like the dog that bites the hand that feeds it." In such instances, John told me, boundary setting requires a combination of gentle sensitivity and "tough love conversation." He expanded on the need to sit down with the persistent late night caller and say, "This is uncomfortable. This is unfair [to me]. This is really out of control." Once again, in setting the proper boundaries, the contrast between friendship and kinship was invoked with John's declaration, "Yes, I'm a friend who's there for you . . . in the appropriate ways. But I'm a friend, I'm not your family." With a kind of conceptual elegance, John summed up the differing obligations of friendship and kinship as follows:

> I would put [the difference] in the context of choice. I have the freedom to choose how much I want to be involved in my friendship with someone. I have the freedom to choose how much I'm going to take on and not take on. And it's freedom in the biggest sense of the word. I am completely free. I can walk away with no obligations. Now, I have the freedom in how

I choose to relate to my family, but my family might not necessarily think I have a choice. And that obviously makes the dynamic different. Even if I feel I have the freedom to choose how I want to relate to my mother and father, [they] are still connected to me in some [special] way and . . . have their own expectations of that relationship. Whereas a friend is in the same boat as I am. They know I'm a friend. I have the freedom to hit the road if I want to . . . [In families] you have all the roles . . . that are predefined by society. Friendship doesn't have that. I mean, we're just two people, two ships that pass in the night and whether we both . . . drop anchor is our choice.

Another important dimension of friendship relationships opened as John began to describe in some detail how he had negotiated a caring relationship with a woman whom he met some years ago in their workplace. As he portrayed the escalation of self-disclosure in the relationship, I thought to ask how the process being described might be different for male and female friendships. After all, John earlier told me that he has befriended a couple of dozen people with depression. I simply assumed that this group included both men and women. I was, therefore, slightly taken aback when John casually explained, "I haven't done it for men." Good interviewers need to pick up on any suggestive comments that promise new and potentially valuable lines of inquiry. Sometimes these opportunities are not so clear and thus easily missed, but in this case only the most obtuse interviewer would fail to ask, "How do you explain that all of the friends you help are women?"

For the first time in our talk John stumbled a bit and seemed at something of a loss to explain his motives. He began by saying, "Because women can . . . because women are in different places . . . because women. . . ." And finally, "I don't know." Then, after some mutual speculation, John reached firmer explanatory grounds with his observation that "My sense is that men don't have the skills to continue when you start to drop the subtleties. . . . They either pick up on what you're trying to raise and run like hell emotionally in the other direction, or they aren't prepared or skilled enough to pick up on your dropping subtleties."

After still more discussion, John reached a conclusion that has been affirmed by a volume of social science literature. It is that men are good at *sociability*, but not nearly as skilled at *intimacy*.[15] Although, as the movie *When Harry Met Sally* illustrates, it is hard for men and women to have an intimate friendship without the intrusion of sexuality as a compromising factor, deeply intimate friendships between men pose the greatest problems because of widespread male homophobia. John seemed to me right on the mark when he said, "If it's a gay man [whom I'm trying to befriend] he thinks I'm trying to pick him up when I throw out those cues. . . . [Or, if they are heterosexual men] "they might suspect that I'm a gay man and that I'm really interested in them [and they flee]."

In an appendix entitled "Thinking about Sampling," I try to make sense of the fact that only women responded to my newspaper advertisements soliciting interviews with caregivers, *even when the ad explicitly specified men only.* I placed three advertisements asking for male caregivers, one in a newspaper reaching four large communities in the Boston area, a second in the *Boston Phoenix* which reaches a somewhat more culturally diverse audience, and the last in the Boston College student newspaper, *The Heights.* Not one man responded to these requests. I can only conclude from this data that men very rarely take on the caregiver role and, when they do, they are not especially interested in talking about it. It warrants noting that both Marco and John, who did finally come forward, have themselves deeply suffered from depression. It may be that personal experience with the anguish of depression is the *sine qua non* of men's willingness to become caregivers for others afflicted with the illness. And even they may have real difficulty reaching out to male friends whom they suspect are in great emotional turmoil.

It seems reasonable to conclude from John's interview that when individuals *are* able to embark on a helping relationship with a friend, it is generally easier to manage than a caregiving relationship with a family member. The difficulties of negotiating the boundaries of friendships are simply less complicated than those between family members. Therefore, the danger of being engulfed by a friend's depression is normally less than for a family member. At the same time, it is inappropriate to see all family caregiving efforts as equally arduous.

Families, of course, differ in multiple ways and consequently multiple configurations will characterize family caregiving arrangements. We need more refined analyses than could be accomplished in this chapter on the distinctive contingencies faced by husbands, wives, mothers, fathers, and siblings in caregiving roles with each other. Whatever those differences might be, there is no doubt that the millions of people suffering from depression would have a far easier time of it if there were equal numbers of caregivers with John's extraordinary spirit of generosity. That spirit is eloquently captured in his effort to explain why he has chosen to invest the incredible time and energy it takes to help a depressed friend.

> I'm talking about things that make me human, that make me uniquely human and that I value greatly. One of those is relationships with other people, being there for other people. And so in the context of this [interview], it [helping friends with depression] is a labor of love. . . . It may be hours on the phone [and], yeah, it's a pain in the ass. Yeah, it's difficult. And yeah,

I have to rearrange my schedule to deal with it. You know, it might mean that I don't get done the paper that is due for a class [the next day] and I have to skip something in the morning to finish the damn thing. And yeah, it may mean that the paper is not going to be as good as it might. However, you, my friend, were worth it.

ILLNESS AND THE FRAGILITY OF EVERYDAY ENCOUNTERS

Beginning in 1959 with his classic work, *The Presentation of Self in Everyday Life,* Erving Goffman wrote 11 books, each one affirming his unique genius for analyzing the intricacies of everyday social encounters.[16] He was a master ethnographer who brilliantly documented the subtle social rituals through which individuals manage their own identities while protecting those of others. In so doing he showed how we mutually share in the task of sustaining social life itself.

Goffman's description of the strategies used by patients to salvage selves under assault in a mental hospital[17] and his extraordinary insight into the meanings of having a "stigmatized" identity[18] bear the closest kinship with my subject matter. But the range of his thinking informs every chapter in this book because all his work describes how identities are formed, managed, manipulated, protected, changed, and sometimes injured beyond repair. To my mind, though, the most important single legacy of Goffman's scholarship is a deepened appreciation for the fragility of everyday encounters. Together, his writings display just how delicate the social order arising out of human association can sometimes be. He has wryly observed that "life might not be much of a gamble, but social interaction is."[19] This means, I think, that social life as a whole has more stability than our particular everyday encounters where nothing less than our presented identities are at stake.

Goffman's books are filled with virtuoso intellectual performances. He takes readers on dazzling conceptual journeys by inventing a series of ideas for powerfully illuminating the normally taken-for-granted workings of daily interactions. Among these many valuable concepts is the notion of "situational involvement." In his 1963 book *Behavior in Public Places,*[20] Goffman suggests that whenever we enter a social occasion, we must, in order to appear social, proper, and worthwhile, answer correctly the question "Just what level of involvement must I have with others in this situation?" Cocktail parties, business meetings, sporting events, bedrooms, anonymous public places, and classrooms, to name a few contexts,[21] demand very different degrees of involvement from participants.

The notion of situational involvement has been a guiding frame for the choice and presentation of the four case studies that constitute most of this chapter. Aside from the intrinsically dramatic quality of the stories themselves, they illustrate how depressive illness poses distinctive involvement dilemmas for the family and friends of an afflicted person.

As I write about this, it strikes me as surprising that Goffman never took up illness as a focus for extended analysis since the relationship between sick people and those close to them may be the quintessential case for thinking about the moral and social foundations of all human relationships. If a central goal of social science is to understand the basis for social order in everyday life, it is often best to proceed by studying those situations where order breaks down, where normal interactions are thrown into disarray, where the normative arrangements surrounding relationships become opaque. Goffman has, for example, used this strategy in spotlighting embarrassing situations as a way of uncovering the principles of social organization and the bases for successful role performance.[22] In the same way, severe illness, because it so disrupts relationships, illustrates the tenuous nature of everyday life and highlights the taken-for-granted, normally invisible boundaries of social relationships. Prolonged illness makes demands on a partner, family member, or friend that raise directly the question "What do people owe each other in a relationship?" The shortened versions of Rachel's, Anne's, Marco's, and John's experiences demonstrate how delicate a task it is to help someone with depression without being pulled down by their illness.

The four cases were strategically chosen to illustrate how spouses, parents, children, and friends might deal somewhat differently with the problem of extending appropriate sympathy to a depressed person. At various points in this chapter I have been careful to say that the four cases are only sensitizing and suggestive. Among other things, they represent only instances where, despite the strains created by depression, the relationships have endured. It would surely be valuable to learn the dynamics involved in ending a relationship because of illness. Full-scale studies ought also to be done on how depressive illness affects the equilibrium of relationships for different categories of individuals (such as age, gender, race, religion, and social class). For example, might we expect women caregivers to display, on the whole, more porous sympathy and involvement boundaries than men? Would we guess the response to a family member or friend sick with depression to vary in different social classes? And so on.

Were I to venture an initial hypothesis from the 10 interviews with family and friends, I would say that they move through a predictable socialization process. Just as those suffering from depression don't initially know what to make of their feelings, the response of family and friends is at first likely to be bewilderment and consternation. Once it becomes clear that the problem is depression—probably after a dramatic crisis—family and friends go through a period of actively learning about it. This may involve conversations with medical people and sometimes extensive reading. If my interviews and personal experience are at all representative, this learning process is followed by a sometimes lengthy period of heroic efforts to save or cure the depressed person. Heroic measures are undertaken at the outset of a catastrophic illness because sympathy margins remain wide and caregivers may believe that once a depressed person realizes how much he or she is cared about, they will get better. Heroic measures also display strong commitment, something that individuals are expected to show when someone close is in a crisis. Such efforts might continue for some time, even years, but with growing doubts about their efficacy. When it eventually becomes plain that things are not changing for the better and that one's own well-being is seriously jeopardized, the process of retreating from the sick person likely begins.

There is another similarity between Goffman's writings and the level of analysis throughout most of this book. Since this study relies on in-depth interview data, on 50 biographical accounts of an illness experience, I have largely heard how individuals respond to their illness in highly personalized ways and within the domains of their everyday face-to-face encounters. Like Goffman's, my analysis thus far has been on the "micro" level of everyday interaction and has relatively neglected the "macro" dimensions of history, social structure and culture that influence how all of us define the situations of everyday life. However, as a social psychologist, I am well aware that the dramas of daily life occur within larger historical and institutional settings; that "the social does not [simply] 'influence' the private, it dwells within it."[23] Peter and

Brigitte Berger explain the interplay of micro and macro worlds this way:

> First of all, crucially and continuously, we inhabit the *micro-world* of our immediate experience with others in face-to-face relations. Beyond that, with varying degrees of significance and continuity, we inhabit a *macro-world* consisting of much larger structures and involving us in relations with others that are mostly abstract, anonymous and remote. Both worlds are essential to our experience of society, and . . . each world depends upon the other for its meaning to us.[24]

The last chapter, "Sickness, Self, and Society," fills out my thinking by considering the features of the macro structure of American culture that help to explain why so many of us these days are falling ill with depression. I have repeatedly said that medicine's embrace of exclusively biological explanations for depression is theoretically parochial. No illness, including those for which there is an indisputable biological basis, can be understood apart from social context. Location of the pathological condition that causes a difficulty tells us little about the subjective experience of the problem. AIDS and certain forms of cancer, for example, might be equally painful and deadly. However, the meanings attached to these different diseases, and thus the way they are experienced, are quite different. There is, in other words, an intimate connection between the experience of mental and physical symptoms and society. In the case of depression it may be America's cultural chemistry rather than flawed biology that most primarily explains the growing incidence of people who are diagnosed and treated for emotional pain profound enough to make living problematic.

Chapter 7

Sickness, Self, and Society

Nowadays men often feel that their lives are a series of traps. They sense that within their everyday worlds, they cannot overcome their troubles, and in this feeling, they are often quite correct. . . . Yet men do not usually define the troubles they endure in terms of historical change and institutional contradiction. . . . They do not . . . grasp the interplay of man and society, of biography and history, of self and world. . . . What they need . . . is a quality of mind that will help them to . . . achieve lucid summations of what is going on in the world and of what may be happening within themselves. . . . [T]his quality [of mind] . . . may be called the sociological imagination.

C. Wright Mills, The Sociological Imagination, 1959

My daughter, a senior at Tufts University and a sociology major, asked to read the first chapter of this book. Giving it to her made me feel uneasy, but I knew that eventually my words would be in the public domain and I was certainly curious to learn her reactions. Realizing that some of the incidents described in those pages would be new to her, I sat on the living room couch looking for signs of surprise or distress as she read my "confessions." She seemed absorbed by my account and when she finished I asked for her impressions. She offered two main thoughts. First, probably to allay my concerns, she assured me that my depression has not influenced her as profoundly as I might imagine. Second, she questioned whether culture played as much a part in understanding depression as I seemed to claim. She could appreciate the importance of factors such as class, race, ethnicity, and gender in shaping a number of behaviors, but was hard-pressed to see the appropriateness of cultural explanations for such an obviously *personal* problem as depression. In the largest sense, this last chapter attempts an answer to her question.

Like all human beings, my daughter thinks about the world in causal terms. All of us use cause and effect inferences in trying to understand important features of our lives. As you saw earlier, efforts to come to grips with depression turn on its presumed causes. Directly or indirectly, many of the respondents' comments in earlier chapters represent efforts to satisfactorily complete the statement "I'm depressed because. . . ." In this way, everyone suffering from depression inevitably becomes a theorist as they try to give order and coherence to their situation. With rare exceptions, the theories they generate locate the cause(s) of depression somewhere either in their biographies or their biologies. Occasionally, respondents spin out more complex theories that see depression as resulting from the subtle interplay of personal history, recent life events, and chemical imbalances. However, even those who name situational causes for their emotional problems typically restrict their conceptual vision to the immediate and local circumstances of their lives. Only rarely do sufferers of depression relate their condition to the kinds of broad cultural trends that, I believe, influence our consciousness about everything.

The reach of sociological thinking extends well beyond the immediate milieus of daily life. In fact, exercise of the sociological imagination *requires* analysis of the connections between daily life and larger cultural arrangements. As described in chapter 2, the abiding theoretical questions of sociology flow from consideration of the individual-society connection. Sociologists presume an ongoing intersection of personal biographies and the larger arenas of history and social structure. A sociological angle of vision sees an inseparability between the character of culture and even our innermost thoughts and feelings, including, of course, the deeply troubling thoughts and feelings we label as depression. As George Herbert Mead expressed it with the title of his famous book, an adequate *social* psychology of human experience must consider the ways in which *Mind, Self and Society*[1] mutually transform each other. This last chapter focuses on how the structure of contemporary American society may be implicated in the production of increasingly larger numbers of people who complain of and are diagnosed as having diseased minds and selves.

Like many sociologists, one of my favorite examples to illustrate the cultural roots of what initially appears to be an exclusively personal disorder is Emile Durkheim's classic study of suicide[2] that is generally seen as a sociological *tour de force*. Aside from the intrinsic importance of the topic, Durkheim presumably chose to study suicide because, at first glance, it appears explicable *only* in individualistic, psychological terms. However, by testing a series of logically produced, deductive hypotheses linking suicide to such variables as religion, marital status, and membership in the military, Durkheim convincingly demonstrated the connection between suicide *rates* and degrees of *social integration*. Specifically, he argued that modernizing societies, like his own nineteenth-century France, were less successful than earlier agrarian societies in providing sources of integration for their members. Such societies were characterized by what Durkheim termed *anomie*—a state of relative normlessness. His brilliant work verified that anomic societies that fail to integrate their members adequately also fail to insulate them from suicide. Suicide, in short, is as much a social as it is a psychological phenomenon.

Another first-rate sociologist, Kai Erikson, provides a valuable example for illustrating how a sociological perspective is necessary to see social patterns that would be missed if we *only* look at things "up close and personal," as they say on *Wide World of Sports*.[3] He has us imagine that we are walking along 42nd Street near Times Square. At the street level we can clearly see the faces of the thousands of people who pass us. We can see their individual expressions, their particular body idioms, their apparent ages, and so on. At this range, they normally seem to take no notice of anyone around them. Each stranger appears as a solitary atom, buzzing along in a wholly independent way.

Were we, however, to climb to the roof of a nearby 12-story building and look down on the flow of sidewalk traffic, we would see an extraordinary thing. It is true that from this vantage point we miss the particularities of each individual. However, we would instead witness a miraculous pattern—thousands of people moving along the street in an incredibly well-organized, efficient, and cooperative fashion. Moreover, each person on the street would likely be wholly unaware of their contribution to the web of behavior necessary to sustain such an enormously complex social order. It is as if each pedestrian is guided by an invisible social force, a kind of social gravity, about which they have only the vaguest awareness. I am proposing that most people suffering from depression, like street pedestrians, are only dimly aware of how the constitution of culture might be contributing to their depressed condition.

Although estimates of the number of Americans suffering from depression vary, there is general consensus that the number is in the vicinity of 11 million people and that economic losses from poor productivity, lost work days, hospitalization, outpatient care, and so on, is a staggering $43.7 billion dollars a year.[4] More important to my concerns are the data from a range of studies showing tremendous increases in the rates of depression. For example: (1) The incidence of depression among those born after World War II is much higher and the age of onset much earlier than in earlier population cohorts.[5] (2) In recent decades, there has been a continuing rise in depression among young women, but a disproportionate increase of depression among men has been closing the depression gender gap.[6] (3) There has been an absolute explosion of depression among "baby boomers."[7] These and similar findings warrant the conclusion that America is in the grip of a depression epidemic; that we have entered an "age of melancholy."[8]

It may appear from the tone of these opening paragraphs that I am backing away from my promise in chapter 1 not to make claims about the causes of depression. While any search for patterns necessarily suggests cause, I prefer to think about the link between cultural dimensions and depression in probabilistic terms. Epidemiologists, for example, describe poverty as a "risk factor" for a range of health problems. Poverty provides a context that makes individuals more vulnerable to disease. The notion of risk factors implies likelihoods rather than direct causal relationships. In Durkheimian fashion, this last chapter details the cultural dimensions of contemporary American society that provide the context for our collective vulnerability to emotional distress.[9] In particular, my thesis can be expressed as a theoretical equation. It is:

MEDICALIZATION + DISCONNECTION + POSTMODERNIZATION =
PERSONAL DISLOCATION

Since most of the remainder of this last chapter elaborates the relationships among these cultural trends,[10] I will define what I have in mind as each is discussed. Immediately, though, my argument is best advanced by showing how fundamentally the idea of depression is connected to culture. If the features of a particular culture truly influence what is even recognized as an illness, we should expect wide cultural variation in the labeling of particular physical and emotional experiences as health or illness.

CULTURE, HEALTH, AND EMOTION

In a classic article written almost 50 years ago, the medical historian, Erwin H. Ackerknecht argued against the view that disease is a strictly physical phenomenon. Citing the important role played by social factors in the definition and treatment of illness, Ackerknecht maintained that "medicine's practical goal is not primarily a biological one, but that of social adjustment in a given society. . . . Even the notion of disease depends rather on the decisions of society than on objective facts."[11] As the following examples illustrate, societies differ dramatically in their response to the same physical symptoms:

> Pinto (dyschromic spirochetosis), a skin disease, is so common among many South American tribes that the few *healthy* men that *are not* suffering from pinto are regarded as *pathological* to the point of being excluded from marriage. The crippled feet of the traditional Chinese woman, diseased to us, were, of course, normal to the Chinese. Intestinal worms among the African Thongas are not at all regarded as pathological. They are thought to be necessary for digestion.[12]

Not only is the definition of what constitutes an illness or pathological condition subject to cultural variations, but, in an even more far-reaching sense, one's *experience* of bodily symptoms is shaped by social processes and expectations as well. In a now famous study, Mark Zborowski illustrated how responses to pain varied by the respondent's ethnicity.[13] Jewish-American patients, for example, evidenced substantial philosophical concern and anxiety about their condition and were pessimistic about the future course of their illness. Protestant patients felt optimistic about their prospects for recovery while viewing doctors as experts to whom one went for "mending," much like bringing a car to an auto mechanic for repairs. Italian-Americans, by contrast, wanted immediate pain relief, and, unlike Jewish respondents, had little concern about the larger "meanings" of the pain.

We should expect that the same principles apply to emotional pain and there is, indeed, substantial evidence that depression carries quite different meanings in different cultures. In a series of books and articles,[14] Arthur Kleinman, who is both an anthropologist and a physician, has written with eloquence and power on the value of looking at a range of emotional disorders cross culturally. Although he does not posit a particular theory as underlying his inquiries, Kleinman's analysis bears a striking resemblance to "symbolic interaction," which is the guiding perspective of this book. I say this because the underlying motif of his work is the *socially generated meanings of illness,* the importance of appreciating the dialectics of body and culture, symptom and society. In fact, Kleinman's mission seems nothing short of reforming the teaching and practice of medicine. By dismissing how illness carries very different symbolic meanings in different cultural settings, Western medicine, based nearly exclusively on a biomedical model, falls short in both its modes of diagnosis and treatment.

Like other medical anthropologists, Kleinman's thinking rests on the fundamental distinction between *illness* and *disease*. Throughout I have used these words interchangeably because that is how they are employed in everyday discourse. However, distinguishing the two words helps to make plain the difference between the subjective experience of bodily or emotional distress (illness) and the presumed biological cause of the distress (disease).

When first becoming sick we begin an interpretive process about the meaning of symptoms. We make assessments about the severity of our discomfort, and, usually in consultation with family and friends, assess the significance of our trouble, deciding what to name it and how to respond to it. The point here is that these interpretations can be rooted in widely varying normative orders and cultural symbol systems. Such culturally induced interpretations, moreover, "orient us to how to act when ill, how to communicate distress, how to diagnose and treat, how to regard and manage the life problems illness creates, how to negotiate this social reality and interpret its meaning for ourselves and for others."[15] Disease, in contrast to illness, is "what the practitioner creates in the recasting of illness in terms of theories of disorder."[16] In Western medicine this typically means identifying the biological dysfunction presumably giving rise to the symptoms described by the patient.

Once we recognize the critical importance of cultural meanings in how symptoms are experienced and dealt with, we can also pinpoint a fundamental difficulty with the practice of Western medicine. American medicine is primarily concerned with disease and pays little attention to the patient's illness. The nearly single-minded efforts of physicians to quickly locate the presumed biological dysfunctions associated with symptoms leads to a problematic disjunction between what patients want from doctors and what they get. Evidence from a recent poll on dissatisfaction with conventional medicine[17] suggests that patients want to be heard by physicians and feel alienated when the full context of their illness experience is defined as irrelevant to their treatment. As a result, patients are seeking treatment from "alternative" healers in ever increasing numbers. Not incidentally, anxiety and depression rank one and two among the problems for which alternative help is sought.

Because of bureaucratic time imperatives[18] and physicians' felt need to quickly diagnose the patient's disease, most doctor/patient encounters in the United States are very short. While initial visits to a doctor might range up to 30 minutes, the average length of doctor/patient encounters is typically between 5 and 10 minutes. In a recent *Newsweek* story,[19] it was reported that patients' average time spent with psychiatrists in some clinics is an astonishing three minutes! Whether the figure is as low as three or as high as the 17 minutes reported in another study,[20] one thing is plain: Doctors are normally uninterested in hearing patients' illness experience—they listen only insofar as the information provided helps them to make a diagnosis. In fact, to let the patient "go on" about their symptoms and feelings is often seen as an obstacle to "good" medicine.[21] The medical historian David Rothman provides a telling anecdote of a doctor examining a patient with his stethoscope.[22] As he was doing this, the patient began to ask a question. Without thinking, Rothman's friend, ordinarily a compassionate and sensitive physician, told the patient, "Stop talking so I can hear you."

An anthropologically informed view sees diagnosis and treatment in very different terms. Illness narratives are deemed critical for appreciating precisely what physicians typically leave out of the picture—namely, how culturally prescribed meanings shape illness realities and, therefore, patients' likely responses to different modes of treatment. Just as patients' experiences of symptoms arise out of particular symbol systems, so also must the likely efficacy of treatments be understood in cultural context. Nowhere is this line of thinking more apparently true than in psychiatry where emotional feelings define the problem and where the discovery of a clear disease entity is most elusive. Kleinman and his colleague Byron Good state with wonderful clarity what a cross-cultural perspective on depression teaches us. Based on a range of investigations, they say

> It is simply not tenable ... to argue that dysphoric emotion and depressive illness are invariant across cultures. When culture is treated as a constant ... it is relatively easy to view depression as [exclusively] a biological disorder. ... From this perspective, culture appears epiphenomenal; cultural differences may exist, but they are not considered essential to the phenomenon itself. However, when culture is treated as a significant variable ... many of our assumptions about the nature of emotions and illness are cast into sharp relief. Dramatic differences are found across cultures in the social organization, personal experience, and consequences of such emotions as sadness, grief, and anger, of behaviors such as withdrawal or aggression, and of psychological characteristics such as passivity and helplessness. ... Dysphoria, even the pervasive loss of pleasure ... is associated with quite different symptoms of distress and has widely varied consequences for the sufferer. ... Depressive illness and dysphoria are thus not only interpreted differently in non-Western societies and across cultures; they are constituted as fundamentally different forms of social reality.[23]

The essential finding of Kleinman's work and a number of other anthropologically oriented investigations on depression is that biological, psychological, and social processes are intricately woven together in creating the depression phenomenon. While there does appear to be a core syndrome of depression that can be observed universally across cultures, the equally clear findings of comparative research show wide variation in the experience of depression. Depressive disorders, in other words, display both universal and culture-specific properties.

Psychiatric medicine in the United States, with its heavily scientific bias, largely presumes biochemical pathology as the ultimate source of depressive disorders everywhere. Such a view is sustained despite the existence of "impressive data that there is no such thing as depression that occurs solely from biological causes."[24] To be sure, it would be equally plausible to say that real-world experiences produce depression by altering biochemistry and thus stand first in the hierarchy of depression's causes. Right now, though, it would be as presumptuous to make this claim as it is of American medicine to claim biology as the absolute foundation of depressive disorders. The truth is that there is no way to untangle the intersection of cultural and biological factors and, consequently, no sure way to claim the greater significance of either nature or nurture in causing depression. Despite this epistemological problem, the role of culture and the contributions of social science in understanding the course of illness remain very much at the margins of American medical training and practice.

This discussion asserts wide cultural variation in the incidence, meaning, and experience of psychiatric disorders, but is not grounded with concrete examples. To get specific, I can report that historically the best predictor of rates of admission to mental hospitals and suicides in North America is the health of the economy (the worse the economy the greater the rates); that the incidence and course of schizophrenia is tied to a society's level of technology (the more modernized a society the greater is the incidence of intractable schizophrenia); that a diagnostic category such as "narcissistic personality disorder," increasingly common in the United States, is virtually unheard of elsewhere; that in certain Asian societies "semen loss" resulting from nocturnal discharge is viewed with great alarm and anguish because sperm contains "qi" (vital energy), seen as absolutely necessary for health; that eating disorders such as anorexia and bulimia are most thoroughly characteristic of capitalist economies; that lack of joy, a central criterion for defining someone as depressed in the United States, would never be mentioned as a problem in Buddhist cultures such as Sri Lanka; that it is considered perfectly normal for American Indians grieving the loss of a spouse literally to hear the voices of the dead; and that the linguistic equivalents of anxiety and depression simply do not exist in many languages.[25]

In several of his books, Kleinman singles out China to illustrate how cultural sentiments influence the way doctors and their patients respond to the complex of feelings American doctors would unmistakably call depression. In contrast to the United States, depression is an infrequent diagnosis in China. Instead, patients suffering from a combination of such symptoms as anxiety, general debility, headaches, backaches, sadness, irritability, insomnia, poor appetite, and sexual dysfunction are diagnosed as suffering from "neurasthenia." Ironically, neurasthenia as a diagnostic category originated in the United States and was once thought of as "the American disease." Now, it is virtually never used in this country, just as the depression diagnosis is very rarely used in China. The choice of the neurasthenia diagnosis turns on cultural preferences. In China, where mental illness is deeply stigmatizing for both sick individuals and their families, doctors and patients find congenial a diagnosis—neurasthenia—that traces the disease to a neurological weakness rather than a mental disorder. In other words, the same symptoms are labeled, interpreted, responded to, and experienced quite differently in the two cultures. It would be proper to say that, although suffering from nominally the same symptoms, the illness realities of Chinese and Americans are truly worlds apart.

MEDICALIZATION

The foregoing discussion implies that a necessary condition for widespread depressive illness is a culturally induced readiness to view emotional pain as a disease requiring medical intervention. The grounds for interpreting pain as an abnormal medical condition have been largely established through the increasing incursion of medical and other therapeutic experts into literally every aspect of our lives. Doctors in particular have become explorers, discovering every conceivable aspect of the human condition as potentially problematic and warranting their intervention. Such a "medicalization" process[26] has dramatically increased the number of uncomfortable or disliked feelings and behaviors that we now see as illnesses.

The so-called medical model is based on two apparently unassailable premises: (1) Normalcy is preferable to abnormalcy, and (2) normalcy is a synonym for health and abnormalcy a synonym for pathology. Definitions of health and pathology, in turn, are derived from laboratory research that is presumed to be thoroughly objective. In this way, medical definitions of health gain the status of scientific facts instead of merely collectively agreed on cultural designations.

Because it is better to be healthy than to be sick, the medical model legitimizes physicians' intervention, whether requested or not, to determine one's health status. No other profession provides for the extensive access to a person's body, mind, and self as do physical and psychiatric medicine. By defining certain features of the human condition as illnesses to be cured, physicians give themselves the right to explore every part of the human anatomy, to prescribe a myriad of curative agents, and even to compel treatment.

The term *healthy,* as used in the medical model, can be equated with *conformity.* In societies where it predominates, the medical model often supersedes legal or religious commandments in regulating behavior. "Peculiar" individuals who were once viewed as possessed or as agents of the devil are now classified as emotionally ill. In the name of science, the advice of medical experts is used in the courts to determine whether certain actions should be defined as crimes. Medicine, especially psychiatric medicine, is often used to "treat" individuals whose behaviors do not conform to the expectations of the powerful or impinge on their moral sensitivities.

There can be little dispute that behavior in today's "postindustrial" society is dominated by "experts." Experts follow us through the life course, advising us on virtually every aspect of existence. They are there when we are born and accompany us each step along the way until we die. Among other things, we rely on experts to tell us how to maintain health, how to become educated, how to make love, how to raise children, and how to age correctly. Most relevant here is that experts now tell us when our "selves" need repair and the proper procedures for doing it. Some years ago, Eliot Freidson, a student of the medical profession, wisely pointed out the dangers of the expanded role of professionals in our lives.

> Due to the increased complexity of the technological, economic, and social foundations of our society, we are on the brink of changes in the structure of our society which will have a massive effect on the quality of the lives of the individuals who compose it. *The relationship of the expert to modern society seems in fact to be one of the central problems of our time, for at its heart lie the issues of democracy and freedom and the degree to which [people] can shape the character of their own lives.*[27]

You might also understand that this dependence on therapeutic experts arises out of the distinctive problems posed by modern life. Every generation, because of its unique historical situation, experiences the world differently than its predecessors. Whatever the historical conditions into which people are born, however, one problem remains constant: Human beings need a coherent framework for comprehending life and death. In some historical periods the traditional meanings transmitted from one generation to the next adequately perform this function. In other epochs, meaning coherence is not so easily established. As Peter Berger and Thomas Luckmann note, the current moment in the Western world appears to be one in which many individuals experience particular difficulty in understanding themselves. They say that "In societies with a very simple division of labor ... there is ... no problem of identity. The question 'Who am I?' is unlikely to arise in consciousness, since the socially defined answer is massively real subjectively and consistently confirmed in all significant social interaction."[28]

When people come together and collectively act on their definitions of injustice, a social movement is born. In Ralph Turner's words, "The phenomenon of a man crying out with indignation because his society has not supplied him with a sense of personal worth and identity is the distinctive new feature of our era. The idea that a man who does not feel worthy and cannot find his proper place in life is to be pitied is an old one. The notion that he is indeed a victim of injustice is the new idea."[29] Today, alienation, previously seen as only a work-related phenomenon, has a much broader connotation. In the present era, alienation refers to a psychological condition in which people are unable to locate a clear conception of self and feel a sense of wholeness. In the context of such alienation, the "therapeutic state" has triumphed.[30]

As a more personalized conception of alienation has been taking root in American society, popular writings by psychiatrists, psychologists, and advice columnists have become increasingly influential. Television appearances have made "mind-tinkerers" such as Leo Buscaglia, "Dr. Ruth," Marianne Williamson, and John Bradshaw national celebrities. Their appeal attests to a pervasive anxiety about questions of identity and psychological well-being in the society. Such experts are constantly dispensing prescriptions for happiness, sexual fulfillment, and mental health.

The movement toward an all-embracing concern with psychological health and personal identity has been accompanied by a corresponding transformation in our explanations of human behavior. When people act in a way we consider deviant, our first impulse is to question their mental health and to probe their psychological make-up. Are they normal? Why are they doing that? What is wrong with them? Because of the medicalization process, such behaviors as alcoholism that years ago were viewed as evidence of sinfulness or moral degeneracy are now explained as illness. A "sickness vocabulary" has replaced a "sin vocabulary." For instance, the so-called "abuse excuse" as used in the celebrated trials of Erik and Lyle Menendez for murdering their parents has resulted in two hung juries. I would guess the same result would be virtually impossible had the Menendez brothers committed their crime 20 years ago.

Preoccupied with their disease, huge numbers of Americans purchase the time and expertise of professionals in order to discover more about themselves. With the aid of the helping professions that have emerged as a major cultural force in the last few decades (among them psychiatrists, psychologists, therapists, and social workers), an increasing proportion of the population has set out to feel better, to "get their acts together," "to get their heads straight." We are in an era that has been characterized as the *age of narcissism*[31] and Americans are said to have constructed a "me, myself, and I" society. The availability of thousands of self-help books alone suggests that ours is a culture intensively absorbed with questions of self-fulfillment and self-realization.

The transformation in our self-conceptions has not been accomplished by mental health experts alone. Their orientation toward life is complemented by other self-oriented, self-discovery groups and movements. For example, large numbers of Americans continue to be involved in various fundamentalist and Eastern religious groups, as well as quasi-religious "personal growth" movements like Scientology and Transcendental Meditation.[32] Groups of this sort provide guidance for self-searching pilgrims, often by supplying absolutely definitive answers to the questions "Who am I and where do I fit in?" "New" religions thrive by providing world views alternative to the kind of scientific and bureaucratic rationality that insinuates even the innermost preserves of our everyday lives. The widespread interest in astrology, dianetics, and the paranormal is explicable as a reaction to a world in which science and technology have portrayed the universe as barren and bereft of meaning.

Yet another "revolution" directed toward the search for and repair of broken selves has been occurring in the last decade or so. In many ways, the springing up of self-help and support groups for dealing with almost every imaginable human trouble represents a combination of many of the elements I have been describing. The self-help revolution reflects the full flowering of a therapeutic culture in America. In self-help groups people turn to others afflicted with the same personal troubles and try, through conversation, to "heal" themselves of what they perceive to be their shared illness. An illness rhetoric (often implying biological causation), is sometimes joined with a spiritual vocabulary (as in programs like Alcoholics Anonymous) positing that "recovery" requires surrendering to a higher power. The self-help phenomenon thus derives its allure by combining elements of therapy with elements of religion and science. It is a powerful brew that has drawn the faith of millions.[33]

The magnitude of the self-help movement is suggested by the estimate that during any given week some 15 million Americans will attend one of about 500,000 support group meetings.[34] Moreover, the number of these organizations has quadrupled in the last decade. Today, in any major city, you can attend groups to deal with such diverse problems as alcoholism, mental illness, gambling, spouse abuse, drug addiction, impotence, cross-dressing, and overeating. As might be expected, the response of mental health professionals to the self-help phenomenon has been lukewarm.[35] While many mental health professionals are legitimately concerned about the wisdom of laypersons treating themselves, we should not miss the point that the self-help idea threatens their own claim to exclusive expertise about a number of mental health problems.

Recently a self-help backlash has developed. While people may individually feel better through participation in them, critics say that their collective effect may be the production of a national mentality in which virtually everyone perceives themselves as suffering from some sort of illness and as the "victim" of circumstances beyond their control. Dissidents wonder whether claims such as the one made by John Bradshaw, a leader of the "recovery movement," that 96 percent of American families are "dysfunctional," trivializes such real abuses as incest by grouping them with an enormous range of experiences that are somehow deemed as damaging people. Critics worry that the underlying illness ideology of support groups furthers the view—distinctly a product of the modern world—that individuals do not bear ultimate responsibility for their life problems and personal behaviors. Along these lines, the sociologist Edwin Shur pointed out several years ago that increased personal consciousness is too often achieved at the expense of a diminished social consciousness.[36]

As a final observation about the emergence of a therapeutic culture, I would add that self-absorption is consistent with the emphasis on self-satisfaction fostered by capitalism in general and advertising in particular. In the industrial age, society was primarily organized around the world of work. A person who did not work, for any reason other than physical disability, was defined as immoral, lazy, and worthless. This perspective on work was beautifully captured in Max Weber's notion of the Protestant Ethic which defines work as intrinsically valuable.[37] It appears, however, that the moral restraints of the work ethic have fundamentally been undermined by a consumption ethic. If workers imbued with the Protestant Ethic lived to work, now most of us work to consume.

The shift toward the social production of consumer-oriented selves has had far-reaching consequences. Since material posses-sions alone cannot ensure feelings of meaningfulness and satisfac-tion, many today find themselves caught up in an endless quest for personal significance; a quest made even more illusive by the built-in obsolescence of the products produced. There is always a "better" product in the works, and so the flames of advertising are always nearby heating the cauldron of contemporary anxiety.[38] In advanced capitalist societies virtually anything can be made into a commodity for sale, including our selves.

> "Charisma," "Joy," and "Ecstasy" are less expressions of spon-taneity than they are the names of marketing perfumes. "Love" is a United States postage stamp. "Happy face" figures embla-zon bills from electric utility companies. "Self actualization" is not [an] . . . ongoing growth process but an end product mar-keted by awareness-training organizations that are subsidiar-ies of dog food and tobacco companies. Are you only a "three" on our self actualization scale?? Too bad! We can make you a "ten" during one of our weekend seminars in Anaheim, min-utes away from Disneyland, for only a few thousand dollars.[39]

In chapter 3, I explored the process through which individuals come to define themselves as depressed. Without diminishing the very real suffering described earlier by my respondents, the fore-going discussion acknowledges that the experience of depression occurs within a cultural context that has enormously expanded the range of emotions defined as abnormal. Authors like Martin Gross have been skeptical about the legitimacy of such redefinitions. He comments, for example, that "what the psychological society has done is to redefine normality. It has taken the painful reactions to the normal vicissitudes of life . . . despair, anger, frustration—and labelled them as maladjustments. The semantic trick is in equating happiness with normality. By permitting this, we have given up our simple right to be normal and suffering at the same time."[40] While my sense is that such brush stroke observations about the "diseasing of America"[41] are unfair to millions of people whose suffering far exceeds what human beings ought to endure, they do properly sensitize us to an enormously increased readiness to interpret emotional discomfort as disease. Such a cultural mind-set has made it possible for medicine to "discover" depression and for millions of Americans to realize that they suffer from it.

The underlying metaphor for this chapter is of a cultural chemistry that catalyzes depression. Thus far I have outlined one piece of the mix that foments depression, a culturally induced readiness to interpret emotional pain as illness. Like any chemical mix, the elements involved cannot create a particular reaction until they are brought together. A second factor that really gets the depression reaction going is the increasing disconnection that appears to characterize Americans' relations with each other and with society. An elaboration of the social forces diminishing human connection extends my argument earlier in the book that depression, at its root, is a disease of disconnection.

DISCONNECTION

Sigmund Freud was once asked what people needed to be happy. The questioner no doubt expected a long, complicated answer reflecting Freud's years of deep reflection on the matter. His simple response, however, was *"arbeiten und lieben,"*—work and love.

Happy people feel connected to others at work and through their intimate relationships. When those connections are threatened, diminished, or broken, people suffer. Today, millions of Americans are suffering from what my colleague Charles Derber calls "double trouble."[42] Those in double trouble have neither meaningful work nor sustaining intimate ties. The withering of community life in both domains fosters a rootlessness and social disintegration that unquestionably contributes to the growth of emotional disorders.[43]

As discussed in Chapter 2, these ideas have a rich history. Classical sociological theorists (such as Emile Durkheim, Max Weber, and Ferdinand Toennies), fundamentally agreed that the bond between individuals and society had been dangerously weakened in "modern" society.[44] They were unanimous in their view that people were less morally constrained in urban societies because their relationships and commitments to communities of all sorts had become far more tenuous. These nineteenth-century writers feared that the eclipse of community would foreshadow the demise of the family and would, in turn, precipitate an increase in all sorts of human pathologies—from crime to suicide.

Although these sociologists could not have had America in mind when they wrote, their analysis appears prophetic. Even the most optimistic among us must acknowledge that America has extraordinary problems. Each day the newspaper assails us with more bad news about rates of homelessness, poverty, suicide, drug addiction, AIDS, teenage pregnancy, illiteracy, and unemployment. In the midst of great wealth we are increasingly becoming two nations, the haves and the have nots, one nation black and the other white, one comfortable and the other destitute.[45] Racism, sexism, and ageism characterize ever-increasing antagonisms between groups that perceive each other only as adversaries. The focus here is more limited, however. My analysis turns

on this question: "How do the increasingly loose human connections at work and at home contribute to the staggering and growing number of Americans who have fallen sick with depression?"
Although any analytical separation of work and home is artificial
since these life areas extensively affect each other,[46] I choose for
simplicity's sake to discuss them one at a time.

The Work Disconnection

A well-established tradition of sociological literature illustrates the
centrality of work to personal identity.[47] Occupational status may
be the central yardstick by which we assess our own and others'
"social value." In a very fundamental way, we *are* what we *do*. Our
feelings of self-esteem and personal well-being are wrapped up
in our work. Therefore, it is perfectly predictable that a legion of
studies demonstrate how unemployment deprives individuals of
much more than a regular paycheck. Loss of work bears a consistent relationship with serious family and psychiatric problems.[48]
Our mental health unquestionably depends on being able to provide a satisfactory answer to the ubiquitous question "What kind
of work do you do?" Without work, people feel lifeless, rootless,
and marginal.

The disastrous consequences of joblessness for those at the
bottom of the American class structure is an old story. If there is
any news here it is, unfortunately, that things have gotten worse
for the poorest and most marginalized populations in America's
dying inner cities. Perhaps the outstanding fact bearing on this
issue is the increasing concentration of nonwhites in central city
areas. While there has been some modest movement of blacks to
the suburbs since 1970, it has largely been the middle-class segment of the black population that has moved, leaving behind an

increasing concentration of poor blacks within urban ghettoes. Blacks have been greatly overrepresented in inner city areas since their initial migration from the rural South to the urban North beginning in the 1950s. However, according to William Julius Wilson,[49] poor blacks are experiencing ever increasing *social isolation* within central cities.

Such profoundly important demographic transformations in American society cannot be understood apart from the imperatives of corporate capitalism. We have entered into a new round of capitalist accumulation in which older, industrial cities are no longer favorable sites for the accumulation of profit. Corporations, free to move wherever there is cheaper labor and fewer legal restrictions, have largely fled the rustbelt cities of the midwest and the frostbelt cities of the northeast in favor of cities in the south and southwest. In yet another round of moves, corporations are now leaving the country altogether to "exploit" the cheap labor in Third World countries. These processes are part of the general "deindustrialization of America"[50] that has removed almost all meaningful job opportunities for the hyperghettoized minorities trapped in America's once great cities.

Without work, black men become less desirable marriage partners and are unable to support the families they do have. Poor black families are then increasingly headed by young women dependent on welfare or the few available jobs that provide less than bare subsistence wages. As a result, "children are being raised in an institutionless community, where everyone is poor, instability is the norm, and the social and psychological role of fatherhood is nonexistent."[51] Such a situation breeds depression that spreads easily from one generation to the next. The mechanism of transmission acts like this: (1) Unemployed women caring for children at home suffer from rates of depression as high as 40 percent.[52]

(2) Depressed mothers simply cannot provide the care, nurturance, and empathy that is necessary for children to grow up with good emotional health. Understandably, (3) children whose primary caretaker is depressed are themselves at enormously high risk for becoming depressed.[53] (4) Depressed children become depressed adults who pass on their disease to their own children. And so on and on. So, we have another of the vicious cycles associated with depression. This one, however, is pushed along by an obviously dysfunctional *social* rather than biological system.[54]

The poor in America have always lived with occupational instability and its fallout. In contrast, middle-class workers have historically been immune from occupational insecurity. Indeed, achieving the American Dream of middle-class life has until recently been synonymous with tremendous occupational stability. In decades past, middle- to upper-middle-class workers in large organizations could count on being taken care of from "womb to tomb." No more. Today, the catch-words "downsizing" and "reengineering" keep the fear of job loss at the forefront of middle-class workers' collective consciousness. Once again the logic of capitalist accumulation is creating a revolution. This one is qualitatively different than earlier economic restructurings because it directly touches the middle classes in hurtful ways. Instead of the strong bond of commitment and loyalty that organizations and middle-class workers previously felt toward each other, the new economic rules of corporate life emphasize efficiency, whatever the human cost. Knowing that they could be here today, but gone tomorrow, middle-class workers are constantly in "fear of falling."[55]

Along with those middle-class workers who continue to hold full-time jobs, however tenuously, is a growing army of well-educated "contingent workers" who are occupational nomads often working for "temp agencies." By 1988 one quarter of the

American workforce worked on a contingent basis and the numbers are growing so rapidly that they will likely outnumber full-time workers by the turn of the century.[56] Charles Derber writes that "the loosening of permanent employment is, arguably, the most important revolution taking place in American life. It signals a fundamental transformation of the corporation and the most consequential change in employment of the last 50 years. Every American worker and family will feel the ramifications, for the loosening of work . . . threatens the social contract underpinning the middle class and the American Dream."[57] Middle-class contingent workers *feel* contingent for good reason. They are disconnected from work in a way never before witnessed in the United States.

All social life involves a tension between freedom and constraint. Living in a society inevitably involves a trade-off between personal liberty and commitment to others. We judge some societies as immoral because they allow virtually no personal freedoms and others because they seem unable to constrain their members. For much of its history, the glory of American democracy seemed to be that it provided a healthy balance between commitment and freedom. For a long time, the pursuit of personal happiness and individual goals seemed compatible with a set of cultural values that Americans willingly embraced and held them together as a nation.

In the world of work, at least for "white collar" workers, there has been, until recently, a kind of quid pro quo. Organizations provided long-term security and received, in turn, worker loyalty, commitment, and responsibility. Loyalty, responsibility, security, commitment. These are the binding features of social systems, the glue that sustains the bond between individuals and social institutions. Unhappily, America's emerging "post-industrial" economy seems to have fundamentally altered the meaning of work for many by eroding loyalty, commitment, and mutual responsibility between organizations and workers.[58] Because emotional well-being is so unquestionably related to social attachment, the millions of Americans who are becoming occupationally marginal are at increasingly greater risk for being victimized by diseases of disconnection.

This section has sustained attention on how work is being reshaped in America's post-industrial, advanced capitalist society. Critics of capitalism, however, would maintain that the negative effects of capitalism on human relationships are far more inclusive than those in the workplace. In a more general way, the values underpinning capitalism are evident in a large variety of face-to-face encounters.

Competition, for example, is one of the cornerstones of capitalism. Advocates of capitalism maintain that competition is a necessary ingredient in both maintaining organizational efficiency and motivating individuals. On the negative side, however, competition pits individuals against each other, diminishes trust, and generally dehumanizes relationships. As the earlier discussion of advertising also intimates, capitalism contributes to a culture of inauthenticity. In a society where everything and everyone is evaluated by their profit potential, individuals are aware that they are constantly being manipulated, seduced, and conned by those who want to sell them or "take them." In a world held together by appearances and a tissue of illusions and deceptions, everyone becomes an enemy of sorts whose motives cannot be accepted at face value. In short, the abstract values of capitalism "trickle down" to everyday consciousness in a way that induces human beings to distrust and withdraw from each other. Withdrawal and increased isolation, I maintained in chapter 2, are important features of the social dialectics of depression.

The Love Disconnection

Another underlying theme of nineteenth-century theory was the parallel development of capitalism and unbridled individualism. Although each of the classical theorists focused on somewhat different features of the social order, they agreed that while the central unit of earlier societies had been the larger collectivities of family and community, the central unit in their contemporary society had become the individual. Further, as the pursuit of financial gain and personal mobility became ascendant social values, relationships became more rational, impersonal, and contractual. Whereas people in earlier agrarian societies related to each other emotionally, with their hearts, those in the new social order related rationally, with their heads.

While the sociological analysis of individualism extends to the origins of the discipline, the conversation about its significance in understanding American character and social structure has recently been reinvigorated through the writings of Robert Bellah and his colleagues.[59] In 1985 they published a book entitled *Habits of the Heart* that details how individualism fosters self-absorption and guarantees a collective sense of strangeness, isolation, and loneliness. This book has been widely praised as providing lucid, penetrating insights into our current cultural condition and has stimulated multiple responses to its ideas.

Bellah and his co-authors distinguish two forms of individualism, *instrumental individualism* and *expressive individualism*. Instrumental individualism refers to the freedom to pursue financial and career success. This is the kind of individualism celebrated in the maxims of Ben Franklin's "Poor Richard" and in the Horatio Alger "rags to riches" stories. Expressive individualism, in contrast, refers to the deep and abiding concerns that Americans have with personal self-fulfillment, with the idea that one of life's missions is to maximize personal happiness by discovering who you "really" are. This second form of individualism is thoroughly consistent with the "therapeutic culture" described earlier.

The essential problem posed by "excessive" individualism is that it privatizes the goals and pursuits of persons and thereby erodes the social attachments that provide society's moral anchor. Individualism undermines commitment to community since membership in any community (from the family to local community to nation) implies behavioral constraints that people perceive as inconsistent with personal fulfillment. The dilemma posed by the need both for attachment and freedom is beautifully captured in Bellah's analysis of romantic love in America. Americans believe deeply in romantic love as a necessary requirement for self-satisfaction. At the same time, love and marriage, which are based on the free giving of self to another, pose the problem that in sharing too completely with another one might lose oneself. The difficulties that Americans have in maintaining intimate relationships stems in part from the uneasy balance between sharing and being separate. The argument is summed up this way:

> Love, then, creates a dilemma for Americans. In some ways, love is the quintessential experience of individuality and freedom. At the same time, it offers intimacy, mutuality, and sharing. In the ideal love relationship, these two aspects of love are perfectly joined—love is both absolutely free and completely shared. Such moments of perfect harmony among free individuals are rare, however. The sharing and commitment in a love relationship can seem, for some, to swallow up the individual, making her (more often than him) lose sight of her own interests, opinions, and desires. . . . Losing a sense of one's self may

also lead to being exploited, or even abandoned, by the person one loves.[60]

Among the many groups that have emerged as part of the self-help phenomenon, one deserves special mention in the context of this discussion. Across the country these days thousands flock to a group called "Co-Dependents Anonymous," a relatively new "12-stepper." Co-dependency is "a popular new disease, blamed for such diverse disorders as drug abuse, alcoholism, anorexia, child abuse, compulsive gambling, chronic lateness, fear of intimacy, and low self esteem."[61] I find the idea of co-dependence interesting because this newly discovered disorder arises out of widespread confusion about the permissible limits of human closeness. Members come to these groups because they see themselves as unable to sustain reasonable intimacy boundaries and feel overwhelmed by certain relationships. As previously, it would be unfair to minimize the real pain that pushes individuals to cure themselves of overinvolvement. It nevertheless seems clear that co-dependency can arise as a pathological condition only in a society that fosters deep ambivalence about the value of extensive ties.

That Americans have problems with intimacy and commitment is surely reflected in the failure of half the marriages made in the country. Of course, marital problems and failures cannot be linked exclusively to patterns of self-absorption intrinsic to a cultural ethic of individualism. Failed relationships, as I indicated earlier, are also a result of the long-term, institutionalized poverty of some groups and the declining economic fortunes of others. Such difficult circumstances are hardly conducive to maintaining strong family and communal ties. Still, the passionate belief in individualism itself takes its toll. Americans feel incredibly ambivalent about all forms of social attachments. Like moths to the proverbial flame, they are drawn to sources of connection for the comfort they provide, but equally fear what they perceive as the stifling features of all sorts of intimacies. Many are afraid that supportive social bonds will evolve into bondage. They continuously flirt with intimacy and commitment, but in the end often choose a life style that maximizes both freedom and loneliness.

For a time the prevailing wisdom in America was that, on balance, children were better off when poor marriages split up. Yes, certainly there is substantial trauma when a marriage first ends, but children, the thinking went, are enormously resilient and eventually adapt in an emotionally healthy way. Whatever lingering problems they might have would surely have been worse if they too had to endure the bad marriage. Since the divorce revolution did not really begin until the 1970s, only now are we able to learn about the long-term emotional effects of broken marriages on children.

Immediately, let's recognize that children most usually live with their mothers after a divorce. This fact, coupled with compelling data on the "feminization of poverty"[62] post divorce, suggest the possible initiation of the same type of depression cycle earlier described as existing among poor inner city, female-headed households. In addition, recent data on the long-term effects of divorce debunk the notion that the negative emotional effects of divorce on children are short-lived. The 50 percent divorce rate seems instead to have produced an adult population with persistent and severe emotional problems, depression among them.[63] Among the few issues that political conservatives and liberals agree on these days is that the disintegration of the traditional family across all social classes may be producing just the kinds of problems nineteenth-century theorists presciently imagined.

It is said that when people on their death beds review their lives they rarely say they should have worked harder in order to own even more things than they do. Presumably, most regrets center on relationships that could have been better nurtured and more fulfilling. However, as Bellah's analysis maintains, to live a life that truly centers on the quality of relations with others is exceedingly difficult for many, maybe most, Americans. The cultural pull away from others is often too powerful to resist. A culture that prizes individual self-realization above all else becomes a world held together by only the barest and most tenuous social connections. More and more Americans, identifying individual achievement as the primary medium for personal fulfillment, join the "lonely crowd" identified years ago by David Riesman.[64] To be part of the lonely crowd means being connected to many in general and few in particular. Having opted for loose intimate connections, increasing numbers of people then wonder why they feel the stirrings of emotional discontent that often evolves into the more dramatic malaise of depression.

THE POSTMODERN SELF

Much of this chapter's discussion has been on the ways that Americans go about the elusive search for themselves. The hopeful premise of my comments is that somewhere a true and satisfying self can be found. These days, however, a style of thinking questions the assumption of unitary, coherent selves. Writers working within a wide range of disciplines—from literature to law to sociology—describe a cultural revolution underway in advanced capitalist societies. They say that we are in the midst of a social transformation that will have as dramatic implications for future selves as did the changes wrought by the industrial revolution for earlier generations. We are now entering into a "post-industrial" society dominated by information technologies and characterized by rapid, often bewildering social change. In the early 1970s the "futurologist" Alvin Toffler described the acceleration of change as "a concrete force that reaches deep into our personal lives, compels us to act out new roles, and confronts us with the danger of a new and powerfully upsetting psychological disease" that he called *future shock*.[65] Disorientation, irrationality, and "free-floating violence" arise, Toffler thought, from people's inability to adapt to change.

In the wake of such transformations, social scientists have raised troubling questions about the future. Does a postmodern society, with its emphasis on technical information, services, and consumption, require a different conception of self than the one that fit in the eras of agricultural and industrial production? Will individuals be able to make the self-adaptations required in a complex, rapidly evolving society?

In his book of the same title, Kenneth Gergen refers to the *saturated self*.[66] He means to convey with this term that the pace of communications and life itself has virtually overtaken us and that as a result our selves are "under siege." We may be reaching a point of social saturation that has far-reaching consequences for the ways we conceptualize the human self and its place in the social world. Gergen's distressing notion is that our identities are so fragmented in the postmodern world that they have become incoherent. In the condition of postmodernity, the very concept of the self becomes uncertain and "the fully saturated self becomes no self at all."[67] Gergen comments that "Under postmodern conditions, persons exist in a state of continuous construction and reconstruction; it is a world where anything goes that can be negotiated. Each reality of self gives way to reflexive questioning, irony, and ultimately the playful probing of yet another reality."[68]

In an emerging postmodern world the construction and maintenance of an integrated self becomes deeply problematic because the social structures necessary to anchor the self have themselves become unstable and ephemeral. Postmodern societies are defined by increasingly short-lived and superficial relationships, geographical mobility that diminishes our commitment to place, and a mass media that confronts us with multiple and contradictory points of view on nearly everything. In such a world all values become radically relativized.[69] In effect, contemporary American society gives us very little to grab onto and to believe in. Whatever values, rituals, or beliefs do exist provide only temporary comfort since their validity is constantly open to question and their longevity unlikely. The imagery of impermanence and fantastically rapid social change makes the metaphors used by several respondents in chapter 2 sensible. You may remember that some individuals, in trying to describe their feelings of depression, spoke of being adrift at sea, as anchorless, cut-off, lonely, and awash in an ocean of meaninglessness.

All social life involves elements of both trust and doubt. There is, for example, always an element of doubt in our relations with others since we can never be certain what they are thinking and feeling; we can never be certain about their "true" motives and intentions. At the same time, ordered social life requires a norm of trust that allows us to presume that, most of the time, others are essentially what they claim and appear to be. At the level of individual psychology, Erik Erikson teaches us,[70] the production of healthy human beings requires that individuals come to have a basic trust in others and the world at large. Unhappily, the constantly shifting and elusive social arrangements characteristic of the postmodern world foster massive doubt rather than trust. The collapse of reliable meaning structures for ordering both social and personal life creates, many postmodern theorists say, an "ontological insecurity"[71] that makes all of us increasingly vulnerable to a range of emotional disorders.

The cultural critic Todd Gitlin describes the postmodern consciousness as blank, pessimistic, affectless, and cynical.[72] My colleague at Boston College, Stephen Pfohl[73] characterizes American society as a "panic scene" and Anthony Giddens[74] writes that "personal meaninglessness—the feeling that life has nothing worthwhile to offer—becomes a fundamental psychic problem in circumstances of late modernity." Years ago, during the height of the countercultural movement of the 1960s, "hippies" were deeply disillusioned by America's political and cultural structure. However alienated they were, their agenda of social revolution implied an underlying optimism that things could change for the better. In contrast, the countercultural orientation of the 1990s "Freaks" is "fueled by an internal disposition which is pessimistic and exhausted, cynical and hopeless, a disposition that expresses the end of trust, faith, and belief."[75]

As a person with depression, I am sometimes inclined to embrace such an unrelievedly negative view of America's present and future. I do, in fact, agree with the general direction of the argument I have been summarizing. The postmodern condition unquestionably contributes to a collective identity crisis since a culturally fragmented society produces fractured and diseased selves. At the same time, my theoretical impulse as a symbolic interactionist is to say that the case has been overstated. I have tremendous faith in the capacity of human beings ultimately to refashion themselves and thereby also the world now denying them the conditions for good mental health. I think Robert

Jay Lifton is correct when he maintains that human selves are remarkably resilient and will ultimately adapt positively to the current age of cultural fragmentation.[76]

My particular version of social psychology presumes a mutable,[77] highly adaptive self. When individuals find their lives becoming too impersonal and rational, they will inject into them some sentiment, some passion. When social life becomes too routinized, people will collectively find ways to experience novelty. When they find their lives becoming too unpredictable, on the other hand, they will find ways to introduce ritual and routine into their daily activity.

I expect that the contingencies faced in a postmodern world will eventually require people to question the ideology of individualism described earlier in this chapter. Faced with a blinding rate of social change creating destructive disattachments, I have faith that we will ultimately be smart enough to redefine ourselves in *relational* rather than individualistic terms. Along with a growing number of social scientists, I am fully persuaded that we need to rediscover community as the very best medicine for many of our ills, including the sadness of depression.[78] Unfortunately, it will likely take a great deal more human suffering before we are prompted to reinvent a more healthy society. Of course, we will never eradicate depression because life inevitably involves a degree of suffering. The question for our collective future is whether we will have the wisdom to re-form America in ways that maximize our humanity by minimizing the pains of disconnection.

Postscript

Sociology, Spirituality, and Suffering

During the course of writing this book I have spoken with many people in many different contexts about my work and the perspective I bring to studying depression. Whether at a family gathering, a dinner with friends, or a professional meeting of sociologists, I arrived ready to answer questions about what I was doing. When asked, I normally gave only a two- or three-sentence description because most people don't want any more than that. Usually, the few sentences would go like this: "I'm not primarily interested in explaining what causes depression or how to cure it because I don't think anyone can answer those questions. Instead, I'm interested in how depressed individuals make sense of an inherently ambiguous life situation. I'm interested in how a depression consciousness unfolds over time, how people think about psychiatry and medications, and how they deal with family and friends."

Occasionally, after my few brief descriptive comments, someone might ask questions that I found much harder to answer. They might want to know, for example, whether doing the interviews influenced my own depression, what I had learned about myself by listening to others' stories, or, still more difficult, how the experience of talking to depressed people and writing the book has changed me. I could always come up with something that seemed credible, but I was never really persuaded by my own answers. I found the question about personal change particularly worth considering since I agree with Shulamit Reinharz that research should be self-reflexive and that researchers ought therefore to be somehow transformed by their work.[1] The more I weighed the personal impact of this study, the more I realized that the primary change in my thinking has less to do with sociology exactly than with a heightened respect for the value of spirituality in responding to sickness.

The role of religion and spirituality has always been slight in my life. I grew up Jewish, admire many of the cultural aspects of Judaism, especially the value placed on learning, but know next to nothing about the theology of Judaism. Although I have always been interested in broadly philosophical questions and very much like discussing them, my orientation to such issues has been cerebral, rational, and highly analytical. I certainly would not have classified myself as a "spiritual" person since this has always conveyed for me something mystical and nonrational, if not irrational. As a social "scientist," I have always maintained a skeptical attitude toward explanations of human behavior that could not be supported by systematic data. Guided by such a view, matters of faith have been of little consequence in my life.

During the beginning stages of this research I took a course offered by the Philosophy Foundation in Boston.[2] My interest in the course had nothing to do with this project. I was just looking for a "night out" and had heard others speak well of the school's "practical" orientation toward philosophy. For two semesters I participated in a small class with other beginners and really enjoyed the combination of philosophical debate and meditation exercises. The ideas we discussed came largely from Eastern religious philosophies and I appreciated what my classmates had to say about the nature of wisdom, truth, beauty, and, more concretely, about everyday living.

Although many of the ideas I heard were too abstract and purely speculative for my taste, I liked what seemed to be the central messages of the class. I understood them to be that one should strive to live in the present and that we are misled in identifying ourselves exclusively with our worldly successes or failures. In a much larger way, the teacher maintained, everyone and everything in the universe is connected as in a seamless web. This last idea, although aesthetically pleasant, never really took hold for me during the course.

While studying practical philosophy I was in the middle of interviewing people for this book. As mentioned in chapter 5, I was initially puzzled by the number of respondents who spontaneously spoke about the role of spirituality in their lives. During the early stages of the data collection, however, spirituality meant no more or less to me than any of a large number of issues that were coming out of the interviews. At a certain point, though, enough people spoke about spirituality that I began routinely to ask everyone about it. Certainly there were many who had little to say, and some who claimed no interest in spirituality, but the question often elicited an outpouring of talk. After 25 or so interviews, it seemed dear that my anticipated chapter on coping and adapting would have to pay at least some attention to the role of spirituality.

At the same time that my conceptual consciousness was being raised about the connection between spirituality and depression, I was leaving many of my interviews awed by the courage and grace with which certain people faced unimaginable pain and loss. I was especially impressed with those who spoke of their depression as a gift from which they had learned valuable lessons. While

I could not relate emotionally or intellectually with visions of rein-carnation or explanations of depression as central to a God-given life mission, I left many interviews with a sense that spiritually engaged individuals were in touch with *something* important. The issue was not a matter of evaluating the truth of their particular brand of spirituality. What I felt was a measure of envy of those who displayed an acceptance that seemed to me incongruous with accounts of exceptional pain. These people possessed or knew something that I didn't.

One of my favorite pastimes, happily legitimated by any of my research projects, is wandering around bookstores. During one of my visits to a local store to check for anything new and relevant to this study, I came across Kat Duff's book entitled *The Alchemy of Illness.*[3] This short, beautifully written book captures universal features of the illness experience. It combines description of many of the nitty-gritty emotional and physical dimensions of pain with an articulate explanation of how the author's battle with Chronic Fatigue Syndrome has transformed her self.

The book succeeds, I think, because it shows the value of ill-ness for personal transformations without romanticizing pain in the slightest. It also helped me to comprehend more fully how my own discomfort with Western medicine's response to depression related to the messages I was hearing in my philosophy class and from many of my interviewees. Duff writes, for example, that we have much "to learn, as individuals and as societies, from our ill-nesses and the sacred spaces we inhabit in pain. . . . Cosmopolitan medicine banishes that knowledge by insisting that suffering is without meaning, and unnecessary, because pain can be techni-cally eliminated. Symptoms are divorced from the person who has them and the situations that surround them, secularized as mechanical mishaps, and so stripped of their stories, the spiritual ramifications and missing pieces of history that make meaning."[4] In one of those striking reversals of conventional [Western] wisdom that turns your thinking upside down, *The Alchemy of Illness* is dedicated to the Buddhist idea that illness is an opportunity for enlightenment; that, seen the right way, we do not cure illnesses—instead, they have the potential to cure us. This happens when we realize that illness is "not so much a state of being as a process of transformation."[5]

Although much of this sort of discussion is inspired by religious texts, Eastern mysticism, and Native American cultural beliefs, it resonates well with the principles of social psychology. After all, the essential idea of symbolic interaction theory is that all objects, events, and situations derive their meanings through human interpretation. We are ultimately free to define anything as we choose, including illness. The kinds of spiritual ideas about illness articulated by Duff simply arise from the refusal to see sickness as intrinsically bad.

Duff's book began to persuade me that there is no necessary contradiction between sociological and spiritual thinking. In fact, as I finished her book and then others, such as Thomas Moore's bestseller, *Care of the Soul*,[6] I found a strong compatibility between certain spiritual ideas offered and conventional sociological ideas. In chapter 5, before I had read any materials on spirituality, I concluded from the interview data that a final stage of adaptation (which I call "incorporation") follows the realization that depression is unlikely to be cured. I commented that once individuals realize that medical treatment is unlikely to fix their problem, their thinking moves away from the medical language of cure and toward the spiritual language of transformation. With that interpretation I was speaking only as a sociologist trying to see patterns in data. Several weeks later I read a nearly identical idea in Moore's book. Moore, a theologian and philosopher writes that "A major difference between care and cure is that cure implies the end of trouble. . . . But care has a sense of ongoing attention. There is no end. Conflicts may never be fully resolved. Your character will never change radically, although it may go through some interesting transformations. Awareness can change, of course, but problems persist and never go away. . . . Care of the soul . . . appreciates the mystery of human suffering and does not offer the illusion of a problem-free life."[7]

It turns out that Moore devotes a whole chapter to the "Gifts of Depression." As the title implies, he takes issue with the prevailing medical view that depression is an enemy to be beaten at all costs. Consistent with the main theme of "care" for the soul, Moore sustains the argument that we ought not to pathologize depression. He makes the interesting point that the word "depression" itself shapes the way we think about the human condition it describes. Today, consistent with a medically dominated view of emotional pain, we prefer the more clinical and serious word depression to the more human words "melancholy" or "sadness." This observation is entirely consistent with labeling theory in social psychology that ties the construction of our identities to the labels others apply to us and that we ourselves ultimately adopt.

Moreover, both Duff and Moore entertain the notion that illness is not the private state of the sufferer, but truly a collective problem. The Iroquois Indians, for example, believed that when any single person suffered it reflected the suffering of nature, of the whole world, in fact. By now, this idea had a tone of familiarity. It sounded like my philosophy teacher's effort to let me understand that everyone and everything is connected. Put more sociologically, the idea is that medical diagnoses may cover up social problems; that our presumably personal illnesses are really symptoms of a sick society suffering from humanly produced wounds to the social fabric. In effect, the Iroquois' spiritual belief about illness is essentially indistinguishable from my argument in chapter 7 that depression is related to dysfunctional features of American culture. The link between personal and social illness is most easily seen in the case of illnesses such as emphysema that thrive in the environments we have most badly polluted. But isn't the linkage between our "depressed" cities and "depressed" economy and widespread depressive illness also obvious?

I have always felt that one of the dilemmas of sociological analyses focused on macroscopic ideas like social structure and culture is that they do not yield clear policy recommendations for social change. For example, throughout this book, but in chapter 7 particularly, I maintain that the social disconnection generated by an ethic of individualism is an important element in the proliferation of affective disorders in America. Assuming that position is correct, what can we do about it concretely? Are there really any social policies that can alter such a basic feature of culture, a cultural dimension that has evolved over decades, even centuries? In this regard, psychologists and physicians have something of an advantage over sociologists since it seems so much easier to change people than to affect remote, anonymous, intangible features of a society.

Certainly I am not advocating that sociologists give up on interesting ideas for reforming social ills. In her book *Within Our Reach: Breaking the Cycle of Disadvantage*,[8] Lisbeth Schorr provides clear evidence that a wide range of programs in areas such as prenatal care for low-income mothers, child health services, family support, and the strengthening of schools have made appreciable differences in the lives of the less fortunate. In addition, social movements that are often animated in part by the writings of social scientists have fundamentally altered social structures. For instance, the work of activists no doubt hastened the end of the Vietnam War and, while great gender inequities still exist, changes in legislation, directly the result of the women's movement, have created a more just society.

There is an old joke that asks, "How many psychiatrists does it take to change a light bulb?" The answer—"Only one, but the light bulb has to really want to change." While the joke is meant to poke fun at psychiatrists, it also points to a more serious and important truth—certain changes cannot be forced. Whatever have been the successes of concerted change efforts, it seems clear to me that fundamental changes in the character of a culture are possible only when a society is ready to adopt a new collective consciousness. As an example, Carl Degler points out in his sweeping history of Darwinian thought that biological explanations of human nature dominated America's thinking at the turn of the century, but then fell into disfavor for decades.[9] Within the last 30 or 40 years, as the discussion of psychotropic drugs in this book suggests, biological explanations of human behavior are making a big comeback.

Degler's history of the decline and revival of Darwinian thought reveals another feature of social change that has a place in several famous theories of history. It is that change happens in a cyclical fashion. Here one is easily reminded of Arnold Toynbee's well-known theory that history follows pendulum-like shifts.[10] In sociology, Pitirim Sorokin argued that societies move through predictable cycles distinguished by definable "cultural mentalities."[11] These ideas, I want to maintain, apply to Americans' willingness to recalibrate the ongoing cultural tension between individualism and commitment to community. I see signs that we may be at a cultural turning point in the way that Americans think about the appropriate role of religion, family, and community in their lives. In short, we may be at a juncture where we are ready as a culture to see the wisdom in the spiritual idea that our individual well-being is inseparable from that seamless web of connections my philosophy teacher wanted me to understand.

Another change analogy that seems applicable here is the often heard idea that alcoholics cannot commit themselves to sobriety until they "hit bottom." While it is impossible to know where the bottom is, we have to be pretty close to hitting cultural bottom. Americans, as the saying goes, appear to be "sick and tired of being sick and tired." The incredible range of social ills that characterize American society today seems to be having an effect on everyone, regardless of their politics. Americans may now commonly feel that things are so bad that something has to happen. To be certain, depression is only one of the cultural ailments in a mosaic of ills that has become so widespread that the culture is ripe for change.

I find it interesting that sociologists have always claimed the importance of community to a healthy society. Questions of community are at the core of the discipline. Yet it is only in the last few years that calls for a revitalization of community are being heard at all. There is now even a "communitarian movement" that is flourishing in sociology and gaining attention in the press and at the highest levels of government. The idea of communitarianism, like Darwinism, might be on the cusp of a culture-wide resurgence. One of the gurus of the communitarian movement, Amitai Etzioni, refers to the need for a basic reorientation of cultural values when he says, "What America needs, above all, is a change in the way we approach things, what we value and what we devalue, a *change of heart*."[12] I think people are beginning to listen to Etzioni and his colleagues, not because they are so much more eloquent than earlier writers in stating their case, but because America is ready for a change of heart.

Interestingly, one useful barometer for assessing America's changing values is the number of students studying sociology. As a discipline, sociology prospers when the world is in a state of turmoil. During difficult historical moments students become greatly concerned with the way society is put together and how it might be changed for the better. Therefore, from the late 1960s through the mid-1970s when the Vietnam War and the "Black Revolution" had American society virtually unraveled, huge numbers of students flocked to sociology courses.

During the Reagan and Bush era of the 1980s, America's culture heroes were people like Donald Trump and Michael Milken who did anything necessary to beat their financial competitors. Theirs was a credo of unvarnished entrepreneurial gamesmanship summed up by Gordon Gekko, the main character in the movie *Wall Street,* who declared, "Greed is good." During those years the number of sociology majors dwindled as students abandoned the humanities and social sciences in favor of business-related courses. For the last several years, however, the number of sociology majors has been sharply rising as young people seem fed up with the excesses of economic individualism. The growing numbers of students drawn to careers of social service may be a harbinger of a transition from the "Me" to a "We" society.

The estimated 11 to 15 million people suffering from depression and the millions more with anxiety disorders are the victims of a society that has lost sight of what I now see as a shared sociological and spiritual message. It is that our individual emotional health and the health of society are inseparable. If we do not nourish society by realizing our individual responsibilities to it, we pay the price in terms of individual illness. In this way, those millions pained by affective disorders are part of a dialectical process in which the extent of collective suffering eventually creates an urge to change the social structures that have made so many of us ill. During this current moment of cultural discontent we may be better able to appreciate the spiritual message that all of us are connected to and responsible for each other. Although we can never return to the small, intimate communities of the nineteenth century, such a communitarian vision is the necessary starting place for efforts at social reconnection and thereby the creation of a more generally happy society.

APPENDIX

Thinking about Sampling

As described in chapter 1, I contacted the respondents for this study in a variety of ways. At the beginning of the research, I sought interviewees from among friends and acquaintances whom I knew suffered from depression. By the end of the study these personal contacts accounted for 11 of the 50 individuals whose words constitute the core of this study. These persons referred another four people to me who then became part of the sample. When personal contacts and referrals dried up, I began putting advertisements in a local newspaper. Each time an advertisement appeared it yielded between five and seven responses. I should mention that these advertisements appeared in the "Help Wanted" section of the newspaper and this may partly explain the number of persons who were unemployed at the time of the interview. Eventually, 30 individuals were recruited through the advertisements. Another four people volunteered to talk to me after I described my work at a depression self-help group. Finally, one of the interviewees was a contributor to an Internet depression support group and was recruited via electronic mail.

Rarely can social scientists doing in-depth interviews claim their samples to be statistically representative of the populations of people to whom they would like to generalize their findings. I can say, however, that the current sample contains variation by gender (18 males, 32 females); age (20s = 12, 30s = 18, 40s = 14, 50s = 4, 60s = 2); occupation (12 professionals, 14 white collar workers, 8 blue collar workers, 5 students, 11 unemployed persons); and religion (16 Jews, 23 Catholics, 9 Protestants, 1 Buddhist, 1 Quaker). Thirty-eight of the respondents are college educated and all, with the exception of an East Indian, are white. Twenty-nine of the fifty have been hospitalized at least once for their depression.

Thirty-four are single and never married, five are single and divorced, and the remaining 11 are married.

Although I tried to recruit respondents from a range of social class positions, my sample is skewed toward well-educated individuals. These are the persons most likely to have medical knowledge of depression and access to the health care system. It is, therefore, worth repeating the caveat offered in chapter 3 that the processes described in this book fit only the experiences of those who have come to frame their problem in medical terms. There are, no doubt, millions of people, probably clustered at the lower ends of America's stratification system, who never define their bad feelings as a disease warranting medical intervention. Although there are obvious and substantial methodological problems, social scientists should find ways to chart the "careers" of people with emotionally troubled lives who seek solace and care outside the medical system.

One question that I have been frequently asked, especially at professional meetings, is "How does your sample break down in terms of the kind of depression people have experienced?" Those familiar with psychiatric lingo might want to know, for example, how many of those interviewed could be categorized as having suffered major depression, dysthymic conditions, exogenous depressions, endogenous depressions, and so on. Since part of my thinking about depression includes the arbitrariness and socially constructed character of psychiatric diagnoses, I tell questioners that I am only interested in how persons come to be placed and place themselves in one or another category. Consequently, the only criterion for inclusion in the sample was that a person had been "officially" diagnosed as depressed by a physician. What I can say is that the majority were sick enough to spend time in hospitals, and there is no question in my mind that all 50 persons have endured pain that *they* consider well beyond normal limits.

From among the several attributes distinguishing respondents, I want particularly to comment on the way in which the gender distribution in the sample evolved. As the study moved along, the number of women responding to my advertisements began significantly to outnumber the men. Since I assumed that depression occurred far more frequently among women, this imbalance did not disturb me initially. However, after the fortieth interview or so, I calculated that the women constituted much more than two-thirds of the sample to that point. Therefore, I made a concerted effort toward the end of the study to recruit more men. Anxious to complete the data collection, I placed an advertisement offering men $25 for the interview. Only the last four interviews were "bought" this way to raise the final proportion of men to 36 percent ($n = 18$). As a result, the ratio of men to women in my sample approximates the reported gender rates of depression for the whole country.

The relative unwillingness of men and the eagerness of women to volunteer for this study is instructive. Although I was aware of the gender differences throughout the study, the difficulty of recruiting men did not sharply stand out until I began to gather data for the chapter on family and friends. Initially, four of the 10 people interviewed for chapter 6 were women and since I also wanted to hear from men who were close to depressed persons, I explicitly advertised for them. The advertisement was placed in a weekly newspaper that reaches four large Massachusetts communities—Boston, Cambridge, Newton, and Brookline—and read as follows:

CLOSE TO SOMEONE WITH DEPRESSION?
I am a sociologist at Boston College writing a book on depression. If you are a man who is a child of a depressed parent or a close friend to a depressed person, I would like to hear your story. For more information call David Karp (552-4137).

To be sure that there was no confusion, the word "man" was highlighted in the advertisement. I was, therefore, nonplussed when four women, but no men replied. When I asked the women whether they had understood my request properly, two were uncertain. The other two indicated they knew I was asking for men, but still called because, as one said, "I thought you might want to talk with me anyway." What an interesting datum! Women caregivers are apparently so anxious to talk about their concerns for a friend or family member that they call even when not invited, while men won't respond at all.

In discussing this "finding" with a colleague we quickly agreed that women have always been socialized to be caregivers and feel far more comfortable with that role than men. Beyond that, though, my friend cited Deborah Tannen's observation that when it comes to human relations problems, men are solution-oriented whereas women are sympathy-oriented.[1] Perhaps, she reasoned, men quickly "burn out" as caregivers. Men, she hypothesized, can make an early commitment to help a depressed friend or family member. However, when it becomes apparent that proposed solutions for the problem do not work, they quickly give up. Women, on the other hand, who do not approach their commitment to a sick friend or family member in solution terms are, compared to men, far more tolerant caregivers. Women, in other words, might be more involved caregivers than men because they are trained for that role and because their commitment to caregiving is not contingent on the eradication of the problem.

There are other dimensions to sampling that are too rarely discussed in studies based on qualitative data. For example, as the data are collected, researchers using an inductive logic of inquiry[2] scour the materials for emerging patterns. The search for patterns raises at least two interesting methodological questions. How many respondents need to make similar comments before deciding that a clear pattern exists? And, once having settled on a pattern worth writing about, what criteria are used in deciding on the particular data to illustrate the theme?

I have always felt that one of the most difficult tasks associated with analyzing in-depth interviews is to uncover regularities across all the cases while respecting the complexity and diversity of each person's feelings and experiences. Of course, if there were no consistencies to the way individuals experience depression, there wouldn't be much of a sociological analysis to provide. Sometimes a pattern in the data is easy to spot because it is virtually universal. As described in chapter 3, for instance, nearly every single person moved through a period during which they could not associate their bad feelings with the word depression. In other cases, the regularity was "strong," but clearly variable as in the clear majority of individuals who initially resisted taking antidepressant medications. Then there are interesting regularities of perception and behavior among only a minority in the sample that nevertheless seem important to write about. For example, although only about a dozen of the 50 persons sampled had become significantly involved with Buddhist teachings, this number among a group of Americans seemed extraordinary to me and worth explaining.

I am suggesting the inappropriateness of using strict numerical guidelines in choosing whether a theme is worth writing about. Although numbers surely matter, the choice is often guided as much by subjective judgments that some things respondents say are more noteworthy than others. Sometimes this is so because these comments are deeply revealing of the phenomena investigated or because they help to sustain a line of thinking that, although speculative, feels valuable, novel, or insightful. Seen this way, all analysis requires artful selectivity. A thoroughly unanalytical approach to some phenomenon would require reporting every feature of the situation without evaluating the relative importance of things. It would be the sociological equivalent of one of Andy Warhol's movies that simply recorded people sleeping for eight hours without any commentary.

While the selection of themes for discussion inevitably involves subjective choices, researchers cannot disregard materials that do not conform to the pattern they wish to highlight. In the end, good social science presumes honest researchers who go out of their way to look for cases that do not fit an emerging pattern and then to acknowledge them in the writing. There are some social scientists who see negative cases as threatening to their analysis. In contrast, because my version of social psychology emphasizes human beings' unlimited capacity for interpreting their worlds in multiple ways, I expect significant variation. I am, therefore, not frightened by diversity of response. Instead, I see such variation as an opportunity for comparative analysis, as a way of disciplining and refining my thinking about the patterns I do see.

A related methodological problem involves decisions about how many and which quotes to use when exemplifying a theme. You may have noted that I rarely presented more than three or four data "specimens" each time I made a point. The numbers of quotes used normally varied with the significance of a particular theme to my overall analysis. However, I was also sensitive to the balance between my own writing and data presentation. I sometimes judged that presenting several more quotes would not make a more compelling case. These decisions aside, I could have provided many more illustrations for every point made in this book. Therefore, another sampling issue involved decisions about which respondents got to speak and with what frequency.

A complicating factor to data presentation in qualitative research is that some respondents are far more articulate, interesting, and eloquent than others. Often, as I listened to an individual speak during an interview, I was thinking, "Wow, this is great data and just has to find a place somewhere in the book." In other cases, alternatively, I felt that the interview was not very good because the individuals offered clipped responses to my questions or generally did not express themselves very well. Since every author wants to engage readers, the urge is to let some people speak much more than others. The thinking goes, "Why not let this person speak for others since he or she is just expressing their sentiment, but in a more compelling way?" While you have, in fact, heard from some of the individuals in my sample more frequently than others, I have generally tried to democratize the frequency with which respondents are quoted. Additionally, I have been attentive to the frequencies with which men's and women's voices are heard. The result of these efforts is that the proportion of male and female quotes are nearly identical to their percentages in the sample.

Finally, discussions of sampling nearly always occur in the context of evaluating how widely findings can be generalized. The conventional wisdom in the social sciences is that only studies utilizing large sample sizes meet the criteria for valid generalization. For that reason, the argument is often made that qualitative studies, with their characteristically small samples, are useful only for sensitizing researchers to the issues that are then best studied with large-scale survey studies that often sample thousands of individuals.

I have always felt that relegating small sample qualitative studies to a kind of helpful, but secondary role in making important generalizations about social life is unfair and just plain wrong. Remember that this study was motivated in the first instance by the failure of survey research to provide exactly the kind of experiential understanding of depression that can only be obtained by learning in-depth what persons think, feel, and experience. Therefore, I might very well say that for me the statistical findings of survey research served the sensitizing function. The hundreds of studies reporting an enormous range of statistical correlations provided a sense of the magnitude and complexity of the problem. However, only qualitative data can catch at the meanings people attach to depression and thereby give a deeper, and I would say more valid, sense of what the experience is like for individuals.

Some years ago I published a paper on the experience of aging during the 50- to 60-year decade in a journal that rarely publishes qualitative studies based on small samples.[3] In his preface to the journal's contents, the editor felt obliged to explain that although my study used a "non-standard" methodology, he and other readers found that it truly captured their own life experience. While I was put off by the methodological parochialism of the comment, I was, of course, pleased that the work accomplished what all good qualitative research ought to. Sociology is filled with examples of studies based on observation of single cases or interviews with small numbers of people that provide powerful generalizations about underlying forms of social life.[4] One does not need huge sample sizes to discover underlying and repeating forms of social life that, once described, offer new levels of insight for people. For me, the test of this study's validity has nothing to do with arcane discussions of scientific epistemology. My goal has been to evoke in readers the same "aha" response that apparently prompted the journal editor to publish my earlier work on aging.

The ultimate test of a study's worth is that the findings ring true to people and let them see things in new ways. In this case, I hope those personally familiar with depression recognize themselves in the words of my respondents and feel that that my analysis illuminates their life situations. Aside from the scientific worth of what I have done, such a response is important to me because I believe that knowledge and understanding are the fundamental preconditions for positive change.

NOTES

Introduction

1. Representative works in those areas include D. Karp, G. Stone, and W. Yoels, *Being Urban: A Sociology of City Life*, 2nd ed. (New York: Praeger Publishers, 1991); J. Clair, D. Karp, and W. Yoels, *Experiencing the Life Cycle: A Sociology of Aging* (Springfield, Illinois: Charles Thomas Co., 1993); D. Karp, L. Holmstrom, and P. Gray, "Of roots and wings. Letting go of the college-bound child," *Symbolic Interaction* 27 (2004): 357–382.

2. D. Karp, *The Burden of Sympathy: How Families Cope with Mental Illness* (New York: Oxford University Press, 2001); D. Karp, *Is It Me or My Meds? Living with Antidepressants* (Cambridge, Mass.: Harvard University Press, 2006); D. Karp and G. Sisson (eds.), *Voices from the Inside: Readings on the Sociology of Mental Health and Illness* (New York: Oxford University Press, 2010).

3. For a description and analysis of the Chicago School of Sociology and its legacy, see G. Fine, *A Second Chicago School? The Development of a Postwar American Sociology* (Chicago: University of Chicago Press, 1995).

4. See N. Anderson, *The Hobo; The Sociology of the Homeless Man* (Chicago: University of Chicago Press, 1923); H. Zorbaugh, *The Gold Coast and the Slum: A Sociological Study of Chicago's Near North Side* (Chicago: University of Chicago Press, 1929); E. Sutherland, *Professional Thief, by a Professional Thief* (Chicago: University of Chicago Press, 1937); F. Thrasher, *The Gang: A Study of 1,313 Gangs in Chicago* (Chicago: University of Chicago Press, 1927); W. I. Thomas and F. Znaniecki, *The Polish Peasant in Europe and America; Monograph of an Immigrant Group* (Chicago: The University of Chicago Press, 1918).

5. The idea of the conceptual value of looking at social structures from the point of view of marginalized groups is captured by Peter Berger's observation that much sociological work reflects what he terms an "unrespectability motif." See P. Berger, *Invitation to Sociology: A Humanistic Perspective* (Garden City, N.Y.: Doubleday, 1963). A similar idea is argued in H. Becker, "Whose side are we on?," *Social Problems* 14 (1967): 239–247.

6. A. Frank, *The Wounded Storyteller: Body, Illness, and Ethics* (Chicago: University of Chicago Press, 1995), p. 25. See also A. Frank, *Letting Stories Breathe: A Socio-Narratology* (Chicago: University of Chicago Press, 2010).

7. The local organization changed its name several years ago to DBSA, The Depression and Bipolar Support Alliance. I suspect that this name change was motivated, in part, by the negative connotations attached to the "manic depression" diagnosis. DBSA is a national organization with multiple groups across the United States.

8. Although I finally settled on the title *Speaking of Sadness*, I have sometimes felt slightly uncomfortable that the choice of the word "sadness" does an injustice to the profound pain of severe depression. Gloria Steinem offered an interesting distinction between the words sadness and depression during a 2006 television interview. When asked about the depth of her sadness after the loss of her husband, she responded with the observation that "In depression you care about nothing. In sadness you care about everything."

9. The President at the time, Steve Lappen, provided me a copy of his unpublished address.

10. D. Karp, "Illness ambiguity and the search for meaning: A case study of a self-help group for affective disorders," *Journal of Contemporary Ethnography* 21 (1992): 139–170.

11. A few examples of well-known mental illness memoirs would include K. Jamison, *An Unquiet Mind* (New York: A.A. Knopf, 1995); M. Vonnegut, *The Eden Express* (New York: Praeger, 1975); K. Millett, *The Loony-Bin Trip* (New York: Simon and Schuster, 1995); L. Slater, *Prozac Diary* (New York: Random House, 1998); S. Kayson, *Girl Interrupted* (New York: Turtle Bay Books, 1993).

12. Karl Marx famously maintained that capitalism "contained the seeds of its own destruction." As part of his argument, he maintained that the Industrial Revolution and capitalism could not emerge without rapid urbanization. Cities were required to maintain a large pool of workers for the new urban factories. At the same time, the close proximity of workers in urban places allowed them to talk with each other about their collective exploitation by the factory owners (the bourgeoisie) and thus to develop a working-class political consciousness. Although Marx's predictions about an eventual proletariat revolution and the emergence of a one-class socialist society have not

come to pass, his analysis nevertheless affirms the linkage between shared stories and the development of class consciousnesses.

13. See E. Hughes, *Men and their Work* (New York: Free Press, 1958).

14. A. Strauss, "Turning points in identity." In C. Clark and H. Robboy (eds.), *Social Interaction* (New York: St. Martin's, 1992).

15. See P. Conrad, *The Medicalization of Society: On the Transformation of Human Conditions into Treatable Disorders* (Baltimore: Johns Hopkins University Press, 2007).

16. This argument is more fully explored in D. Karp, "Social science, progress, and the ethnographer's craft," *Journal of Contemporary Ethnography* 28 (1999): 597–609.

17. D. Karp, 2006, op. cit.

18. See R. Whitaker, *Anatomy of an Epidemic: Magic Bullets, Psychiatric Drugs, and the Astonishing Rise of Mental Illness in America* (New York: Random House, 2010a), p. 130.

19. We should be mindful of the fact that persons can also experience adverse effects from such alternative treatments.

20. E. Freidson, *Profession of Medicine* (New York: Harper and Row, 1970), p. 336.

21. P. Kramer, *Listening to Prozac: A Psychiatrist Explores Antidepressant Drugs and the Remaking of the Self* (New York: Penguin Books, 1993).

22. See C. Barber, *Comfortably Numb: How Psychiatry is Medicating A Nation* (New York: Vintage Books, 2008).

23. M. Foucault, *Madness and Civilization: A History of Insanity in the Age of Reason*. Translated from the French by Richard Howard (New York: Vintage Books, 1973).

24. For a complete description of the history of the tortuous mistreatment of the hospitalized mentally ill, see R. Whitaker, *Mad In America: Bad Science, Bad Medicine, and the Enduring Mistreatment of the Mentally Ill* (New York: Basic Books, 2010b).

25. Despite the widespread rejection of "psychosurgery," there remain those researchers who argue that carefully controlled neurosurgical interventions can have an ameliorative affect in those cases of especially severe, chronic, and disabling affective and obsessive compulsive disorders. See G. Cosgrove's and S. Rauch's advocacy of psychosurgery on the website of Boston's prestigious Massachusetts General Hospital. The electronic address is http://neurosurgery.mgh.harvard.edu/functional/psysurg.htm.

26. See, for example, Whitaker, 2010a, op. cit.; D. Healy, *The Anti-Depressant Era* (Cambridge, Mass.: Harvard University Press, 1995); D. Healy, *The Creation of Psychopharmacology* (Cambridge, Mass.: Harvard University Press, 2002).

27. Among the names most fully associated with the anti-psychiatry move-
ment, especially during the 1960s and 1970s, are the following: E. Goffman,
Asylums: Essays on the Social Situation of Mental Patients (Garden City,
N.Y.: Doubleday Anchor, 1961a); T. Szasz, *Ideology and Insanity: Essays
on the Psychiatric Dehumanization of Man* (Garden City, N.Y.: Anchor
Books, 1970); T. Szasz, *The Myth of Mental Illness: Foundations of a Theory
of Personal Conduct* (London, Paladin, 1972); R. Laing, *The Politics of
Experience* (New York: Ballantine Books, 1967); T. Scheff, *Being Mentally
Ill: A Sociological Theory* (Chicago: Aldine, 1966).

28. T. Szasz, Ibid., *Myth of Mental Illness*.

29. The documentary *Titicut Follies*, directed by Frederick Wiseman, was produced in 1967. It exposed the brutal treatment of inmates at Bridgewater
State Hospital for the criminally insane. The film provoked debates about
censorship because the state of Massachusetts tried to prevent its release,
claiming that patients' rights to privacy were abridged. The film received
a number of prestigious awards for its powerful and consciousness-raising
portrayal of the horrific conditions at Bridgewater State Hospital. The film is
easily found in many libraries and is also available for purchase on a variety
of websites.

30. G. Greenberg, *The Book of Woe* (New York: Blue Rider Group, Penguin
Books, 2013), p. 167.

31. A. Frances, *Saving Normal: An Insider's Revolt Against Out-of-Control
Psychiatric Diagnosis, DSM-5, Big Pharma, and the Medicalization of Ordinary
Life* (New York: HarperCollins Publishers, 2013), p. 67.

32. Allen Frances devotes a whole chapter in his book *Saving Normal* to what he
terms "diagnostic inflation." A. Frances, Ibid., pp. 77–113.

33. M. Scott Peck, *The Road Less Traveled: A New Psychology of Love, Traditional
Values, and Spiritual Growth* (New York: Simon and Schuster, 1978).

34. A. Horwitz and J. Wakefield, *The Loss of Sadness: How Psychiatry Transformed
Normal Sorrow into Depressive Disorder* (New York: Oxford University Press,
2007), p. 6.

35. For a detailed analysis of the fundamental transformation in American psychiatry, see T. M. Luhrmann, *Of 2 Minds: The Growing Disorder in American
Psychiatry* (New York: Alfred A. Knopf, 2000).

36. T. Szasz, *Pharmacracy: Medicine and Politics in America* (Westport,
CN: Praeger, 2001), p. 25.

37. S. Kirk, T. Gomory, and D. Cohen, *Mad Science: Psychiatric Coercion,
Diagnosis, and Drugs* (New Brunswick, N.J.: Transaction Publishers, 2013).

38. I. Kirsch, *The Emperor's New Drugs: Exploding the Antidepressant Myth*
(New York: Basic Books, 2010).

39. D. Healy, 2002, op. cit.

40. I. Kirsch, op. cit., p. 97.

41. M. Angell, *The Truth About the Drug Companies: How They Deceive Us and What to Do About It* (New York: Random House, 2005); J. Abramson, *Overdo$ed America: The Broken Promise of American Medicine: How the Pharmaceutical Companies Distort Medical Knowledge, Mislead Doctors, and Compromise Your Health* (New York: HarperCollins, 2004); J. Cohen, *Overdose: The Case Against the Drug Companies* (New York: PenguinPutnam, Inc., 2001).

42. R. Whitaker, 2010a, op. cit.

43. R. Whitaker, Ibid., p. 7.

44. R. Whitaker, Ibid. The first chapter in *The Anatomy of an Epidemic* is entitled "A Modern Plague."

45. Plainly, Whitaker is using the word "storytelling" differently than I use it throughout this chapter. In the context of this quote, storytelling conveys the idea of creating fictions.

46. R. Whitaker, Ibid, p. 312.

47. The ideas expressed in the following section parallel those discussed in an earlier essay. See D. Karp and L. Birk, "Listening to voices: Patient experience and the meanings of mental illness." In C. Aneshensel et al., *The Handbook of the Sociology of Mental Health* (New York: Springer Publishing Company, 2013). My coauthor Lara Birk was especially helpful in more fully sensitizing me to the conceptual linkages among feminist, disability, race, and psychiatric survivor movements.

48. D. Solorzanon and T. Yosso, "Critical race methodology: Counter-storytelling as an analytical framework for education research," *Qualitative Inquiry* 8 (2002): p. 25.

49. Howard Becker was among the first to argue that the "creation" of deviance must consider questions of power. His ideas, central to the evolution of "labeling theory," require that we consider those who both make social rules and then decide which rule breakers should be defined as deviants. See H. Becker, *Outsiders: Studies in the Sociology of Deviance* (London: Free Press of Glencoe, 1963). The notion that all social realities, including definitions of deviance, are social construction is also advanced in P. Berger and T. Luckman, *The Social Construction of Reality: A Treatise in the Sociology of Knowledge* (Garden City, N.Y.: Doubleday, 1966).

50. This quote, originally appearing in Sander Gilman's book entitled *Disease and Representation: Images of Illness from Madness to AIDS* (Ithaca, N.Y.: Cornell University Press, 1988, p. 11), was taken from O. Wahl, *Media Madness: Public Images of Mental Illness* (New Brunswick, N.J.: Rutgers University Press, 1995), p. 125.

51. See G. Hornstein, *Agnes's Jacket: A Psychologist's Search for the Meanings of Madness* (New York: Rodale, Distributed to the trade by MacMillan, 2009), p. xii.

52. G. Hornstein, Ibid.

53. B. Friedan, *The Feminine Mystique* (New York: Norton, 1963).

54. J. Chamberlin, *On Our Own: Patient-Controlled Alternatives to the Mental Health System* (New York: Hawthorn Books, 1978).

55. J. Chamberlin, "The ex-patient movement: Where we've been and where we are going," *The Journal of Mind and Behavior* 11 (1990): 323–336. This article was reprinted on the following website: http://www.power2u.org/articles/history-project/ex-patients.html. The quote used is on the third page.

56. See, for example, E. Speed, "Patients, consumers, and survivors: A case study of mental health service user discourse," *Social Science and Medicine* 62 (2006): 28–38.

57. Ibid., p. 30.

58. Ibid., p. 29.

59. R. Whitaker, 2010a, op. cit.

60. You can find several of Laura Delano's blogs on the Mad in America website. The edited version of the one offered here can be found at the following web address: http://www.madinamerica.com/2014/05/alive/. You may also want to consult her own website at www.recoveringfrompsychiatry.com.

61. See P. Berger, 1963, op. cit.

62. G. H. Mead, *Mind, Self and Society from the Standpoint of a Social Behaviorist*. Edited by Charles W. Morris (Chicago: University of Chicago Press, 1934).

63. J. Chamberlin, "Rehabilitating ourselves: The psychiatric survivor movement," *International Journal of Mental Health* 24 (1995), p. 45.

Chapter 1

1. Here, as throughout the book, all names have been changed to protect the anonymity of my interviewees. To fully ensure that anonymity I have also either left out or changed the names of places and organizations that could even remotely compromise a respondent's identity.

2. In the 1960s and 1970s, social scientists such as Erving Goffman and Thomas Scheff, along with psychiatrists like Thomas Szasz and R. D. Laing, challenged the notion of "mental illness." The power of their analyses notwithstanding, there has been a virtual revolution in psychiatry in the last ten or fifteen years resulting in the dominance of biological explanations for affective disorders and a nearly universal consensus among psychiatrists that such disorders are most effectively treated with drugs. See E. Goffman, *Asylums* (New York: Doubleday Anchor, 1961a); T. Scheff, *Being Mentally Ill* (Chicago: Aldine, 1966); T. Szasz, *Ideology and Insanity: Essays on the Psychiatric Dehumanization of Man.* (Garden City, N.Y.: Anchor

Books, 1970); R. D. Laing, *The Politics of Experience* (New York: Ballantine Books, 1967).

3. See P. Kramer, *Listening to Prozac: A psychiatrist Explores Antidepressant Drugs and the Remaking of the Self* (New York, Penguin, 1993).

4. C. W. Mills, *The Sociological Imagination* (New York: Oxford University Press, 1959).

5. The methodology employed in this study could properly be called a form of "autoethnography." In sociology, an emphasis has historically been placed on scientific objectivity and detachment requiring that the writer's own self be somehow minimized and neutralized. However, within the last 15 to 20 years, writers working within feminist and postmodernist frameworks have challenged this view of science. In her book entitled *Social Science and the Self* (New Brunswick, N.J.: Rutgers University Press, 1991), Susan Krieger makes the case that whether researchers admit it or not, their selves are implicated in every observation and analysis they make. Instead of viewing the self as a contaminant, it is more reasonable and honest to recognize that "whenever we discuss others, we are always talking about ourselves" (p. 5). As this first chapter indicates, you will find that I am very present in this text. Every analysis offered in the book, although always disciplined by the data collected, is, at least initially, guided by personal introspection. Among additional publications that argue the importance of autoethnography and the inevitably self-reflexive nature of social science writing, see S. Reinharz, *On Becoming a Social Scientist* (New Brunswick, N.J.: Transaction Books, 1984); L. Richardson, "Writing: A method of inquiry." In N. Denzin and Y. Lincoln (eds.), *Handbook of Qualitative Research* (Thousand Oaks, Calif.: Sage, 1994); C. Ellis, *Final Negotiations* (Philadelphia: Temple University Press, 1994); Patricia Adler and Peter Adler, "Observational techniques." In N. Denzin and Y. Lincoln (eds.), *Handbook of Qualitative Research* (Thousand Oaks, Calif.: Sage, 1994).

6. These numbers were reported on in P. Breggin, *Toxic Psychiatry* (New York: St. Martin's Press, 1991).

7. As an example, see P. Conrad and J. Schneider, *Deviance and Medicalization* (St. Louis: Mosby, 1980).

8. See, for example, J. Newmann, "Gender, life strains, and depression," *Journal of Health and Social Behavior* 27 (1986): 161–178; S. Nolen-Hocksema, "Sex differences in unipolar depression: Evidence and theory," *Psychological Bulletin* 101 (1987): 259–282; R. Schafer and P. Keith, "Equity and depression among married couples," *Social Psychological Quarterly* 43 (1980): 430–435. A notable exception to the exclusively statistical studies based on large-scale survey research data is D. Jack, *Silencing the Self: Women and Depression* (Cambridge, Mass.: Harvard University Press, 1991). This book is based on life histories of 12 women.

9. See, for example, C. Aneshensel, R. Frerichs, and G. Huba, "Depression and physical illness: A multiwave, nonrecursive causal model," *Journal of Health and Social Behavior* 25 (1984): 350–371; D. Benson and C. Ritter, "Belief in a just world, job loss, and depression," *Sociological Focus* 23 (1990): 49–63; A. Dean, B. Kolody, and P. Wood, "Effects of social support from various sources on depression in elderly persons," *Journal of Health and Social Behavior* 31 (1990): 148–161; G. Kennedy, H. Kelman, and C. Thomas, "The emergence of depressive symptoms in late life: The importance of declining health and increasing disability," *Journal of Community Health* 15 (1990): 93–104; R. Kessler, J. House, and J. Blake, "Unemployment and health in a community sample," *Journal of Health and Social Behavior* 28 (1987): 51–59.

10. S. Plath, *The Bell Jar* (New York: Bantam, 1972); N. Mairs, *Plaintext Essays* (Tucson: University of Arizona Press, 1986); W. Styron, *Darkness Visible: A Memoir of Madness* (New York: Random House, 1990); E. Wurtzel, *Prozac Nation* (Boston: Houghton Mifflin Co., 1994).

11. See the appendix entitled "Thinking about Sampling" for a fuller discussion of the characteristics of this study's sample.

12. See, for example, H. Blumer, *Symbolic Interaction: Perspective and Method* (Englewood Cliffs, N.J.: Prentice-Hall, 1969); D. Karp and W. Yoels, *Sociology in Everyday Life* (Itasca, Ill.: F. E. Peacock, 1993).

13. See J. Comaroff and P. Maguire, "Ambiguity and the search for meaning: Childhood leukaemia in the modern clinical context." In P. Conrad and R. Kern (eds.), *The Sociology of Health and Illness* (New York: St. Martin's, 1986); J. Schneider and P. Conrad, "In the closet with epilepsy: Epilepsy, stigma potential and information control." In P. Conrad and R. Kern (eds.), *The Sociology of Health and Illness* (New York: St. Martin's, 1986); D. Stewart and T. Sullivan, "Illness behavior and the sick role in chronic disease: The case of multiple sclerosis," *Social Science and Medicine* 16 (1982) 1397–1404.

14. D. Jack, op. cit.

15. A. Strauss, "Turning points in identity." In C. Clark and H. Robboy (eds.), *Social Interaction* (New York; St. Martin's, 1992).

16. E. Hughes, *Men and Their Work* (New York: Free Press, 1958).

17. C. W. Mills, op. cit.

18. William Julius Wilson, *The Truly Disadvantaged* (Chicago: University of Chicago Press, 1987).

19. C. Lasch, *Haven in A Heartless World* (New York: Basic Books, 1977).

20. R. Bellah et al., *Habits of the Heart: Individualism and Commitment in American Life* (Berkeley: University of California Press, 1985).

21. E. Becker, *The Birth and Death of Meaning* (Glencoe, Ill.: Free Press, 1962).

22. Particularly impressive is the work of Arthur Kleinman. Among his books demonstrating cross-cultural variation in the meanings of affective disorders are A. Kleinman and B. Good (eds.), *Culture and Depression: Studies*

in the Anthropology and the Cross-Cultural Psychiatry of Affect and Disorder (Berkeley: University of California Press, 1985); A. Kleinman, *Social Origins of Distress and Disease* (New Haven, Conn.: Yale University Press, 1986); *Rethinking Psychiatry* (New York: Free Press, 1988); and *The Illness Narratives* (New York: Basic Books, 1988).

23. The cover story for the July 6, 1992, issue of *Time Magazine* was entitled "Pills for the mind." The cover story for the February 7, 1994, issue of *Newsweek Magazine* was entitled "Beyond Prozac—How science will let you change your personality with a pill."

Chapter 2

1. See, for example, W. Cockerham, *Medical Sociology* (Englewood Cliffs, N.J.: Prentice-Hall, 1992); and P. Conrad and J. Schneider, *Deviance and Medicalization* (St. Louis: C.V. Mosby, 1980).
2. T. Parsons, *Essays in Sociological Theory* (Glencoe, Ill.: The Free Press, 1954).
3. E. Durkheim, *Suicide* (Glencoe, Ill.: The Free Press, 1951).
4. See, for example, C. Derber, *Money, Murder and the American Dream: Wilding from Main to Wall Street* (London: Faber and Faber, 1991); R. Bellah et al., *Habits of the Heart: Individualism and Commitment in American Life* (Berkeley: University of California Press, 1985); R. Bellah et al., *The Good Society* (New York: Alfred Knopf, 1991).
5. See P. Thoits, "Multiple identities and psychological well-being: A reformulation and test of the social isolation hypothesis," *American Sociological Review* 48 (1983): 174–187.
6. For example, see K. Erikson, *Everything in Its Path* (New York: Simon and Schuster, 1976).
7. For example, see P. Brown, "Diagnostic conflict and contradiction in psychiatry," *Journal of Health and Social Behavior* 28 (1987): 37–50; A. Kleinman and B. Good (eds.), *Culture and Depression: Studies in the Anthropology and the Cross-Cultural Psychiatry of Affect and Disorder* (Berkeley: University of California, 1985).
8. S. Kirk and H. Kutchins, *The Selling of DSM: The Rhetoric of Science in Psychiatry* (New York: Aldine de Gruyter, 1992).
9. See B. Bettelheim, *Surviving and Other Essays* (New York: Knopf, 1979); and J. Rosenberg, "Female Experiences During the Holocaust" (Master's thesis, Boston College, 1993).
10. See, for example, J. Puig-Antich et al., "The psychosocial functioning and family environment of depressed adolescents," *Journal of the American Academy of Child and Adolescent Psychiatry* 32 (1993): 244–253; I. Miller, G. Keitner, and M. Whisman, "Depressed patients with dysfunctional families: Description and course of illness," *Journal of Abnormal Psychology* 101

(1992): 637–646; K. Sternberg, M. Lamb, and C. Greenbaum, "Effects of domestic violence on children's behavior problems and depression," *Developmental Psychology* 29 (1993): 44–52.

11. M. Rosenberg, "A symbolic interactionist view of psychosis," *Journal of Health and Social Behavior* 25 (1984): 289–302.

12. G. Simmel, "The stranger." In K. Wolff (ed.), *The Sociology of Georg Simmel* (Glencoe, Ill.: The Free Press, 1950b).

13. The phrase "lived world" is drawn from A. Schutz, *Collected Papers* (The Hague, Netherlands: M. Nijhoff, 1962).

14. A. Hochschild, *The Managed Heart: Commercialization of Human Feeling* (Berkeley: University of California Press, 1983).

15. A. Strauss, "Turning points in identity." In C. Clark and H. Robboy (eds.), *Social Interaction* (New York: St. Martin's, 1992).

16. P. Rieff, *Triumph of the Therapeutic* (New York: Harper and Row, 1966).

17. E. Goffman, *Stigma: Notes on the Management of Spoiled Identity* (Englewood Cliffs, N.J.: Prentice-Hall, 1963b).

18. As examples, see G. Frank, "Beyond stigma: Visibility and self-empowerment of persons with congenital limb deficiencies," *Journal of Social Issues* 44 (1988): 95–115; N. Gerstel, "Divorce and stigma," *Social Problems* 34 (1987): 172–185; P. Luken, "Social identity in later life: A situational approach to understanding old age stigma," *International Journal of Aging and Human Development* 25 (1987): 177–193; J. Moneymaker, "The social significance of short stature: A study of the problems of dwarfs and midgets," *Loss, Grief and Care* 3 (1989): 3–4, 183–189.

19. R. Anspach, "From stigma to identity politics: Political activism among the physically disabled and former mental patients," *Social Science and Medicine* 13A (1979): 765–774.

Chapter 3

1. P. Berger and T. Luckmann, *The Social Construction of Reality* (Garden City, N.Y.: Doubleday, 1966).

2. See A. Solzhenitsyn, *The Gulag Archipelago, 1918–1956; An Experiment in Literary Investigation* (New York: Harper and Row, 1974); also, T. Szasz, *Cruel Compassion: Psychiatric Control of Society's Unwanted* (New York: John Wiley and Sons, 1994).

3. S. Kirk and H. Kutchins, *The Selling of DSM: The Rhetoric of Science in Psychiatry* (New York: Aldine, 1992).

4. See M. Foucault, *Madness and Civilization: A History of Insanity in the Age of Reason.* Translated from the French by Richard Howard (New York: Vintage Books, 1973).

5. E. Hughes, *Men and Their Work* (New York: Free Press, 1958).
6. Although the notion of "stage" is difficult to avoid, I want to suggest that in much social science literature the term conveys a determinism that I find unfortunate. Stages imply that, for whatever process being described, everyone must move through them in a predictably timed sequence. Hence, I often use the terms "moment," "benchmark," or "juncture" in the depression career to suggest a process that is more fluid than the stage idea.
7. A. Strauss, "Turning points in identity." In C. Clark and H. Robboy (eds.), *Social Interaction* (New York: St. Martin's, 1992). The identity transitions described in the pages to follow bear an instructive resemblance to the idea of biographical "epiphanies" developed by Norman Denzin in a number of important books. See N. Denzin, *The Alcoholic Self* (Newbury Park, Calif.: Sage Publishing Co., 1987); N. Denzin, *Interpretive Interactionism* (Newbury Park, Calif.: Sage Publishing Co., 1989b); N. Denzin, *Interpretive Biography* (Newbury Park, Calif.: Sage Publishing Co., 1989a).
8. See D. Karp and W. Yoels, "Work, careers, and aging," *Qualitative Sociology* 4 (1981): 145–166.
9. R. Emerson and S. Messinger, "The micro-politics of trouble," *Social Problems* 25 (1977): 121–133. For another formulation of the trouble idea, see the early work of Charlotte Schwartz. Schwartz's doctoral dissertation studied how 30 people who sought help at a university psychiatric service conceptualized their problem. Her interview data suggested that informants distinguished three mutually exclusive subjective states of trouble. She calls them *exigencies of living* (or momentary difficulties), *normal trouble* (ordinary trouble), and *special trouble* (serious problems). An elaboration of these categories can be found in her work entitled *Clients' Perspectives on Psychiatric Troubles in a College Setting* (unpublished doctoral dissertation, Brandeis University, 1976). See also her article with Merton Kahne entitled "The social construction of trouble and its implications for psychiatrists working in college settings," *Journal of the American College Health Association* 25 (February, 1977): 194–197.
10. R. Emerson and S. Messinger, op. cit., p. 122.
11. Ibid.
12. Ibid.
13. P. Berger and H. Kellner, "Marriage and the construction of reality," *Diogenes* 46 (1964): 1–25.
14. D. Vaughan, *Uncoupling: Turning Points in Intimate Relationships* (New York: Oxford University Press, 1986).
15. Social scientists have been critical of the meaning of psychiatric diagnoses and the processes through which they are established. For examples, see P. Brown, "Diagnostic conflict and contradiction in psychiatry," *Journal of Health and Social Behavior* 28 (1987): 37–50; M. Rosenberg, "A symbolic

interactionist view of psychosis," *Journal of Health and Social Behavior* 25 (1984): 289–302.

16. See, for example, A. Stanton and M. Schwartz, *The Mental Hospital* (New York: Basic Books, 1954); E. Goffman, *Asylums* (Garden City, N.Y.: Doubleday Anchor, 1961a); and W. Gove, *Deviance and Mental Illness* (Beverly Hills, Calif.: Sage, 1982).

17. D. L. Rosenhan, "On being sane in insane places." In C. Clark and H. Robboy (eds.), *Social Interaction* (New York: St. Martin's, 1992).

18. Ibid., pp. 333–334.

19. Ibid., p. 336.

20. See S. Kaysen, *Girl, Interrupted* (New York: Vintage Books, 1994); N. Mairs, *Plaintext Essays* (Tucson: University of Arizona Press, 1986); L. Shiller, *The Quiet Room* (New York: Warner Books, 1994). Another recent book by Jeffrey Geller and Maxine Harris entitled *Women of the Asylum: Voices from Behind the Walls, 1840–1845* (New York: Doubleday, 1994), offers a broader historical perspective by using a variety of first-person accounts to document the plight of women committed to asylums against their will. For a look at life inside McLean's Hospital in Massachusetts see *Under Observation: Life Inside a Psychiatric Hospital* (New York: Ticknor and Fields, 1994) by Lisa Berger and Alexander Vuckovic. Vuckovic is a physician at the hospital.

21. J. Holstein and G. Miller, "Rethinking victimization: An interactional approach to victimology," *Symbolic Interaction* 13 (1990): 103–122.

22. Susanna Kaysen develops this notion in her book entitled *Girl, Interrupted*, op. cit.

Chapter 4

1. See, for example, J. Gabe and M. Bury, "Tranquilisers as a social problem," *Sociological Review* 36 (1988): 320–352.

2. The psychiatrist Peter Breggin has recently written a rejoinder to Kramer's book in which he makes the unsettling argument that Prozac and other antidepressant medications are dangerous drugs. See P. Breggin, *Talking Back to Prozac* (New York: St. Martin's Press, 1994). For another critique of Kramer's book see S. Nuland, "The pill of pills," *The New York Review of Books* (June 9, 1994, pp. 4, 6–8). Nuland notes in his review that despite theories about the relationship of the neurotransmitter serotonin to depression, the causes of depression are still extremely unclear. He says, "Unfortunately for what would at first glance appear to be a tidy theory, it remains anything but certain that clinical depression is, in fact, caused by a decrease in serotonin or its fellows at the synapse. The truth is that the basic causes of the disease called depression are still unknown" (p. 6).

3. M. Heirich, "Change of heart: A test of some widely held theories of religious conversion," *American Journal of Sociology* 85 (1977): 673–674. See also D. Snow and R. Machalek, "The sociology of conversion," *Annual Review of Sociology* 10 (1984): 167–190; and A. Greil and D. Rudy, "Social cocoons: Encapsulation and identity transforming organizations," *Sociological Inquiry* 54 (1984): 260–278.

4. A. Lindesmith, *Opiate Addiction* (Bloomington: Indiana University Press, 1947).

5. H. Becker, *Outsiders: Studies in the Sociology of Deviance* (New York: The Free Press of Glencoe, 1963).

6. Although prior research clarified how patients understood and legitimated their use of psychotropic drugs in a global way (e.g., as a resource for helping them to fulfill family and work roles), this research did not explore how meanings attached to psychotropic drugs change over the period of their use. An important premise of symbolic interaction theory is that the meanings of objects, events, and situations are constantly being renegotiated and reinterpreted. Correspondingly, this chapter articulates with the more general depression "career" path described in the last chapter. I see the meanings attached to medications as a critical factor in determining respondents' ongoing redefinitions of self and illness.

7. A. Strauss, "Turning points in identity." In C. Clark and H. Robboy (eds.), *Social Interaction* (New York: St. Martin's, 1992).

8. C. W. Mills, "Situated actions and vocabularies of motive." In J. Manis and B. Meltzer (eds.), *Symbolic Interaction* (Boston: Allyn & Bacon, 1972).

9. S. Lyman and M. Scott, "Accounts," *American Sociological Review* 33 (1968): 46–62.

10. See, for example, Becker, op. cit.; and E. Lemert, *Social Pathology* (New York: McGraw-Hill, 1951).

11. H. Becker, "Notes on the concept of commitment," *American Journal of Sociology* 66 (1960): 32–40.

12. J. Lofland and L. Skonovd, "Patterns of conversion." In E. Barker (ed.), *Of Gods and Men: New Religious Movements in the West* (Macon, Ga.: Mercer University Press, 1983).

13. Ibid., p. 10.

14. M. Weber, *The Theory of Social and Economic Organization*, translated by A. M. Henderson and T. Parsons (New York: Oxford University Press, 1947).

15. P. Berger and T. Luckmann, *The Social Construction of Reality* (Garden City, N.Y.: Doubleday, 1966).

16. P. Conrad, "The meaning of medications: Another look at compliance," *Social Science and Medicine* 20 (1985): 29–37.

17. Ibid., p. 36.

18. See P. Conrad and J. Schneider, *Deviance and Medicalization* (St. Louis: Mosby, 1980).

19. See, for example, C. Derber, W. Schwartz, and Y. Magrass, *Power in the Highest Degree: Professionals and the Rise of the New Mandarin Class* (New York: Oxford University Press, 1990); M. Gross, *The Psychological Society* (New York: Random House, 1978); C. Lasch. "Life in the therapeutic state," *New York Review of Books* (June 12, 1980): 24–31.

20. P. Berger and T. Luckmann, op. cit.

21. Ibid., p. 112.

22. D. Karp, "Illness ambiguity and the search for meaning: A case study of a self-help group for affective disorders," *Journal of Contemporary Ethnography* 21 (1992): 139–170.

23. R. Anspach, "From stigma to identity politics: Political activism among the physically disabled and former mental patients," *Social Science and Medicine* 13A (1979): 765–774.

Chapter 5

1. As with most features of clinical depression, there is a very substantial literature on the related issues of coping and adaptation. However, like most of the writing on depression, this research is largely statistical and devoted to describing how different variables influence the ability to adapt. Consequently, the focus of attention is on such standard demographic variables as age, gender, religion, ethnicity, and marital status. For a sampling of the kind of research relating these factors to different coping strategies, see H. Koenig, H. Cohen, and D. Blazer, "Religious coping and depression among elderly, hospitalized, medically ill men," *American Journal of Psychiatry* 149 (December, 1992): 1693–1700; D. McDaniel and C. Richards, "Coping with dysphoria: Gender differences in college students," *Journal of Clinical Psychology* 46 (November, 1990): 896–899; K. Glyshaw, L. Cohen, and L. Towbes, "Coping strategies and psychological distress: Perspective and analyses of early and middle adolescents," *American Journal of Community Psychology* 17 (October, 1989): 607–623; W. Vega, B. Kolody, and R. Valle, "Marital strain, coping and depression among Mexican-American women," *Journal of Marriage and the Family* 50 (May, 1988): 391–403; R. Kessler and M. Essex, "Marital status and depression: The importance of coping resources," *Social Forces* 61 (December, 1982): 484–507.

2. K. Charmaz, *Good Days, Bad Days* (New Brunswick, N.J.: Rutgers University Press, 1991).

3. S. Kaysen, *Girl, Interrupted* (New York: Vintage Books, 1993).

4. S. Rothman, *Living in the Shadow of Death: Tuberculosis and the Social Experience of Illness in American Society* (New York: Basic Books, 1994).

5. See C. Clark, "Sympathy biography and sympathy margin," *American Journal of Sociology* 93 (1987): 290–321.

6. The classic statement on the nature of the "sick role" was offered some years ago by Talcott Parsons in his book *Essays on Sociological Theory* (Glencoe, Ill.: The Free Press, 1954). Parsons essentially looks at being ill as a special form of deviance since individuals are withdrawn from society and unable to perform their usual social functions. For this reason, Parsons argues, people are expected to occupy the sick role for as little time as possible. Parsons's conceptualization has been criticized on the grounds that it applies only to the experience of acute illnesses from which people fully recover and neglects the special contingencies associated with chronic illness from which persons, by definition, do not recover.

7. In his book entitled *The Illness Narratives* (New York: Basic Books, 1988), Arthur Kleinman writes (p. 57), "If there is a single experience shared by virtually all chronic pain sufferers it is that at some point those around them—chiefly practitioners, but also at times family members—come to question the authenticity of the patients experience of pain."

8. This process bears a similarity to other "stage theories" describing how people come to acceptance of difficult life conditions, including even that their illness will eventuate in their death. The most famous of these "theories" is the one described by Elizabeth Kubler-Ross in her book *On Death and Dying* (New York: Macmillan, 1969). However, as previously, I want to sound a note of caution about the flexibility of the process I am describing here. It would be a mistake to think that there is something inevitable about the movement from diversion to incorporation, or that all persons with depression arrive, over time, at a more spiritual understanding of their suffering. The processes described in this and other chapters should be viewed as "sensitizing." My goal is to describe regularities in the data, although avoiding the position that individuals with depression march in a lock-step fashion through inevitable stages.

9. Marx's argument, of course, was that a proletarian revolution could only occur when those oppressed by capitalism developed a "class consciousness" that rested on a clear and collectively shared understanding of the sources of their common exploitation by the bourgeoisie, the owners and controllers of the emerging factories of the nineteenth century.

10. See especially R. Emerson and S. Messinger, "The micro-politics of trouble," *Social Problems* 25 (1977): 121–133.

11. It is probably fair to say that among social scientists, two in particular are responsible for having "discovered" and then described the extent of family violence. Beginning in the late 1970s, Murray Straus and Richard Gelles published a series of books that have, in turn, generated a flood of research on family violence. In particular, readers may want to look at these

books: M. Straus, R. Gelles, and S. Steinmetz, *Behind Closed Doors: Violence in the American Family* (Garden City, N.Y.: Doubleday, 1980); R. Gelles and M. Straus, *Intimate Violence in Families* (Beverly Hills, Calif.: Sage, 1985); R. Gelles and M. Straus, *Intimate Violence* (New York: Simon and Schuster, 1988); R. Gelles, *Family Violence* (Beverly Hills, Calif.: Sage, 1987). See also, R. Gelles and D. Loseke (eds.), *Current Controversies on Family Violence* (Newbury Park, Calif.: Sage, 1993).

12. For example, J. Kashani, A. Daniel and A. Dandoy, "Family violence: Impact on children," *Journal of the American Academy of Child and Adolescent Psychiatry* 31 (March, 1992): 181–189.

13. I first realized how significant those suffering from affective disorders considered the labels applied to them as I listened to conversations on that issue in a self-help group for people with depression. At one meeting, for example, the question of labels came up as a topic of discussion. People around the room expressed their preferences, with some wishing to avoid the word illness altogether. They spoke about having a "chemical imbalance" or "emotional disorder." Some found the words disease and illness appropriate, but tried to avoid the word "mental," referring instead to their "emotional" illness or disease. These data are reported in my article entitled "Illness ambiguity and the search for meaning: A case study of a self-help group for affective disorders," *Journal of Contemporary Ethnography* 21 (July, 1992): 139–170. Plainly, people suffering from depression intuitively understand the validity of "labeling theory" in sociology. Although labeling theory has been used to study the development of all sorts of deviant identities, it has been most thoroughly applied to consider the effects of the "mental illness" label.

For a general discussion of labeling theory see H. Becker, *Outsiders: Studies in the Sociology of Deviance* (New York: Free Press, 1963); E. Lemert, *Social Pathology* (New York: McGraw-Hill, 1951); E. Goffman, *Stigma: Notes on the Management of Spoiled Identity* (Englewood Cliffs, N.J.: Prentice-Hall, 1963b). To see how labeling theory has been more specifically applied to the case of mental illness, see E. Goffman, *Asylums: Essays on the Social Situation of Mental Patients and Other Inmates* (Garden City, N.Y.: Doubleday, 1961a); T. Szasz, *The Myth of Mental Illness* (London: Paladin, 1972); B. Link, F. Cullen, J. Frank, and J. Wozniak, "The social rejection of former mental patients: Understanding why labels matter," *American Journal of Sociology* 92 (1987): 1461–1500.

14. J. Bernard, *The Future of Marriage* (New York: Basic Books, 1972).

15. See F. Ritchie, W. Yoels, J. Clair, and R. Allman, "Competing medical and social ideologies and communication accuracy in medical encounters," *Research in the Sociology of Health Care* 12 (1995): 189–211; and W. Yoels, J. Clair, F. Ritchie, and R. Allman, "Role-taking accuracy in medical encounters: A test of two theories," *Sociological Focus* 26 (1993): 183–201.

16. The "romantic love ideal," formulated in France and Germany during the twelfth century, filtered down from the nobility to the lower classes over the centuries. In its pure form, the ideal of romantic love involves the notion that there is only one person in all the world that we are meant to love: Although "love is blind," we will eventually recognize our "true love." The role of *fate* is a strong feature of the romantic ideal. From adolescence on, we wait for that moment when "that old black magic has us in its spell." Soren Kierkegaard has this to say about the mental tricks required to maintain the purity of the romantic love ideal:

> The proposition that the first love is the true love is very accommodating and can come to the aid of mankind in various ways. If a man is not fortunate enough to get possession of what he desires, then he still has the sweetness of the first love. If a man is so fortunate to love many times, each time is still the first love. . . . One loves many times, and each time one denies the validity of the preceding times, and one still maintains the correctness of the proposition that one loves only once.

    See S. Kierkegaard, *Either/Or* (Garden City, N.Y.: Doubleday, 1959), p. 252.

17. The results of this survey were reported in the *Boston Globe* on Thursday, January 28, 1993, p. 11, in an article entitled "Unconventional treatments tried most for what ails us."

18. G. Simmel, "The metropolis and mental life." In *The Sociology of Georg Simmel*, translated and edited by K. Wolff (Glencoe, Ill.: The Free Press, 1950a), p. 414.

19. In something of a startling move, even the drug company Eli Lilly which, of course, has made untold millions of dollars from the sale of Prozac, launched an unusual ad campaign in March 1994 to deplore the role of the media in exaggerating the drug's power. See "Listening to Eli Lilly: Prozac hysteria has gone too far," *The Wall Street Journal*, Thursday, March 31 (1994): B1ff. Recent discussions of Prozac's effectiveness have been stimulated by the claims made for the drug in Peter Kramer's best-selling book, *Listening to Prozac: A Psychiatrist Explores Antidepressant Drugs and the Remaking of the Self* (New York: Penguin, 1993). For recent critical responses to Kramer's book, see D. Rothman, "Shiny Happy People," *The New Republic*, February 14 (1994): 34ff; and S. Nuland, "The pill of pills," *The New York Review of Books*, June 9 (1994): 4, 6–8. In his review, Nuland points out that Prozac is, in fact, no more effective in lifting depression than the tricyclic antidepressant medications that have been used since the 1950s.

20. Discussions of the connection between frustration and aggression can be found in virtually any standard textbook in social psychology. See, for example, chapter 5, entitled "Human aggression" in E. Aronson, *The Social Animal*, 5th ed. (New York: W. H. Freeman, 1988).

21. See, for example, D. Stewart and T. Sullivan, "Illness behavior and the sick role in chronic disease: The case of multiple sclerosis, " *Social Science and Medicine* 16 (1982): 1397–1404. The authors report on multiple sclerosis patients who, as their "initial confidence in their physician's skills waned . . . began to see them as 'evasive', 'non-supportive', 'insensitive', 'uncaring', and 'dishonest' " (p. 1400).

22. Among the several studies that explore how self-help groups provide a coherent ideology about the cause and cure of their members' afflictions, see P. Antze, "Role of ideologies in peer psychotherapy groups" and B. Sherman, "Emergence of ideology in a bereaved parents group." Both of these articles appear in M. Lieberman and L. Borman (eds.), *Self-Help Groups for Dealing with Crisis* (San Francisco: Jossey-Bass, 1979). For an illustration of the quasi-religious character of a self-help group formed to deal with problems of mental illness, see R. Omark, "The dilemma of membership in Recovery, Inc.: A self-help ex-mental patient organization," *Psychological Reports* 44 (1979): 1119–1125; and H. Wechsler, "The self-help organization in the mental health field: Recovery, Inc., a case study," *Journal of Nervous and Mental Disease* 25 (1960): 297–314.

23. D. Rudy, *Becoming Alcoholic: Alcoholics Anonymous and the Reality of Alcoholism* (Carbondale: Southern Illinois University Press, 1986).

24. See A. Haynal, *Depression and Creativity* (New York: International Universities Press, 1985). I should note that particular attention has been given to the connection between bi-polar or manic-depression and creativity. See, for example, K. Jamison, *Touched with Fire: Manic-Depressive Illness and the Artistic Temperament* (New York: Free Press, 1993); C. Holden, "Manic depression and creativity," *Science* 233 (August 15, 1986): 725; B. Bower, "Manic depression: Risk and creativity," *Science News* 134 (September 3, 1988): 151. The connection between mental illness and creativity has also been explored in the popular media. See C. Simon, "Diagnosing the muse: Science struggles to find a link between creativity and madness," *The Boston Globe Magazine*, April 3 (1994): 10–11, 24–26.

25. The radical psychiatrist Ronald Laing argued some years ago that "going crazy" might very well arise from seeing clearly the character of social reality. See R. Laing, *The Politics of Experience* (New York: Pantheon, 1967); and *Self and Others* (New York: Penguin, 1969). Along these same lines, Shelley Taylor maintains in her book entitled *Positive Illusions* (New York: Basic Books, 1989, p. xi) that mental health may require "benign fictions about the self, the world, and the future."

26. See J. Thorne, *You Are Not Alone: Words of Experience and Hope for the Journey Through Depression* (New York: HarperCollins, 1993); and K. Cronkite, *At the Edge of Darkness: Conversations about Conquering Depression* (New York: Doubleday, 1994). Of these two books, Cronkite's is the more

detailed and even-handed. However, neither one, in my view, sustains a meaningful analysis about the illness experience.

27. W. Abbott, "Begin by shooting the poet," *Nation*, August 2 (1975): 88–89.

28. Although there are a number of important books detailing the underlying assumptions of symbolic interaction theory, Herbert Blumer's book entitled *Symbolic Interaction: Perspective and Method* (Englewood Cliffs, N.J.: Prentice-Hall, 1969) is still considered among the most sophisticated treatments of the implications of George Herbert Mead's thinking. Mead was a philosopher at the University of Chicago whose ideas later became the basis for the theory that Blumer himself termed symbolic interaction. Throughout his career, Blumer was the major American spokesman for the ways Mead's work applied to the development of a sociologically informed social psychology.

29. The metaphor of others as mirrors in which we see ourselves reflected was first developed by an early twentieth-century theorist named Charles Horton Cooley. In his book entitled *Human Nature and the Social Order* (New York: Schocken, 1964) Cooley presented the concept of the "looking glass self." His idea was that our selves are a product of three elements: our imagination of how we appear to others, our imagination of the evaluations others are making of us, and the self-feelings (e.g., pride, mortification) that arise from these imaginings.

Chapter 6

1. See A. Strauss, *Negotiations: Varieties, Contexts, Processes, and Social Order* (San Francisco: Jossey-Bass, 1978).

2. K. Duff, *The Alchemy of Illness* (New York: Bell Tower, 1993), p. 83.

3. C. Clark, "Sympathy biography and sympathy margin," *American Journal of Sociology* 93 (1987): 290–321.

4. Decisions about data collection in this chapter were prompted by strategic, theoretical considerations and, therefore, I have done "purposive" or "theoretical sampling" in a fashion consistent with the discussion of this technique in a number of books on qualitative methods. Among those authors who discuss the merits of theoretical sampling are B. Glaser and A. Strauss, *The Discovery of Grounded Theory* (Chicago: Aldine, 1967); and Y. Lincoln and E. Guba, *Naturalistic Inquiry* (Newbury Park, Calif.: Sage, 1985).

5. See D. Karp, "Gender, academic careers, and the social psychology of aging," *Qualitative Sociology* 8 (Spring, 1985): 9–28. Also, L. Holmstrom, *The Two Career Family* (Cambridge, Mass.: Schenkman, 1972); and H. Papaneck, "Men, women and work: Reflections on the two person career," *American Journal of Sociology* 78 (1973): 852–872.

6. A. Hochschild, *Second Shift: Working Parents and the Revolution at Home* (New York: Viking Penguin, 1989).

7. B. Spock, *Baby and Child Care* (New York: Pocket Books, 1968).

8. P. Slater, *The Pursuit of Loneliness* (Boston: Beacon Press, 1970), p. 68.

9. In their 1973 book entitled *The Hidden Injuries of Class,* Richard Sennett and Jonathan Cobb relate the well-documented pattern of male authoritarianism in working-class families to their relative powerlessness at work.

10. See A. Daniels, "Invisible work," *Social Problems* 34 (1987): 403–415. For a more general discussion of women's work see S. Hesse-Biber and M. Fox, *Women at Work* (Belmont, Calif.: Mayfield, 1984).

11. Exchange theory, a social psychological perspective arising from principles of behavioral psychology, assumes an underlying norm of reciprocity. See G. Homans, *Human Behavior: Its Elementary Forms* (New York: Harcourt, Brace, 1961); and P. Blau, *Exchange and Power in Social Life* (New York: John Wiley and Sons, 1964).

12. See M. Olson's two books, *The Logic of Collective Action: Public Goods and the Theory of Groups* (Cambridge, Mass.: Harvard University Press, 1965); and *The Rise and Decline of Nations: Economic Growth, Stagflation, and Social Rigidities* (New Haven, Conn.: Yale University Press, 1982).

13. L. Rubin, *Just Friends: The Role of Friendship in Our Lives* (New York: Harper and. Row, 1985).

14. Rubin, ibid., p. 21.

15. See, for example, G. Allen, *Friendship* (Boulder, Colo.: Westview, 1989); B. Thorne and Z. Luria, "Sexuality and gender in children's daily worlds," *Social Problems* 33 (1986): 176–190; M. Kimmel and M. Messner (eds.), *Men's Lives* (New York: Macmillan, 1989).

16. In order of their publication, Goffman has written the following books: *The Presentation of Self in Everyday Life* (New York: Doubleday Anchor, 1959); *Asylums: Essays on the Social Situation of Mental Patients and Other Inmates* (Garden City, N.Y.: Doubleday Anchor, 1961a); *Encounters: Two Studies in the Sociology of Interaction* (Indianapolis, Ind.: Bobbs-Merrill, 1961b); *Behavior in Public Places: Notes on the Social Organization of Gatherings* (New York: The Free Press, 1963a); *Stigma: Notes on the Management of Spoiled Identity* (Englewood Cliffs, N.J.: Prentice-Hall, 1963b); *Interaction Ritual: Essays on Face-to-Face Behavior* (New York: Anchor, 1967); *Strategic Interaction* (Philadelphia: University of Pennsylvania Press, 1969); *Relations in Public: Microstudies of Public Order* (New York: Basic Books, 1971); *Frame Analysis: An Essay on the Organization of Experience* (New York: Harper and Row, 1974); *Gender Advertisements* (New York: Harper and Row, 1979); *Forms of Talk* (Oxford: Basil Blackwell, 1981). Goffman also wrote too large a number of essays to be mentioned here.

17. E. Goffman, *Asylums,* op. cit.

18. E. Goffman, *Stigma,* op. cit.

19. E. Goffman, *The Presentation of Self in Everyday Life,* op. cit., p. 243.

20. E. Goffman, *Behavior in Public Places,* op. cit.

21. I have used Goffman's notion of "situational involvement" to think about the character of interaction in college classrooms and urban public places. See D. Karp and W. Yoels, "The college classroom: Some observations on the meanings of student participation," *Sociology and Social Research* 60 (July, 1976): 421–439; D. Karp, "Hiding in pornographic bookstores: A reconsideration of the nature of urban anonymity," *Urban Life and Culture* 4 (1973): 427–451. See also chapter 4, "The social organization of everyday city life," in D. Karp, G. Stone, and W. Yoels, *Being Urban: A Sociology of City Life,* 2nd ed. (New York: Praeger, 1991).

22. E. Goffman, "Embarrassment and social organization," *American Journal of Sociology* 62 (1956): 264–271.

23. R. Jacoby, *Social Amnesia* (Boston: Beacon Press, 1975), quoted in L. Rubin, *Intimate Strangers: Men and Women Together* (New York: HarperCollins, 1983), p. 4.

24. P. Berger and B. Berger, *Sociology: A Biographical Approach* (New York: Basic Books, 1975), p. 8.

Chapter 7

1. George Herbert Mead, *Mind, Self and Society* (Chicago: University of Chicago, 1934).

2. E. Durkheim, *Suicide* (Glencoe, Ill.: The Free Press, 1951).

3. K. Erikson, "On sociological prose," *The Yale Review* 78 (1989): 525–538.

4. M. Miller, "Dark days, the staggering cost of depression," *The Wall Street Journal,* Thursday, December 2 (1993): B1, 6.

5. G. Klerman, "Evidence for increases in rates of depression in North America and Western Europe in recent decades." In H. Hippius, G. Klerman, and N. Matussek (eds.), *New Results in Depression Research* (Berlin, Germany: Springer Verlag, 1986).

6. J. Brody, "Recognizing demons of depression, in either sex," *New York Times,* Wednesday, December 18 (1991): C21.

7. See G. Klerman et al., *Interpersonal Psychotherapy of Depression* (New York: Basic Books, 1984); B. Felton, "Cohort variation in happiness," *International Journal of Aging and Human Development* 25 (1987): 27–42; D. Regier et al., "One month prevalence of mental disorders in the United States," *Archives of General Psychiatry* 45 (1988): 977–986.

8. T. Maher, "The withering of community life and the growth of emotional disorders." *Journal of Sociology and Social Welfare* 19 (1992): 138.

9. Although the context of the discussion here, as throughout the book, is on the ways social context shapes the depression experience, the broad social and cultural arrangements described in this chapter do not relate exclusively to depression. As indicated in the text, to pin generic features of American culture to depression alone would be like relating poverty in America to one social problem only. Just as poverty bears a strong relationship to a whole host of human difficulties, the features of American society that foster loneliness, depersonalization, distrust, inauthenticity, mutual indifference, and social disconnection are associated with multiple emotional illnesses. A whole range of disorders from anxiety to depression to paranoia to schizophrenia flourish in societies and situations that maximize the kinds of personal dislocations arising out of social disattachment.

10. The following discussion represents an elaboration of ideas previously developed in two of my earlier books. See, especially, the chapter entitled "The therapeutic state and the problem of aging" in J. Clair, D. Karp and W. Yoels, *Experiencing the Life Cycle: A Social Psychology of Aging* (Springfield, Ill.: Charles Thomas, 1993); and the chapter entitled "Social change and the search for self" in D. Karp and W. Yoels, *Sociology in Everyday Life*, 2nd ed. (Itasca, Ill.: F. E. Peacock, 1993).

11. E. Ackerknecht, "The role of medical history in medical education," *Bulletin of the History of Medicine* 21 (1947): 142–143.

12. Ibid., p. 143.

13. M. Zborowski, "Cultural components in responses to pain." In C. Clark and H. Robboy (eds.), *Social Interaction* (New York: St. Martin's. 1992).

14. Among his work demonstrating cross-cultural variation in the meanings of affective disorders see A. Kleinman and B. Good (eds.), *Culture and Depression: Studies in the Anthropology and the Cross-Cultural Psychiatry of Affect and Disorder* (Berkeley: University of California Press, 1985); A. Kleinman, *Social Origins of Distress and Disease* (New Haven, Conn.: Yale University Press, 1986); *Rethinking Psychiatry* (New York: Free Press, 1988); and *The Illness Narratives* (New York: Basic Books, 1988).

15. A. Kleinman, *Social Origins of Distress and Disease,* op. cit., p. 145.

16. A. Kleinman, *The Illness Narratives,* op. cit., p. 5.

17. The results of this survey were reported in the *Boston Globe* on Thursday, January 28, 1993, p. 11.

18. See W. Yoels and J. Clair, "Never enough time: How medical residents manage a scarce resource," *The Journal of Contemporary Ethnography* 23 (1994): 185–213.

19. G. Cowley, "The culture of Prozac," *Newsweek*, February 7 (1994), p. 42.

20. H. Waitzkin, *The Politics of Medical Encounters: How Patients and Doctors Deal with Social Problems* (New Haven, Conn.: Yale University Press, 1991).

21. W. Yoels and W. Clair, op. cit.
22. D. Rothman, "Shiny happy people," *The New Republic*, February 14 (1994).
23. A. Kleinman and B. Good, op. cit., p. 492.
24. A. Kleinman, *Rethinking Psychiatry*, op. cit., p. 73.
25. These and similar examples are found throughout the works of Arthur Kleinman noted previously.
26. For a complete discussion of the medicalization process and particularly the medicalization of deviance, see P. Conrad and J. Schneider, *Deviance and Medicalization* (St. Louis: C.V. Mosby, 1980).
27. E. Freidson, *Profession of Medicine* (New York: Harper and Row, 1970), p. 336; emphasis added.
28. P. Berger and T. Luckmann, *The Social Construction of Reality: A Treatise in the Sociology of Knowledge* (Garden City, N.Y.: Doubleday, 1966), p. 164.
29. R. Turner, "The theme of contemporary social movements," *British Journal of Sociology* 20 (1969): 395.
30. See P. Rieff, *Triumph of the Therapeutic* (New York: Harper and Row, 1966).
31. C. Lasch, *The Culture of Narcissism* (New York: W.W. Norton, 1978).
32. For a broadly based discussion of such groups see R. Wuthnow, "Religious movements and counter-movements in North America." In J. Beckford (ed.), *New Religious Movements and Rapid Social Change* (London: Sage, 1986).
33. In his recent book entitled *Sharing the Journey Together: Support Groups and America's New Quest for Community* (New York: The Free Press, 1994), Robert Wuthnow argues that the ever proliferating range of support groups now constitute the primary mechanism through which Americans achieve a sense of community and connection.
34. *Newsweek*, "Unite and Conquer," February 5 (1990): 50–55.
35. See T. Powell, *Self Help Organizations and Professional Practice* (Silver Spring, Md.: National Association of Social Workers, 1987); and T. Powell (ed.), *Working with Self Help* (Silver Spring, Md.: National Association of Social Workers, 1990).
36. E. Schur, *The Awareness Trap* (New York: McGraw-Hill, 1976).
37. M. Weber, *The Protestant Ethic and the Spirit of Capitalism*, translated by T. Parsons (New York: Scribner, 1930).
38. Among those who have written about the relationship between capitalism and advertising, the work of Stewart Ewen is particularly cogent. Sec Ewen's two books entitled *Captains of Consciousness* (New York: McGraw-Hill, 1976) and *All Consuming Images* (New York: Basic Books, 1988).
39. L. Zurcher, "The bureaucratizing of impulse: The self-conception of the 1980s," *Symbolic Interaction* 9 (1986): 169–178.
40. M. Gross, *The Psychological Society* (New York: Random House, 1978), p. 6.
41. S. Peele, *Diseasing of America: Addiction Treatment Out of Control* (Lexington, Mass.: Lexington Books, 1989).

42. Personal conversation.

43. See T. Maher, "The withering of community life and the growth of emotional disorders," *Journal of Sociology and Social Welfare* 19 (1992): 125–146.

44. For a discussion of how nineteenth-century theorists considered the changing nature of the social bond with the advent of urban industrialization, see D. Karp, G. Stone, and W. Yoels, *Being Urban: A Sociology of City Life,* 2nd ed. (New York: Praeger, 1991).

45. A. Hacker, *Two Nations: Black and White, Separate, Hostile, Unequal* (New York: Scribner's, 1992).

46. R. Sennett and J. Cobb demonstrate, as an example, how the powerlessness of working-class men on their jobs helps to explain the widely observed pattern of male authoritarianism in working class homes. This analysis is found in their book *The Hidden Injuries of Class* (New York: Random House, 1973).

47. See, for example, H. Becker and A. Strauss, "Careers, personality, and adult socialization," *American Journal of Sociology* 62 (1956): 253–263; and E. Hughes, *Men and Their Work* (New York: The Free Press, 1958).

48. See R. Cohn, "The effects of employment status change on self attitudes," *Social Psychology* 41 (1978): 81–93; R. Coles, "Work and self-respect." In E. Erikson (ed.), *Adulthood* (New York: W.W. Norton, 1978); R. Rothman, *Working: Sociological Perspectives* (Englewood Cliffs, N.J.: Prentice-Hall, 1987).

49. W. Wilson, *The Truly Disadvantaged* (Chicago: University of Chicago Press, 1987).

50. B. Bluestone and B. Harrison, *The Deindustrialization of America* (New York: Basic Books, 1982).

51. T. Maher, op. cit., p. 134.

52. Reported in T. Maher, op. cit.

53. Reported in T. Maher, op. cit.

54. If anything, the rate of severe depression among America's underclass is probably underestimated since this population segment is the most invisible, has the least access to information about depression, and has effectively been abandoned by the health care system.

55. B. Ehrenreich, *Fear of Falling: The Inner Life of the Middle Class* (New York: Pantheon, 1989).

56. *Time,* "Temping of America," March 29 (1993): 41–44, 46–47.

57. C. Derber, "The loosening of America: Contingent work and the temporary life" (unpublished working paper), p. 5.

58. See, for example, C. Davies, "The throwaway culture: Job detachment and depression," *The Gerontologist* 25 (1985): 228–231.

59. R. Bellah et al., *Habits of the Heart: Individualism and Commitment in American Life* (Berkeley: University of California Press, 1985).

60. Ibid., p. 93.

61. W. Kaminer, "Chances are you're co-dependent too," *New York Times Book Review*, February 11 (1990): 1, 26ff.

62. L. Weitzman, *The Divorce Revolution: The Unexpected Social and Economic Consequences in America* (New York: Free Press, 1985).

63. J. Wallerstein and S. Blakeulee, *Second Chances: Men, Women and Children: A Decade After Divorce* (New York: Ticknor and Fields, 1989).

64. D. Riesman et al., *The Lonely Crowd: A Study of the Changing American Character* (New Haven, Conn.: Yale University Press, 1950).

65. A. Toffler, *Future Shock* (New York: Bantam Books, 1973). Toffler has also made prognostications about the future in *The Third Wave* (New York: Bantam Books, 1984).

66. K. Gergen, *The Saturated Self: Dilemmas of Identity in Modern Life* (New York: Basic Books, 1991).

67. Ibid., p. 7.

68. Ibid.

69. For a good descriptive, critical overview of the way postmodern theorists view the self, see M. Schwalbe, "Goffman against postmodernism: Emotion and the reality of the self," *Symbolic Interaction* 16 (1993): 333–350.

70. E. Erikson, *Childhood and Society* (New York: W.W. Norton, 1963).

71. See A. Giddens, *Modernity and Self-Identity* (Stanford, Calif.: Stanford University Press, 1991).

72. T. Gitlin, "Post-modernism: Roots and politics," *Dissent* (Winter, 1989): 110–118.

73. S. Pfohl, *Death at the Parasite Cafe* (New York: St. Martin's Press, 1992).

74. Giddens, op. cit., p. 9.

75. S. Gottschalk, "Uncomfortably numb: Countercultural impulses in the postmodern era," *Symbolic Interaction* 16 (1993): 369.

76. R. Lifton, *The Protean Self: Human Resistance in an Age of Fragmentation* (New York: Basic Books, 1993).

77. See L. Zurcher, *The Mutable Self* (Beverly Hills, Calif.: Sage, 1977).

78. See, for example, A. Etzioni, *The Spirit of Community* (New York: Simon and Schuster, 1993).

Postscript

1. S. Reinharz, *On Becoming a Social Scientist* (New Brunswick, N.J.: Transaction Books, 1984).

2. The Philosophy Foundation exists worldwide. Many of the people I met in the Boston branch have been members of the "school" for as long as 20 or more years.

3. K. Duff, *The Alchemy of Illness* (New York: Bell Tower, 1993).

4. Ibid., pp. 45–46.

5. Ibid., p. 78.

6. T. Moore, *Care of the Soul* (New York: HarperCollins, 1992).

7. Ibid., pp. 18–19.

8. L. Schorr, *Within Our Reach: Breaking the Cycle of Disadvantage* (New York: Anchor Books, 1989).

9. C. Degler, *In Search of Human Nature* (New York: Oxford University Press, 1991).

10. See, for example, A. Toynbee, *A Study of History* (New York: Oxford University Press, 1947).

11. See P. Allen (ed.), *Pitirim Sorokin in Review* (Durham, N.C.: Duke University Press, 1963).

12. A. Etzioni, *The Spirit of Community* (New York: Simon and Schuster, 1993), p. 18.

Appendix

1. D. Tannen, *You Just Don't Understand: Men and Women in Conversation* (New York: Morrow, 1990).

2. For materials on the logic of analytic induction see Y. Lincoln and E. Guba, *Naturalistic Inquiry* (Newbury Park, Calif.: Sage, 1985); B. Glaser and A. Strauss, *The Discovery of Grounded Theory* (Chicago: Aldine, 1967); K. Charmaz, "The grounded theory method: An explication and interpretation." In R. Emerson (ed.), *Contemporary Field Research* (Boston: Little, Brown, 1983); J. Katz, "A theory of qualitative methodology: The social system of analytic fieldwork." In R. Emerson (ed.), *Contemporary Field Research* (Boston: Little, Brown, 1983).

3. D. Karp, "A decade of reminders: Age consciousness between fifty and sixty years old," *The Gerontologist* 6 (1988): 727–738.

4. The notion that sociological analysis should seek to illuminate underlying social forms was first offered by the classical theorist Georg Simmel who argued for what he termed a "formal sociology." See G. Simmel, "The study of societal forms." In K. Wolff (ed.), *The Sociology of Georg Simmel* (Glencoe, Ill.: The Free Press, 1950c). Examples of case studies that make powerful generalizations about social forms abound in sociology. A few examples are G. Fine, *With the Boys: Little League Baseball and Preadolescent Culture*

(Chicago: University of Chicago Press, 1987); H. Becker, *Outsiders: Studies in the Sociology of Deviance* (New York: Free Press, 1963); F. Hunter, *Community Power Structure* (Chapel Hill: University of North Carolina Press, 1953); W. Whyte, *Street Corner Society* (Chicago: University of Chicago Press, 1943).

REFERENCES

Abbott, W. 1975. "Begin by shooting the poet." *Nation*, August 2: 88–89.

Abramson, J. 2004. *Overdo$ed America: The Broken Promise of American Medicine: How the Pharmaceutical Companies Distort Medical Knowledge, Mislead Doctors, and Compromise Your Health.* New York: HarperCollins.

Ackerknecht, E. 1947. "The role of medical history in medical education." *Bulletin of the History of Medicine* 21: 142–143.

Adler, P and P. Adler. 1994. "Observational techniques." In N. Denzin and Y. Lincoln (eds.), *Handbook of Qualitative Research.* Thousand Oaks, Calif.: Sage.

Allen, G. 1989. *Friendship.* Boulder, Colo.: Westview.

Allen, P. (ed.). 1963. *Pitirim Sorokin in Review.* Durham, N.C.: Duke University Press.

Anderson, N. 1923. *The Hobo.* Chicago: University of Chicago Press.

Aneshensel, C., R. Frerichs, and G. Huba. 1984. "Depression and physical illness: A multiwave, nonrecursive causal model." *Journal of Health and Social Behavior* 25: 350–371.

Angell, M. 2005. *The Truth about the Drug Companies: How They Deceive Us and What to Do about It.* New York: Random House.

Anspach, R. 1979. "From stigma to identity politics: Political activism among the physically disabled and former mental patients." *Social Science and Medicine* 13A: 765–774.

Antze, P. 1979. "Role of ideologies in peer psychotherapy groups." In M. Lieberman and L. Borman (eds.), *Self-Help Groups for Dealing with Crisis.* San Francisco: Jossey-Bass.

Aronson, E. 1988. "Human aggression." In *The Social Animal,* 5th edition. New York: W. H. Freeman.

REFERENCES

Barber, C. 2008. *Comfortably Numb: How Psychiatry is Medicating A Nation.* New York: Vintage Books.

Becker, E. 1962. *The Birth and Death of Meaning.* Glencoe, Ill.: Free Press.

Becker, H. 1960. "Notes on the concept of commitment." *American Journal of Sociology* 66: 32–40.

Becker, H. 1963. *Outsiders: Studies in the Sociology of Deviance.* New York: Free Press.

Becker, H. 1967. "Whose side are we on." *Social Problems* 14: 239–247.

Becker, H. and A. Strauss. 1956. "Careers, personality, and adult socialization." *American Journal of Sociology* 62: 253–263.

Bellah, R. et al. 1985. *Habits of the Heart: Individualism and Commitment in American Life.* Berkeley: University of California Press.

Bellah, R. et al. 1991. *The Good Society.* New York: Alfred Knopf.

Benson, D. and C. Ritter. 1990. "Belief in a just world, job loss, and depression." *Sociological Focus* 23: 49–63.

Berger, L. and A. Vuckovic. 1994. *Under Observation: Life Inside a Psychiatric Hospital.* New York: Ticknor and Fields.

Berger, P. 1963. *Invitation to Sociology: A Humanistic Perspective.* Garden City, N.Y.: Doubleday.

Berger, P. and B. Berger. 1975. *Sociology: A Biographical Approach.* New York: Basic Books.

Berger, P. and H. Kellner. 1964. "Marriage and the construction of reality." *Diogenes* 46: 1–25.

Berger, P. and T. Luckmann. 1966. *The Social Construction of Reality: A Treatise in the Sociology of Knowledge.* Garden City, N.Y.: Doubleday.

Bernard, J. 1972. *The Future of Marriage.* New York: Basic Books.

Bettelheim, B. 1979. *Surviving and Other Essays.* New York: Knopf.

"Beyond Prozac—How science will let you change your personality with a pill." 1994. *Newsweek Magazine,* February 7.

Blau, P. 1964. *Exchange and Power in Social Life.* New York: John Wiley and Sons.

Bluestone, B. and B. Harrison. 1982. *The Deindustrialization of America.* New York: Basic Books.

Blumer, H. 1969. *Symbolic Interaction: Perspective and Method.* Englewood Cliffs, N.J.: Prentice-Hall.

Bower, B. 1988. "Manic depression: Risk and creativity." *Science News* 134 (September 3): 151.

Breggin, P. 1991. *Toxic Psychiatry.* New York: St. Martin's Press.

Breggin, P. 1994. *Talking Back to Prozac.* New York: St. Martin's Press.

Brody, J. 1991. "Recognizing demons of depression, in either sex," *New York Times,* December 18: C21.

Brown, P. 1987. "Diagnostic conflict and contradiction in psychiatry." *Journal of Health and Social Behavior* 28: 37–50.

Chamberlin, J. 1978. *On Our Own: Patient-Controlled Alternatives to the Mental Health System.* New York: Hawthorn Books.

Chamberlin, J. 1990. "The ex-patient movement: Where we've been and where we are going." *The Journal of Mind and Behavior* 11: 323–336.

Chamberlin, J. 1995. "Rehabilitating ourselves: The psychiatric survivor movement." *International Journal of Mental Health* 24: 39–46.

Charmaz, K. 1983. "The grounded theory method: An explication and interpretation." In R. Emerson (ed.), *Contemporary Field Research.* Boston: Little, Brown.

Charmaz, K. 1991. *Good Days, Bad Days.* New Brunswick, N.J.: Rutgers University Press.

Clair, J., D. Karp, and W. Yoels. 1993. *Experiencing the Life Cycle: A Social Psychology of Aging,* 2nd edition. Springfield, Ill.: Charles C. Thomas.

Clark, C. 1987. "Sympathy biography and sympathy margin." *American Journal of Sociology* 93: 290–321.

Cockerham, W. 1992. *Medical Sociology.* Englewood Cliffs, N.J.: Prentice-Hall.

Cohen, J. 2001. *Overdose: The Case Against the Drug Companies.* New York: PenguinPutnam.

Cohn, R. 1978. "The effects of employment status change on self attitudes." *Social Psychology* 41: 81–93.

Coles, R. 1978. "Work and self-respect." In E. Erikson (ed.), *Adulthood.* New York: W. W. Norton

Comaroff, J. and P. Maguire. 1986. "Ambiguity and the search for meaning: Childhood leukaemia in the modern clinical context." In P. Conrad and R. Kern (eds.), *The Sociology of Health and Illness.* New York: St. Martin's.

Conrad, P. 1985. "The meaning of medications: Another look at compliance." *Social Science and Medicine* 20: 29–37.

Conrad, P. 2007. *The Medicalization of Society: On the Transformation of Human Conditions into Treatable Disorders.* Baltimore: Johns Hopkins University Press.

Conrad, P. and R. Kern (eds.). 1986. *The Sociology of Health and Illness.* New York: St. Martin's.

Conrad, P. and J. Schneider. 1980. *Deviance and Medicalization.* St. Louis: Mosby.

Cooley, C. 1964. *Human Nature and the Social Order.* New York: Schocken.

Cowley, G. 1994. "The culture of Prozac," *Newsweek,* February 7: 41–42.

Cronkite, K. 1994. *At the Edge of Darkness: Conversations about Conquering Depression.* New York: Doubleday.

Daniels, A. 1987. "Invisible work." *Social Problems* 34: 403–415.

Davies, C. 1985. "The throwaway culture: Job detachment and depression." *The Gerontologist* 25: 228–231.

Dean, A., B. Kolody, and P. Wood. 1990. "Effects of social support from various sources on depression in elderly persons." *Journal of Health and Social Behavior* 31: 148–161.

Degler, C. 1991. *In Search of Human Nature*. New York: Oxford University Press.

Denzin, N. 1987. *The Alcoholic Self*. Newbury Park, Calif.: Sage.

Denzin, N. 1989a. *Interpretive Biography*. Newbury Park, Calif.: Sage.

Denzin, N. 1989b. *Interpretive Interactionism*. Newbury Park, Calif.: Sage.

Derber, C. 1991. *Money, Murder and the American Dream: Wilding from Main Street to Wall Street*. London: Faber and Faber.

Derber, C. 1994. "The loosening of America: Contingent work and the temporary life" (unpublished working paper).

Derber, C., W. Schwartz, and Y. Magrass. 1990. *Power in the Highest Degree: Professionals and the Rise of the New Mandarin Class*. New York: Oxford University Press.

Duff, K. 1993. *The Alchemy of Illness*. New York: Bell Tower.

Durkheim, E. 1951. *Suicide*. Glencoe, Ill.: The Free Press.

Ehrenreich, B. 1989. *Fear of Falling: The Inner Life of the Middle Class*. New York: Pantheon.

Ellis, C. 1994. *Final Negotiations*. Philadelphia: Temple University Press.

Emerson, R. and S. Messinger. 1977. "The micro-politics of trouble." *Social Problems* 25: 121–133.

Erikson, E. 1963. *Childhood and Society*. New York: W.W. Norton.

Erikson, K. 1976. *Everything in Its Path*. New York: Simon and Schuster.

Erikson, K. 1989. "On sociological prose." *The Yale Review* 78: 525–538.

Etzioni, A. 1993. *The Spirit of Community*. New York: Simon and Schuster.

Ewen, S. 1976. *Captains of Consciousness*. New York: McGraw-Hill.

Ewen, S. 1988. *All Consuming Images*. New York: Basic Books.

Felton, B. 1987. "Cohort variation in happiness." *International Journal of Aging and Human Development* 25: 27–42.

Fine, G. 1987. *With the Boys: Little League Baseball and Preadolescent Culture*. Chicago: University of Chicago Press.

Fine, G. 1995. *A Second Chicago School? The Development of a Post War American Sociology*. Chicago: University of Chicago Press.

Foucault, M. 1973. *Madness and Civilization: A History of Insanity in the Age of Reason*. Translated from the French by Richard Howard. New York: Vintage Books.

Frances, A. 2013. *Saving Normal: An Insider's Revolt Against Out-of-Control Psychiatric Diagnosis, DSM-5, Big Pharma, and the Medicalization of Ordinary Life*. New York: HarperCollins Publishers.

Frank, A. 1995. *The Wounded Storyteller: Body, Illness, and Ethics*. Chicago; University of Chicago Press.

Frank, A. 2010. *Letting Stories Breathe: A Socio-Narratology*. Chicago: University of Chicago Press.

Frank, G. 1988. "Beyond stigma: Visibility and self-empowerment of persons with congenital limb deficiencies." *Journal of Social Issues* 44: 95–115.

Freidson, E. 1970. *Profession of Medicine.* New York: Harper and Row.

Friedan, B. 1963. *The Feminine Mystique.* New York: Norton.

Gabe, J. and M. Bury. 1988. "Tranquilisers as a social problem." *Sociological Review* 36: 320–352.

Geller, J. and M. Harris. 1994. *Women of the Asylum: Voices from Behind the Walls, 1840–1845.* New York: Doubleday.

Gelles, R. 1987. *Family Violence.* Beverly Hills, Calif.: Sage.

Gelles, R. and D. Loseke (eds.). 1993. *Current Controversies on Family Violence.* Newbury Park, Calif.: Sage.

Gelles, R. and M. Straus. 1985. *Intimate Violence in Families.* Beverly Hills, Calif.: Sage.

Gelles, R. and M. Straus. 1988. *Intimate Violence.* New York: Simon and Schuster.

Gergen, K. 1991. *The Saturated Self: Dilemmas of Identity in Modern Life.* New York: Basic Books.

Gerstel, N. 1987. "Divorce and stigma." *Social Problems* 34: 172–185.

Giddens, A. 1991. *Modernity and Self-Identity.* Stanford, Calif.: Stanford University Press.

Gilman, S. 1988. *Disease and Representation: Images of Illness from Madness to AIDS.* Ithaca, N.Y.: Cornell University Press.

Gitlin, T. 1989. "Post-modernism: Roots and politics." *Dissent* (Winter): 110–118.

Glaser, B. and A. Strauss. 1967. *The Discovery of Grounded Theory.* Chicago: Aldine.

Clyohaw, K., L. Cohen, and L. Towbes. 1989. "Coping strategies and psychological distress: Perspective and analyses of early and middle adolescents." *American Journal of Community Psychology* 17 (October): 607–623.

Goffman, E. 1956. "Embarrassment and social organization." *American Journal of Sociology* 62: 264–271.

Goffman, E. 1959. *The Presentation of Self in Everyday Life.* New York: Doubleday Anchor.

Goffman, E. 1961a. *Asylums: Essays on the Social Situation of Mental Patients and Other Inmates.* Garden City, N.Y.: Doubleday Anchor.

Goffman, E. 1961b. *Encounters: Two Studies in the Sociology of Interaction.* Indianapolis, Ind.: Bobbs-Merrill.

Goffman, E. 1963a. *Behavior in Public Places: Notes on the Social Organization of Gatherings.* New York: Free Press.

Goffman, E. 1963b. *Stigma: Notes on the Management of Spoiled Identity.* Englewood Cliffs, N.J.: Prentice-Hall.

Goffman, E. 1967. *Interaction Ritual: Essays on Face-to-Face Behavior.* New York: Doubleday Anchor.

Goffman, E. 1969. *Strategic Interaction.* Philadelphia: University of Pennsylvania Press.

Goffman, E. 1971. *Relations in Public: Microstudies of Public Order.* New York: Basic Books.

Goffman, E. 1974. *Frame Analysis: An Essay on the Organization of Experience.* New York: Harper and Row.

Goffman, E. 1979. *Gender Advertisements.* New York: Harper and Row.

Goffman, E. 1981. *Forms of Talk.* Oxford: Basil Blackwell.

Gottschalk, S. 1993. "Uncomfortably numb: Countercultural impulses in the postmodern era." *Symbolic Interaction* 16: 351–378.

Gove, W. 1982. *Deviance and Mental Illness.* Beverly Hills, Calif.: Sage.

Greenberg, G. 2013. *The Book of Woe.* New York: Blue Rider Group, Penguin Books.

Greil, A. and D. Rudy. 1984. "Social cocoons: Encapsulation and identity transforming organizations." *Sociological Inquiry* 54: 260–278.

Gross, M. 1978. *The Psychological Society.* New York: Random House.

Hacker, A. 1992. *Two Nations: Black and White, Separate, Hostile, Unequal.* New York: Scribner's.

Haynal, A. 1985. *Depression and Creativity.* New York: International Universities Press.

Healy, D. 1995. *The Anti-Depressant Era.* Cambridge, Mass.: Harvard University Press.

Healy, D. 2002. *The Creation of Psychopharmacology.* Cambridge, Mass.: Harvard University Press.

Heirich, M. 1977. "Change of heart: A test of some widely held theories of religious conversion." *American Journal of Sociology* 85: 653–680.

Hesse-Biber, S. and M. Fox. 1984. *Women at Work.* Belmont, Calif.: Mayfield.

Hochschild, A. 1983. *The Managed Heart: Commercialization of Human Feeling.* Berkeley: University of California Press.

Hochschild, A. 1989. *Second Shift: Working Parents and the Revolution at Home.* New York: Viking Penguin.

Holden, C. 1986. "Manic depression and creativity." *Science* 233 (August 15): 725.

Holmstrom, L. 1972. *The Two Career Family.* Cambridge, Mass.: Schenkman.

Holstein, J. and G. Miller. 1990. "Rethinking victimization: An interactional approach to victimology." *Symbolic Interaction* 13: 103–122.

Homans, G. 1961. *Human Behavior: Its Elementary Forms.* New York: Harcourt, Brace.

Hornstein, G. 2009. *Agnes's Jacket: A Psychologist's Search for the Meanings of Madness.* New York: Rodale, Distributed to the trade by MacMillan.

Horwitz, A. and J. Wakefield. 2007. *The Loss of Sadness: How Psychiatry Transformed Normal Sorrow into Depressive Disorder.* New York: Oxford University Press.

Hughes, E. 1958. *Men and Their Work.* New York: Free Press.

Hunter, F. 1953. *Community Power Structure.* Chapel Hill: University of North Carolina Press.

Jack, D. 1991. *Silencing the Self: Women and Depression.* Cambridge, Mass.: Harvard University Press.

Jacoby, R. 1975. *Social Amnesia*. Boston: Beacon Press.

Jamison, K. 1993. *Touched With Fire: Manic-Depressive Illness and the Artistic Temperament*. New York: Free Press.

Jamison, K. 1995. *An Unquiet Mind*. New York: A. A. Knopf.

Kaminer, W. 1990. "Chances are you're co-dependent too." *New York Times Book Review*, February 11: 1, 26ff.

Karp, D. 1973. "Hiding in pornographic bookstores: A reconsideration of the nature of urban anonymity." *Urban Life and Culture* 4: 427–451.

Karp, D. 1985. "Gender, academic careers, and the social psychology of aging." *Qualitative Sociology* 8 (Spring, 1985): 9–28.

Karp, D. 1988. "A decade of reminders: Age consciousness between fifty and sixty years old." *The Gerontologist* 6: 727–738.

Karp, D. 1992. "Illness ambiguity and the search for meaning: A case study of a self-help group for affective disorders." *Journal of Contemporary Ethnography* 21: 139–170.

Karp, D. 1999. "Social science, progress, and the ethnographer's craft." *Journal of Contemporary Ethnography* 28: 597–609.

Karp, D. 2001. *The Burden of Sympathy: How Families Cope with Mental Illness*. New York: Oxford University Press.

Karp, D. 2006. *Is It Me or My Meds? Living with Antidepressants*. Cambridge, Mass.: Harvard University Press.

Karp, D. and L. Birk. 2013. "Listening to voices: Patient experience and the meanings of mental illness." In C. Aneshensel et al., *The Handbook of the Sociology of Mental Health*. New York: Springer Publishing Company.

Karp, D., L. Holmstrom, and P. Gray. 2004. "Of roots and wings: Letting go of the college-bound child." *Symbolic Interaction* 27: 357–382.

Karp, D. and G. Sisson (eds.). 2010. *Voices from the Inside: Readings on the Sociology of Mental Health and Illness*. New York: Oxford University Press.

Karp, D., G. Stone, and W. Yoels. 1991. *Being Urban: A Sociology of City Life,* 2nd edition. New York: Praeger.

Karp, D. and W. Yoels. 1976. "The college classroom: Some observations on the meanings of student participation." *Sociology and Social Research* 60: 421–439.

Karp, D. and W. Yoels. 1981. "Work, careers, and aging." *Qualitative Sociology* 4: 145–166.

Karp, D. and W. Yoels. 1993. *Sociology in Everyday Life,* 2nd edition. Itasca, Ill.: F. E. Peacock.

Kashani, J., A. Daniel, and A. Dandoy. 1992. "Family violence: Impact on children." *Journal of the American Academy of Child and Adolescent Psychiatry* 31 (March): 181–189.

Katz, J. 1983. "A theory of qualitative methodology: The social system of analytic fieldwork." In R. Emerson (ed.), *Contemporary Field Research*. Boston: Little, Brown.

Kaysen, S. 1994. *Girl, Interrupted.* New York: Vintage Books.

Kennedy, G., H. Kelman, and C. Thomas. 1990. "The emergence of depressive symptoms in late life: The importance of declining health and increasing disability." *Journal of Community Health* 15: 93–104.

Kessler, R. and M. Essex. 1982. "Marital status and depression: The importance of coping resources." *Social Forces* 61 (December): 484–507.

Kessler, R., J. House, and J. Blake. 1987. "Unemployment and health in a community sample." *Journal of Health and Social Behavior* 28: 51–59.

Kierkegaard, S. 1959. *Either/Or.* Garden City, N.Y.: Doubleday.

Kimmel, M. and M. Messner (eds.). 1989. *Men's Lives.* New York: Macmillan.

Kirk, S., T. Gomory, and D. Cohen. 2013. *Mad Science: Psychiatric Coercion, Diagnosis, and Drugs.* New Brunswick, N.J.: Transaction Publishers.

Kirk, S. and H. Kutchins. 1992. *The Selling of DSM: The Rhetoric of Science in Psychiatry.* New York: Aldine de Gruyter.

Kirsch, I. 2010. *The Emperor's New Drugs: Exploding the Antidepressant Myth.* New York: Basic Books.

Kleinman, A. 1986. *Social Origins of Distress and Disease: Depression, Neurasthenia, and Pain in Modern China.* New Haven, Conn.: Yale University Press.

Kleinman, A. 1988. *Rethinking Psychiatry.* New York: The Free Press.

Kleinman, A. 1988. *The Illness Narratives.* New York: Basic Books.

Kleinman, A. and B. Good. (eds.). 1985. *Culture and Depression: Studies in the Anthropology and the Cross-Cultural Psychiatry of Affect and Disorder.* Berkeley: University of California.

Klerman, G. 1986. "Evidence for increases in rates of depression in North America and Western Europe in recent decades." In H. Hippius, G. Klerman, and N. Matussek (eds.), *New Results in Depression Research.* Berlin, Germany: Springer Verlag.

Klerman, G. et al. 1984. *Interpersonal Psychotherapy of Depression.* New York: Basic Books.

Koenig, H., H. Cohen, and D. Blazer. 1992. "Religious coping and depression among elderly, hospitalized, medically ill men." *American Journal of Psychiatry* 149 (December): 1693–1700.

Kramer, P. 1993. *Listening to Prozac: A Psychiatrist Explores Antidepressant Drugs and the Remaking of the Self.* New York: Penguin Books.

Krieger, S. 1991. *Social Science and the Self.* New Brunswick, N.J.: Rutgers University Press.

Kubler-Ross, E. 1969. *On Death and Dying.* New York: Macmillan.

Laing, R. 1967. *The Politics of Experience.* New York: Pantheon.

Laing, R. 1969. *Self and Others.* New York: Penguin.

Lasch, C. 1977. *Haven in a Heartless World: The Family Besieged.* New York: Basic Books.

Lasch, C. 1978. *The Culture of Narcissism.* New York: W. W. Norton.

Lasch, C. 1980. "Life in the therapeutic state." *New York Review of Books*, June 12: 24–31.

Lemert, E. 1951. *Social Pathology*. New York: McGraw-Hill.

Lifton, R. 1993. *The Protean Self: Human Resistance in an Age of Fragmentation*. New York: Basic Books.

Lincoln, Y. and E. Guba. 1985. *Naturalistic Inquiry*. Newbury Park, Calif.: Sage.

Lindesmith, A. 1947. *Opiate Addiction*. Bloomington: Indiana University Press.

Link, B., F. Cullen, J. Frank, and J. Wozniak. 1987. "The social rejection of former mental patients: Understanding why labels matter." *American Journal of Sociology* 92: 1461–1500.

"Listening to Eli Lilly: Prozac hysteria has gone too far," 1994. *Wall Street Journal*, March 31: B1ff.

Lofland, J. and L. Skonovd. 1983. "Patterns of conversion." In E. Barker (ed.), *Of Gods and Men: New Religious Movements in the West*. Macon, Ga.: Mercer University Press.

Luhrmann, T. M. 2000. *Of 2 Minds: The Growing Disorder in American Psychiatry*. New York: Alfred A. Knopf.

Luken, P. 1987. "Social identity in later life: A situational approach to understanding old age stigma." *International Journal of Aging and Human Development* 25: 177–193.

Lyman, S. and M. Scott. 1968. "Accounts." *American Sociological Review* 33 (December): 46–62.

Maher, T. 1992. "The withering of community life and the growth of emotional disorders." *Journal of Sociology and Social Welfare* 19(2): 125–146.

Mairs, N. 1986. *Plaintext Essays*. Tucson: University of Arizona Press.

McDaniel, D. and C. Richards. 1990. "Coping with dysphoria: Gender differences in college students." *Journal of Clinical Psychology* 46 (November): 896–899.

Mead, G. H. 1934. *Mind, Self, and Society from the Standpoint of a Social Behaviorist*. Chicago: University of Chicago Press.

Miller, I., G. Keitner, and M. Whisman. 1992. "Depressed patients with dysfunctional families: Description and course of illness." *Journal of Abnormal Psychology* 101: 637–646.

Miller, M. 1993. "Dark days, the staggering cost of depression." *The Wall Street Journal*, December 2: B1, 6.

Millett, M. 1995. *The Loony-Bin Trip*. New York: Simon and Schuster.

Mills, C. W. 1959. *The Sociological Imagination*. New York: Oxford University Press.

Mills, C. W. 1972. "Situated actions and vocabularies of motive." In J. Manis and B. Meltzer (eds.), *Symbolic Interaction*. Boston: Allyn & Bacon.

Moneymaker, J. 1989. "The social significance of short stature: A study of the problems of dwarfs and midgets." *Loss, Grief and Care* 3: 3–4, 183–189.

Moore, T. 1992. *Care of the Soul*. New York: HarperCollins.

Newmann, J. 1986. "Gender, life strains, and depression." *Journal of Health and Social Behavior* 27: 161–178.

Nolen-Hoeksema, S. 1987. "Sex differences in unipolar depression: Evidence and theory." *Psychological Bulletin* 101: 259–282.

Nuland, S. 1994. "The pill of pills." *The New York Review of Books*, June 9: 4, 6–8.

Olson, M. 1965. *The Logic of Collective Action: Public Goods and the Theory of Groups*. Cambridge, Mass.: Harvard University Press.

Olson, M. 1982. *The Rise and Decline of Nations: Economic Growth, Stagflation, and Social Rigidities*. New Haven, Conn.: Yale University Press.

Omark, R. 1979. "The dilemma of membership in Recovery, Inc.: A self-help ex-mental patient organization." *Psychological Reports* 44: 1119–1125.

Papaneck, H. 1973. "Men, women and work: Reflections on the two person career." *American Journal of Sociology* 78: 852–872.

Parsons, T. 1954. *Essays in Sociological Theory*. Glencoe, Ill.: The Free Press.

Peck, M. Scott. 1978. *The Road Less Traveled: A New Psychology of Love, Traditional Values, and Spiritual Growth*. New York: Simon and Schuster.

Peele, S. 1989. *Diseasing of America: Addiction Treatment Out of Control*. Lexington, Mass.: Lexington Books.

Pfohl, S. 1992. *Death at the Parasite Cafe*. New York: St. Martin's Press.

"Pills for the mind." 1992. *Time Magazine*, July 6.

Plath, S. 1972. *The Bell Jar*. New York: Bantam.

Powell, T. 1987. *Self Help Organizations and Professional Practice*. Silver Spring, Md.: National Association of Social Workers.

Powell, T. (ed.). 1990. *Working With Self Help*. Silver Spring, Md.: National Association of Social Workers.

Puig-Antich, J. et al. 1993. "The psychosocial functioning and family environment of depressed adolescents." *Journal of the American Academy of Child and Adolescent Psychiatry* 32: 244–253.

Regier, D. et al. 1988. "One month prevalence of mental disorders in the United States." *Archives of General Psychiatry* 45: 977–986.

Reinharz, S. 1984. *On Becoming a Social Scientist*. New Brunswick, N.J.: Transaction Books.

Richardson, L. 1994. "Writing: A method of inquiry." In N. Denzin and Y. Lincoln (eds.), *Handbook of Qualitative Research*. Thousand Oaks, Calif.: Sage.

Rieff, P. 1966. *Triumph of the Therapeutic*. New York: Harper and Row.

Riesman, D. et al. 1950. *The Lonely Crowd: A Study of the Changing American Character*. New Haven, Conn.: Yale University Press.

Ritchie, F., W. Yoels, J. Clair, and R. Allman. 1995. "Competing medical and social ideologies and communication accuracy in medical encounters." *Research in the Sociology of Health Care* 12: 189–211.

Rosenberg, J. 1993. "Female Experiences During the Holocaust." Master's thesis, Boston College.

Rosenberg, M. 1984. "A symbolic interactionist view of psychosis." *Journal of Health and Social Behavior* 25: 289–302.

Rosenhan, D. L. 1992. "On being sane in insane places." In C. Clark and H. Robboy (eds.), *Social Interaction*. New York: St. Martin's.

Rothman, D. 1994. "Shiny Happy People." *The New Republic*, February 14: 34–36.

Rothman, R. 1987. *Working: Sociological Perspectives*. Englewood Cliffs, N.J.: Prentice-Hall.

Rothman, S. 1994. *Living in the Shadow of Death: Tuberculosis and the Social Experience of Illness in American Society*. New York: Basic Books.

Rubin, L. 1983. *Intimate Strangers: Men and Women Together*. New York: HarperCollins.

Rubin, L. 1985. *Just Friends: The Role of Friendship in Our Lives*. New York: Harper and Row.

Rudy, D. 1986. *Becoming Alcoholic: Alcoholics Anonymous and the Reality of Alcoholism*. Carbondale: Southern Illinois University Press.

Schafer, R. and P. Keith. 1980. "Equity and depression among married couples." *Social Psychological Quarterly* 43: 430–435.

Scheff, T. 1966. *Being Mentally Ill: A Sociological Theory*. Chicago: Aldine.

Schneider, J. and P. Conrad. 1986. "In the closet with epilepsy: Epilepsy, stigma potential and information control." In P. Conrad and R. Kern (eds.), *The Sociology of Health and Illness*. New York: St. Martin's.

Schorr, L. 1989. *Within Our Reach: Breaking the Cycle of Disadvantage*. New York: Anchor Books.

Schur, E. 1976. *The Awareness Trap*. New York: McGraw-Hill.

Schutz, A. 1962. *Collected Papers*. The Hague, Netherlands: M. Nijhoff.

Schwalbe, M. 1993. "Goffman against postmodernism: Emotion and the reality of the self." *Symbolic Interaction* 16: 333–350.

Schwartz, C. 1976. "Clients' Perspectives on Psychiatric Troubles in a College Setting." Unpublished doctoral dissertation, Brandeis University.

Schwartz, C. and M. Kahne. 1977. "The social construction of trouble and its implications for psychiatrists working in college settings." *Journal of the American College Health Association* 25: 194–197.

Sennett, R. and J. Cobb. 1973. *The Hidden Injuries of Class*. New York: Random House.

Sherman, B. 1979. "Emergence of ideology in a bereaved parents group." In M. Lieberman and L. Borman (eds.), *Self-Help Groups for Dealing with Crisis*. San Francisco: Jossey-Bass.

Shiller, L. 1994. *The Quiet Room*. New York: Warner Books.

Simmel, G. 1950a. "The metropolis and mental life." In *The Sociology of Georg Simmel*. Translated and edited by K. Wolff. Glencoe, Ill.: The Free Press.

Simmel, G. 1950b. "The stranger." In *The Sociology of Georg Simmel*. Translated and edited by K. Wolff. Glencoe, Ill.: The Free Press.

Simmel, G. 1950c. "The study of societal forms." In *The Sociology of Georg Simmel*. Translated and edited by K. Wolff. Glencoe, Ill.: The Free Press.

Simon, C. 1994. "Diagnosing the muse: Science struggles to find a link between creativity and madness." *The Boston Globe Magazine*, April 3: 10–11, 24–26.

Slater, L. 1998. *Prozac Diary*. New York: Random House.

Slater, P. 1970. *The Pursuit of Loneliness*. Boston: Beacon Press.

Snow, D. and R. Machalek. 1984. "The sociology of conversion." *Annual Review of Sociology* 10: 167–190.

Solorzanon, D. and T. Yosso. 2002. "Critical race methodology: Counter-storytelling as an analytical framework for education research," *Qualitative Inquiry* 8: 23–44.

Solzhenitsyn, A. 1974. *The Gulag Archipelago, 1918–1956; An Experiment in Literary Investigation*. New York: Harper and Row.

Speed, E. 2006. "Patients, consumers, and survivors: A case study of mental health service user discourse." *Social Science and Medicine* 62: 28–38.

Spock, B. 1968. *Baby and Child Care*. New York: Pocket Books.

Stanton, A. and M. Schwartz. 1954. *The Mental Hospital*. New York: Basic Books.

Sternberg, K., M. Lamb, and C. Greenbaum. 1993. "Effects of domestic violence on children's behavior problems and depression." *Developmental Psychology* 29: 44–52.

Stewart, D. and T. Sullivan. 1982. "Illness behavior and the sick role in chronic disease: The case of multiple sclerosis." *Social Science and Medicine* 16: 1397–1404.

Straus, M., R. Gelles, and S. Steinmetz. 1980. *Behind Closed Doors: Violence in the American Family*. Garden City. N.Y.: Doubleday.

Strauss, A. 1978. *Negotiations: Varieties, Contexts, Processes, and Social Order*. San Francisco: Jossey-Bass.

Strauss, A. 1992. "Turning points in identity." In C. Clark and H. Robboy (eds.), *Social Interaction*. New York: St. Martin's.

Styron, W. 1990. *Darkness Visible: A Memoir of Madness*. New York: Random House.

Sutherland, E. 1937. *Professional Thief, by a Professional Thief*. Chicago: University of Chicago Press.

Szasz, T. 1970. *Ideology and Insanity: Essays on the Psychiatric Dehumanization of Man*. Garden City, N.Y.: Anchor Books.

Szasz, T. 1972. *The Myth of Mental Illness: Foundations of a Theory of Personal Conduct*. London: Paladin.

Szasz, T. 1994. *Cruel Compassion: Psychiatric Control of Society's Unwanted*. New York: John Wiley and Sons.

Szasz, T. 2001. *Pharmacracy: Medicine and Politics in America*. Westport, Conn.: Praeger.

Taylor, S. 1989. *Positive Illusions: Creative Self Deception and the Healthy Mind*. New York: Basic Books.

Tannen, D. 1990. *You Just Don't Understand: Men and Women in Conversation* (New York: Morrow, 1990).

"The temping of America." 1993. *Time Magazine*, March 29: 40–44, 46–47.

Thoits, P. 1983. "Multiple identities and psychological well-being: A reformulation and test of the social isolation hypothesis." *American Sociological Review* 48: 174–187.

Thomas, W. I. and F. Znaniecki. 1918. *The Polish Peasant in Europe and America; Monograph of an Immigrant Group.* Chicago: The University of Chicago Press.

Thorne, B. and Z. Luria. 1986. "Sexuality and gender in children's daily worlds." *Social Problems* 33: 176–190.

Thorne, T. 1993. *You Are Not Alone: Words of Experience and Hope for the Journey Through Depression.* New York: HarperCollins.

Thrasher, F. 1927. *The Gang: A Study of 1,313 Gangs in Chicago.* Chicago: University of Chicago Press.

Toffler, A. 1973. *Future Shock.* New York: Bantam Books.

Toffler, A. 1984. *The Third Wave.* New York: Bantam Books.

Toynbee, A. 1947. *A Study of History.* New York: Oxford University Press.

Turner, R. 1969. "The theme of contemporary social movements." *British Journal of Sociology* 20: 390–405.

"Unconventional treatments tried most for what ails us." 1993. *Boston Globe,* January 28: 11.

"Unite and conquer," 1990. *Newsweek,* February 5. 50–55.

Vaughan, D. 1986. *Uncoupling: Turning Points in Intimate Relationships.* New York: Oxford University Press.

Vega, W., B. Kolody, and R. Valle. 1988. "Marital strain, coping and depression among Mexican-American women." *Journal of Marriage and the Family* 50 (May): 391–403.

Vonnegut, M. 1975. *The Eden Express.* New York: Praeger.

Wahl, O. 1995. *Media Madness: Public Images of Mental Illness.* New Brunswick, N.J.: Rutgers University Press.

Waitzkin, H. 1991. *The Politics of Medical Encounters: How Patients and Doctors Deal with Social Problems.* New Haven, Conn.: Yale University Press.

Wallerstein, J. and S. Blakeulee. 1989. *Second Chances: Men, Women and Children: A Decade After Divorce.* New York: Ticknor and Fields.

Weber, M. 1930. *The Protestant Ethic and the Spirit of Capitalism.* Translated by T. Parsons. New York: Scribner.

Weber, M. 1947. *The Theory of Social and Economic Organization.* Translated by A. M. Henderson and T. Parsons. New York: Oxford University Press.

Wechsler, H. 1960. "The self-help organization in the mental health field: Recovery, Inc., a case study." *Journal of Nervous and Mental Disease* 25: 297–314.

Weitzman, L. 1985. *The Divorce Revolution: The Unexpected Social and Economic Consequences in America.* New York: Free Press.

Whitaker, R. 2010a. *Anatomy of an Epidemic: Magic Bullets, Psychiatric Drugs, and the Astonishing Rise of Mental Illness in America.* New York: Random House.

Whitaker, R. 2010b. *Mad In America: Bad Science, Bad Medicine, and the Enduring Mistreatment of the Mentally Ill.* New York: Basic Books.

Whyte, W. 1943. *Street Corner Society.* Chicago: University of Chicago Press,

Wilson, W. 1987. *The Truly Disadvantaged: The Inner City, the Underclass, and Public Policy.* Chicago: The University of Chicago Press.

Wurtzel, E. 1994. *Prozac Nation.* Boston: Houghton Mifflin Co.

Wuthnow, R. 1986. "Religious movements and counter-movements in North America." In J. Beckford (ed.), *New Religious Movements and Rapid Social Change.* London: Sage.

Wuthnow, R. 1994. *Sharing the Journey Together: Support Groups and America's New Quest for Community.* New York: The Free Press.

Yoels, W. and J. Clair. 1994. "Never enough time: How medical residents manage a scarce resource." *The Journal of Contemporary Ethnography* 23: 185–213.

Yoels, W., J. Clair, F. Ritchie, and R. Allman. 1993. "Role-taking accuracy in medical encounters: A test of two theories." *Sociological Focus* 26: 183–201.

Zborowski, M. 1992. "Cultural components in responses to pain." In C. Clark and H. Robboy (eds.), *Social Interaction.* New York: St. Martin's.

Zorbaugh, H. and H. Chudacoff. 1929. *The Gold Coast and the Slum: A Sociological Study of Chicago's Near North Side.* Chicago: University of Chicago Press.

Zurcher, L. 1977. *The Mutable Self.* Beverly Hills, Calif.: Sage.

Zurcher, L. 1986. "The bureaucratizing of impulse: The self conception of the 1980s." *Symbolic Interaction* 9: 169–178.

INDEX

References to footnotes are denoted by an italicized *n*

Abbott, Ward, 249
abnormalcy, 313
Abramson, John, 35
abuse
    child, 66, 69, 330
    drug, 330
    sexual, 286–87
    spouse, 318
accounts, 188
Ackerknecht, Erwin H., 306
adapting. *See* coping
addiction, Klonopin, 16–17
addictive personality, 176
affective disorders, 3, 77
    America's population, 65
    biological explanation, 169, 188, 360*n*2
    cross-cultural variation, 362*n*22, 376*n*14
    self-help group, 205, 356*n*10, 368*n*22, 370*n*13
    social connection, 89, 91, 343, 347
age of narcissism, 317
aggression
    depression, 310
    frustration and, 236, 371*n*20
Agnes's Jacket (Hornstein), 41
AIDS (acquired immunodeficiency syndrome), 77, 132, 299, 322

Al-Anon meeting, 284
The Alchemy of Illness (Duff), 340–41
Alcoholics Anonymous, 119, 238, 241, 243–44, 318
alcoholism, 108, 138, 244, 268, 316, 318, 330
Alger, Horatio, 328
alienation, 114–15, 316
American Dream, 325–26
American Indians. *See* Native Americans
American medicine, 171, 308, 311
American Psychiatric Association (APA), 25, 27, 47, 65, 358*n*35
Amitriptyline, 55, 194
The Anatomy of an Epidemic (Whitaker), 36, 47
Angell, Marcia, 35
anhedonia, 98
anomie, 303–4
anorexia, 288, 312, 330
antianxiety medications, 168
antidepressants, 14, 34, 74, 190, 225, 235, 261, 283, 366*n*2, 371*n*19
    biology of depression, 80
    brain chemistry, 32–34, 55, 62–63
    era, 24
    feeling dependent on, 168–69, 177

397

antidepressants (*Cont.*)
    overuse of, 172
    pharmaceutical companies, 34–35
    psychiatry, 33–34
    recommendations, 157
    redefinition of self, 202
    resistance to, 181–83, 185, 352
    significance, 166
    suicide attempt, 179
    view of reality, 203
    Xanax, 178
    see also drugs
anti-psychiatry ideology, 205
anti-psychiatry movement, 24,
    132–33, 358*n*27
anxiety, 27, 38, 316, 320
    depression and, 15, 45, 53, 55, 58, 97,
        101, 208, 214, 217, 231, 307, 309,
        312, 376*n*9
    Doxepin, 63
    Klonopin, 16–17, 168
    Trazadone, 192
anxiety disorders, 65, 346
APA. *See* American Psychiatric
    Association (APA)
asylums, 23–24, 40–41, 149, 151–52,
    208, 366*n*20
Ativan, 16
aura of depression, 260, 262–63
autistic spectrum disorder, 29
autoethnography, 361*n*5

Baby and Child Care (Spock), 269
baby boomers, 305
Bean-Bayog, Margaret, 226–27
Becker, Ernest, 79
Becker, Howard, 180, 188, 359*n*49
Becoming Alcoholic (Rudy), 244
Behavior in Public Places (Goffman), 296
"Being Sane in Insane Places"
    (Rosenhan), 150
Bellah, Robert, 77, 328–29, 332
Benadryl, 273
benzodiazepines, 16–17
Berger, Brigitte, 299
Berger, Peter, 144, 198, 204, 298–99,
    315, 356*n*5

Bernard, Jessie, 227
binge eating disorder, 29
biochemical pathology, 311
biological determinism, 80, 161, 365*n*6
biological psychiatry, 27, 33
bipolar disorder, 21, 30, 37
black box medicine, 17
black population, 41, 113, 322–24
Black revolution, 346
Blumer, Herbert, 373*n*28
The Book of Woe (Greenberg), 28
Boston Phoenix (newspaper), 293
Bradshaw, John, 316, 319
brain chemistry, 32, 38
breakdown, 107, 117–18, 262, 270, 279
Bride of Frankenstein (film), 153
Bridgewater State Hospital, 358*n*29
Brodsky, Joseph, 249–50
Buddhism, 30, 195, 242–43, 248, 312, 341,
    349, 352
bulimia, 148, 312
Buscaglia, Leo, 316
Bush, George H. W., 346

cancer, 84, 89–90, 186, 270, 299
capitalism, 319, 324, 327–28, 356*n*12,
    369*n*9, 377*n*38
career, 56, 67
    depression, 73, 107–8, 207–8, 215, 277,
        365*n*6, 367*n*6
    depression experience, 134–63, 350
    drug-taking, 203
    social service, 346
    success, 328
    suffering, 165
caregiving, 277, 284–85, 290, 294, 351
Care of the Soul (Moore), 341
caring
    for depressed child, 272–76
    for depressed friend, 286–95
    for depressed husband, 257–68
    for depressed parent, 276–85
catastrophic thinking, 58, 262
Catholic, 173, 242, 277, 349
cause. *See* depression causes
Celexa, 22
Chamberlin, Judi, 42, 50, 360*n*55, 360*n*63

change of heart, 345–46, 367n3
Charmaz, Kathy, 207–8, 380n2
Chicago School of Sociology, 2
child abuse, 66, 69, 330
childhood bipolar disorder, 30, 37
children, 297
  acting out, 175
  coping strategies, 219–20
  depression, 137
  hospitalization of, 268–74
  influence of depression on, 75–76
  interview of mother of depressed, 268–
    76, 285, 289, 297
  normalcy, 108, 138
  raising, 314, 324–25, 331
  relationships with parents, 256–57, 267
  socialization, 91
  what they owe to parents, 276–86
China, depression in, 312–13
chronic fatigue syndrome, 254, 340
chronic illness, 71, 208, 212–13,
    256, 369n6
Circus World, 55
cities, 1, 76, 323–24, 343, 356n12
Clark, Candace, 255–56
classical sociological theory, 90, 322
classism, 50
clinical depression, 10, 14, 72, 74,
    123, 246
Clinton, Bill, 107
cocaine, 182
co-counseling, 17, 56–57, 60
co-dependency, 330
Co-Dependents Anonymous, 330
cognitive behavioral therapy, 17–18
Cohen, Jay, 35
communication, incommunicability of
    depression, 110–19
communitarian movement, 345, 347
community, 3, 8, 109, 138, 227, 243–45,
    285, 324, 328–29, 336, 344–45
  sense of, 11, 77, 243, 377n33
  withering of, 322, 375n8
concentration, 95, 209, 222, 323–24
confessions, 301
Conrad, Peter, 201
consciousness, 74–75

consciousness-raising process,
    42–43, 358n29
consumption, 210, 319, 333
contingent workers, 325–26
conversion
  disenchantment, 181, 198–202
  drug experience, 181, 191–98
  resistance, 181–88
  trial commitment, 181, 188–90
conversion motifs, 189
Cooley, Charles Horton, 90, 373n29
coping
  children, 219–20
  depression, 207–14
  diversion, 214–20
  exercise, 17, 191, 338
  good and bad days, 208–10
  incorporation, 237–48
  looking for right doctor, 226–36
  psychoanalysis/psychotherapy, 18, 25,
    131, 228, 372n22
  shopping, 79, 216
  spirituality, 179, 224, 242–44, 248–49,
    287, 337–41
  sports, 92, 217, 296
  trying to fix depression, 220–26
  work, 115–16, 142, 207, 217–20
cosmetic psychopharmacology, 172
counter-narratives, 38–40, 44
counter-storytelling, 39
creativity, depression and, 195–96,
    245, 372n24
Crichton, Michael, 209
crisis, 107, 110, 128, 136, 145–64, 184, 186,
    214, 225
cultural chemistry, 38, 299, 321
culture, 250
  American, 299, 341, 343, 376n9
  capitalism, 327
  depression, 302–4, 306, 376n9
  everyday life, 298–99
  health and emotion, 305–13
  medical, 9
  mental illness, 14, 63, 92
  pain, 244
  paradox of, 78, 102
  self-help, 317

culture (*Cont.*)
  self-realization, 332
  social structure, 343–46
  subcultures, 120, 180, 188
  therapeutic, 118, 318–19, 329

Darkness Visible (Styron), 89
Darwinism, 344–45
DBSA (Depression and Bipolar Support
  Alliance), 5, 43, 356n7
death, 23, 30, 41, 93–95, 174, 315, 369n8
deconversion, drugs, 181, 198–202
Degler, Carl, 344
deindustrialization of America, 324
deinstitutionalization process, 152
Delano, Laura, 46, 360n60
democratization, 39, 204
depression
  acceptance of, 44, 144, 160, 164, 189,
    204, 207, 241
  adolescence, 66, 127
  agitated, 54, 97, 102, 147
  ambiguity, 74, 92, 164, 172, 370n13
  analysis of, 3–5
  aura of, 260, 262–63
  biochemical definition, 28, 65, 80, 169,
    181, 189, 200
  biologically reductionist explanation,
    38, 48–49, 80
  career view of, 134–63
  in China, 312–13
  chronicity of, 64, 135, 162
  "clinical" diagnosis, 14
  co-counseling, 17, 56–57, 60
  colors associated with, 95
  complaining about, 150–51, 211, 303
  contagious, 75, 251
  conveying feeling of, 93–95
  core syndrome, 311
  creativity and, 195–96, 245, 372n24
  crisis, 146–57
  cross-cultural perspective, 310–11
  cultural trends and, 302, 306
  denial of, 176
  describing, 92–101
  disconnection, 73, 321
  diversion, 214–20

downward spiral, 91, 96–97, 121
dysthymic, 350
economic losses, 305
empathy and, 86, 106, 118, 211, 226,
  235, 247, 265, 325
endogenous, 350
exogenous, 350
fatalism about, 239, 241
feedback loop, 91, 163
getting beyond, 136–37, 210, 237
as gift, 207, 241, 248, 339, 342
illness "career," 9–10
illness of self, 71, 73
inchoate feelings, 108–9, 136–41, 186
incidence in America, 304–5
incommunicability of, 110–19, 144
incomprehension of others, 11, 72, 114,
  119, 245, 254, 279
invisibility of, 211, 279
isolation, 7–8, 69–70, 73
life chances, 212
life choices, 212, 221
living with, 53–54, 164
major, 27, 30, 81, 92, 212, 272, 350
medical definition, 164–66, 169, 189
medications, 14–15
metaphors for, 66, 164, 321
naming, 107–10
nightmarish therapies, 23–24
normalcy of, 53
paradox of, 101–6
personal experience, 8, 10–12, 45–46,
  66–72, 169, 294, 298, 310
pervasiveness of, 65–67
phenomenology of experience, 75,
  78–79, 89
positive aspects of, 20, 35–36,
  120–21, 195
rates of, 66, 305, 324, 350
relapse, 37, 199
reoccurrence, 162–63
responding to treatment, 13–21
re-visioning experience, 10–11
sampling, 349–54
seeking professional therapy, 19–20
sensitivity, 247
stereotypes of, 40, 83

stigma, secrecy and self-hatred, 119–22
structural factors, 77–78
subjective experience, 50, 80–81,
    299, 308
trying to fix, 220–26
unremitting character, 99–100
depression career
    coming to grips, 136, 158–63
    crisis period, 136, 146–57
    feeling something is really wrong,
        136, 140–46
    inchoate feelings, 108–9, 136–41, 186
depression causes
    biological, 21, 25–28, 30, 32–34, 38, 48,
        62, 80–81, 119, 169–70, 190, 299, 308,
        310–11, 318, 344, 360n2
    cultural, 15, 18, 22–23, 31, 33, 76, 132,
        171–72, 255, 302–3, 305–12, 376n9
    family structure, 66
    gender roles, 66
    medical, 74, 97, 123, 132, 166, 172–73,
        189, 197, 204, 207
    medicalization, 12, 313–21
    powerlessness, 66
    situational, 57, 140, 144, 221, 296,
        302, 375n21
    social, 376n9
depression consciousness, 74, 134,
    143, 337
Derber, Charles, 322, 326
desperation, 60, 63, 173, 186, 225, 273, 287
diagnosis
    American Psychiatric Association, 27
    bi-polar depression, 268, 270, 356n7
    clinical depression, 10, 14, 123, 246
    diagnostic inflation, 29, 358n32
    major depression, 30
    official, 44, 66–67, 145, 148, 350
    schizophrenia, 150, 151
Diagnostic and Statistical Manual of Mental
    Disorders (DSM), 22, 25
    DSM-5, 29–30
    DSM-III, 27–28
    DSM-IV, 29, 30, 132
    methodology, 31–32
disconnection, 321–32
    deepening, 106–22

depression as disease of, 73, 321
equation, 305
love, 328–32
stigma, secrecy and self-hatred,
    119–22
theme, 101
work, 323–27
diseasing of America, 321
disenchantment, drugs, 181, 198–202
Disneyland, 320
Disney World, 55
divorce, 42, 64–65, 119, 257, 290, 331
Dostoyevsky, Fyodor, 53
double trouble, 322
Douglas, Michael, 117
downsizing, 325
Doxepin, 63, 194
Dr. Drew, 20
Dr. Oz, 20
Dr. Phil, 20
Dr. Ruth, 316
drugs
    abuse, 330
    addiction, 69, 318, 322
    antidepressants, 235, 366n2
    attitudes about, 168–69
    benzodiazepines, 16–17
    combination of, 15
    competing, 35–36
    conversion phase, 181, 191–98
    critics of, 37–38
    disease model in psychiatry, 32–33
    disenchantment and deconversion, 181,
        198–202
    interpreting experience of taking,
        180–202
    Klonopin, 16–17, 44, 168–69
    medicalization of depression, 12
    miracle, 15, 33, 64, 161, 173, 181, 191,
        193–94, 197, 199, 241
    patients' feeling about, 157, 161, 166
    psychotropic, 66, 68, 171, 176–77, 180,
        189, 344, 367n6
    resistance stage, 181, 182–88
    selective serotonin reuptake inhibitors
        (SSRIs), 22, 34
    self-medication with street, 175–76

drugs (*Cont.*)
  treating depression, 65–66, 80–81,
    89, 177–78
  trial commitment, 181, 188–90
  US Food and Drug Administration (US
    FDA), 35
  withdrawal, 16–17
  "wonder," 26, 171
  see also Prozac
Duff, Kat, 254, 340–42
Durkheim, Emile, 90, 303, 305, 322
dyschromic spirochetosis, 306
dysfunction
  American culture, 343
  biological, 26, 33, 308, 325
  families, 83, 103, 108, 138, 148, 220,
    319, 363n10
  neurotransmitter, 22
  sexual, 200, 312
  social, 325
dysphoria, 117, 310, 368n1
dysthymia, 350

Eastern mysticism, 341
Eastern religions, 242, 317, 338–39
eating disorders, 29, 148, 312
ECT (electro-convulsive shock) treatments, 45, 133, 153, 155, 274
EKG, 273, 275
Elavil, 191
Eli Lilly, 371n19
Emerson, Robert, 140, 144, 165n9
emotional alienation, 115
emotional economy, 105, 255, 257
emotional labor, 115
empathy, 86, 106, 118, 211, 226, 235, 247,
  265, 325
encephalitis, 257–58
epidemiologists, 305
epilepsy, 71, 169, 201, 259–60, 362n13
Erikson, Erik, 99, 334
Erikson, Kai, 304
escape fantasies, 109, 138
ethnicity, 66, 242, 256, 302, 307, 368n1
Etzioni, Amitai, 345
everyday encounters, fragility of, 295–99
Ewen, Stewart, 377n38

experts, 13, 20
  doctors, 307
  medical, 35, 314–17
  mental health, 66, 148, 317
  psychiatric, 18, 23, 43, 67, 145, 158, 164,
    234, 270
  therapeutic, 14, 66, 68, 136, 157, 226,
    313, 315
expressive individualism, 328–29

Falling Down (film), 117
family
  dysfunction, 83, 103, 108, 138, 148, 220,
    319, 363n10
  friends and, 253–57, 286–95
  illness and everyday
    encounters, 295–99
  marriage, 257–68
  mothers, 268–76
  parents, 276–86
  in sickness and in health, till death do us
    part, 257–68
  violence, 220, 369–70n11
fatalism, 239, 241
fear of falling, 325
feeling powerless, 96, 138
feeling trapped, 45, 86, 94, 109,
  138–39
The Feminine Mystique (Friedan), 42
feminization of poverty, 331
Foster, Vincent, 107
Foucault, Michel, 23
Frances, Allen, 28–29, 358n32
Frank, Arthur, 2
Franklin, Benjamin, 328
Freaks, 335
free-floating violence, 333
Freeman, Walter, 24
free rider problem, 285
Freidson, Eliot, 20, 314
Freud, Sigmund, 25, 131, 321
Friedan, Betty, 42
friends
  family and, 253–57, 286–95
  interview, 286–94, 297
  obligations of friendship, 290–94
friendship, 126, 208, 286, 288–94

frustration
  aggression and, 236, 371*n*20
  depression, 21, 72, 113, 264, 269, 321
future shock, 333, 379*n*65

gambling, 318, 330
Gaudier-Brzeska, Henri, 249–50
gay people, 113, 278, 282–83, 293
gay rights, 39
Gekko, Gordon, 346
Gelles, Richard, 369*n*11
Gergen, Kenneth, 333
Giddens, Anthony, 335
Gitlin, Todd, 335
Goffman, Erving, 119, 295–96, 298,
  360*n*2, 374*n*16, 375*n*21
Good, Byron, 310
Good Days, Bad Days (Charmaz), 208
grand mal seizures, 153, 258
Greenberg, Gary, 28
grief, 54, 58–59, 101, 310
Gross, Martin, 320
guilt, 175, 270

Habits of the Heart (Bellah), 328
halfway houses, 130, 273
Healy, David, 33
The Heights (newspaper), 293
helplessness, sense of, 97–99, 137, 310
heroin addiction, 17, 180
heterosexism, 50
Hill, Anita, 113
hippies, 335
Hippocrates, 1
Hippocratic oath, 16
Hochschild, Arlie Russell, 114–15
Holstein, James, 160
homelessness, 77, 322
hope, 58–60, 62, 64, 91, 161, 171, 204
hopelessness, feeling of, 79, 91, 93–94,
  99, 105, 156, 192, 240, 246, 335
Hornstein, Gail, 41
Horwitz, Allan, 31
hospitalization
  asylums, 23–24, 40–41, 149, 151–52,
    208, 366*n*20
  crisis, 145, 186, 225, 273

depression, 8–9, 60, 68, 84, 89, 117–18,
  161–62, 164
drug experiment, 21
economics of, 305
experience, 259
extended, 212, 268, 283
failure of system, 26
giving up, 156
identity comments about, 155–57
involuntary, 41, 133, 149
mental hospitals, 24–26, 60, 150, 152,
  195, 295, 311
mental illness, 130, 149
multiple, 47, 84, 125, 129, 176, 231, 268
schizophrenia, 150–52
suicide attempts, 117–18
surrender, 156
women as inmates, 40–41
Hughes, Everett, 73, 134
human beings, behavior and experiences,
  13–14, 170
Husserl, Edmund, 163
hyperghettoization, 76, 324
hypersexual disorder, 29

identity
  illness and, 73, 123, 131–34, 158–63
  periodic assessments, 71–72
  personal, 44, 109, 138, 316, 323
  politics, 121, 205, 364*n*19, 368*n*23
  secrecy, 120
  sexual, 280
  shared, 126
  social construction of illness, 131–34
identity turning points, 10, 72, 74, 118,
  123, 128, 134–36, 144, 214
illiteracy, 322
illness
  culture, health and emotion, 306–13
  disease vs., 308
  as metaphor, 66, 93, 158, 164
  narratives, 53, 210, 309–10
illness consciousness, 109, 138, 164, 180
The Illness Narratives (Kleinman),
  53, 369*n*7
Imipramine, 62, 192, 194
impression-management, 115

inchoate feelings, 108–9, 136–41, 186
incommunicability, depression,
    110–19, 144
in-depth interviewing, 67–68, 298,
    349, 351
individualism
    economic, 346
    ethic of, 77, 330, 343–44
    excessive, 329
    expressive, 328–29
    ideology of, 336
    instrumental, 328
    radical, 90
    sociological analysis of, 328
inductive logic, 351
industrial revolution, 333, 356n12
insane literature, 41
insomnia, 16, 55, 97, 312
instrumental individualism, 328
insurance policy, 225
interviews
    crisis, 145
    depression, 5–8, 10, 67–70, 75, 77–78,
        81, 84, 136
    dysfunctional families, 108
    feelings about psychiatrists, 184–85
    feelings of safety, 102
    hospitalization, 151–52
    John and friends, 286–94, 297
    Karen, 125–31, 133, 135–36
    Keith, 223–25
    law student Alex, 237
    Marco, 276–85, 289, 293, 297
    mother, Anne, 268–76, 285, 289, 297
    Nina, 83–85, 89, 93, 126
    Randall, 173–79
    reaction to taking medication, 157,
        161–62, 166
    reconstructing the past, 123
    using own experience in, 238–41
intimacy, 230, 233, 235, 293, 329–31
Iroquois Indians, 342–43
isolation, 6
    affective disorders, 91
    depression as illness of, 7–8, 69–70,
        73, 90–91, 101, 105–7, 110, 114, 123,
        266, 287

poor people and minorities, 76
self-hatred and, 121–22
self-isolation, 103
sense of, 59, 328
social, 324, 363n5

Jews/Jewish, 242, 307, 338, 349
Journal of Affective Disorders (journal), 67
Judaism, 338
Just Friends (Rubin), 290

Kaysen, Susanna, 208, 366n22
Kellner, Hansfried, 144
Kierkegaard, Soren, 71, 371n16
Kirk, Stuart, 33
Kirsch, Irving, 33–34
Kleinman, Arthur, 53, 307–8, 310–12,
    362–63n22, 369n7, 377n25
Klonopin, 16–17, 44, 168–69
Kramer, Peter, 22, 172, 366n2, 371n19
Krieger, Susan, 361n5
Kubler-Ross, Elizabeth, 369n8

labeling, 39, 120, 148, 150, 180, 188, 306
labeling theory, 342, 359n49, 370n13
Laing, Ronald, 360n2, 372n25
Lanchester, Elsa, 153
Lexapro, 22
Librium, 27, 171, 176
Lifton, Robert Jay, 335–36
Lindesmith, Alfred, 180
Listening to Prozac (Kramer), 22,
    171–72, 371n19
lived world, 107, 249, 364n13
lobotomies, 24
Lofland, J., 189
lonely crowd, 332
The Loss of Sadness (Horwitz and
    Wakefield), 31
love disconnection, 328–32
Lozano, Paul, 226–27
LSD, 182
L-tryptophan, 58
Luckmann, Thomas, 198, 204, 315

macro worlds, 49, 299
Mad in America blog (Delano), 46–47, 360n60

madness, 23, 208, 245
Mairs, Nancy, 67
The Managed Heart (Hochschild), 114
manic depression, 3, 268, 356n7, 372n24
Manic Depression and Depression
    Association (MDDA), 3–5
manic psychosis, 270
marihuana, 180, 182
marriage
    black families, 324
    divorce and, 42, 64–65
    everyday life, 212
    health, 306
    love disconnection, 328–32
    Rachel and Ted, 257–67
    relationship, 227, 229, 261, 266–67, 269,
        271, 329–31
    in sickness and in health, till death do us
        part, 257–68
    social construction of, 144
Marx, Karl, 5, 115, 214, 356–57n12, 369n9
masked depression, 165
Massachusetts General Hospital,
    258, 357n25
mass media, 20, 334
McLean's Hospital, 3, 60, 62, 100, 366n20
MDDA. *See* Manic Depression and
    Depression Association (MDDA)
Mead, George Herbert, 49, 90,
    303, 373n28
Mead, Margaret, 244
medicalization
    depressive illness, 12, 313–21
    equation, 305
    society, 203
medical model, psychiatry, 23, 30, 44–45,
    62, 203–4, 313–14
medical version of reality, 74, 97, 123, 166,
    172–73, 189, 204, 207
medications
    depression, 14–15
    interpreting drug experience, 180–202
    meaning of taking, 157, 167–73
    miracle, 15, 33, 64, 161, 173, 181, 191,
        193–94, 197, 199, 241
    see also antidepressants; drugs
melancholy, 54, 214, 305, 342

age of, 305
Menendez, Erik, 317
Menendez, Lyle, 317
mental disorders, biologically reductionist
    explanation, 38, 48–49, 80
mental hospitals, 24–26, 60, 150, 152, 195,
    295, 311
mental illness, 2
    coming to grips with, 158–63
    creativity, 245
    fragility of everyday encounters, 295–99
    illusion, 132
    myth of, 25, 63
    political category, 63
    power and, 132
    social construction, 131–34
    Soviet Union, 132
mentalism, 42
mental patient, being a, 43, 61, 118,
    125, 129
Messinger, Sheldon, 140, 144, 165n9
metaphors
    chemistry catalyzing depression, 321
    describing experience, 168, 334
    illness, 66, 164
    medium of expression, 93
    "miracle" of medication, 193
    others as mirrors, 251, 373n29
    micro worlds, 49
Midler, Bette, 79
Milken, Michael, 346
Miller, Gale, 160
Mills, C. Wright, 64, 76, 301
Miltown, 27
Mind, Self and Society (Mead), 303
minor neurocognitive disorder, 29
miracle, medication as, 15, 33, 64, 161, 173,
    181, 191, 193–94, 197, 199, 241
money economy, 233–34
Moniz, Egas, 24
Moonstruck (movie), 278
Moore, Thomas, 341–42
mothers, function in family, 268–76

narcissistic personality disorder, 312
Native Americans, 312, 341
    Iroquois Indians, 342–43

nature/nurture debate, 63, 78, 97, 190, 311
negotiation, 44, 76, 188–89, 254
nervous breakdowns, 118
neurasthenia, 312–13
neurotransmitter deficiency theory, 32–33
neurotransmitters, 15, 32, 62
norepinephrine, 62
normal appearances, 117–18, 272
normalcy, 53, 64, 101, 104, 108, 138, 313
normal pain, 30, 131
"Notes on the Concept of Commitment"
 (Becker), 188

objectivity, 167–68, 361n5
One Flew Over the Cuckoo's Nest (film), 152
oppression, 43, 50
Orlando, Florida, 55, 63–64
overconsumption, 36

panic scene, 335
parallel world, 165
parents, 276–85, 289, 293, 297
Parsons, Talcott, 89, 369n6
passing, 115, 119
pathology
 depression, 169, 311
 health and, 313
 medicine and illness, 170
 mental health, 44, 133
 pain without, 217
Paxil, 22
Peck, M. Scott, 30
perception, 74–75
 and action, 49, 209, 214
 depression altering, 88, 91, 107
 hopelessness, 99
 identity, 135, 143
 reality, 246
personal introspection, 361n5
personal traumas, divorce, 42, 64–65, 119,
 257, 290, 331
Pfohl, Stephen, 335
pharmaceutical companies, 22, 27–28, 34,
 38, 182
Philosophy Foundation, 338, 380n2
pill paradigm, 21
pill pushers, 185

placebo effect, 33–34
Plath, Sylvia, 67, 245
politics, identity, 121, 205, 364n19, 368n23
poly-pharmacy, 15
postindustrial society, 203, 314
postmodernization, 305
postmodern self, 332–36
poverty, 50, 305, 322, 330–31, 376n9
pregnancy, 277, 322
The Presentation of Self in Everyday Life
 (Goffman), 295
Profession of Medicine (Freidson), 20
Protestant Ethic, 319
Protestants, 242, 307, 319, 349
Prozac
 controversy, 187
 depression and, 182–83, 235, 366n2
 Eli Lilly, 371n19
 experience with, 189, 193, 195–97,
  199, 241
 introduction, 22, 34, 36, 64, 79–80
 prescribing, 171–72
psychiatric experts, 18, 23, 43, 67, 145, 158,
 164, 234, 270
psychiatric liberation movement,
 38, 41, 46
Psychiatric-Pharmaceutical Industrial
 Complex, 48
psychiatric survivors, 45–46, 50, 359n47
psychiatrists, 18, 21, 25–29, 80, 89, 129,
 240, 261, 316–17, 344
 ambivalence about, 130, 177, 225–26
 anger toward, 177, 184–85, 213,
  231–33, 235–36
 as experts, 18, 23, 43, 67, 145, 158, 164,
  234, 270
 finding the right, 226–36
 money and, 279
 power and, 41
 time with, 309
psychiatry, 1, 4, 9, 12, 21, 47–48, 169–70
 ambivalence about, 225–26
 anger toward, 184–85, 232
 anti-psychiatry movement, 132, 205
 big pharma and, 28, 182
 biochemical revolution, 33, 64–65
 critiques of, 133

disillusionment with, 40, 60, 205, 227, 236
feelings about, 232, 310, 337
forced intervention, 42
hierarchical nature of, 230
legitimacy of, 4, 19, 33, 133
medical model, 23, 30, 44–45, 62, 203–4, 313–14
power and, 41
questionable revolution, 22–38
status within medicine, 169
psychopharmacology, 62, 172, 195
psychosis, 23, 32, 106, 270
psychosurgery, 357n25
psychotherapy/psychoanalysis, 18, 25, 131, 228, 372n22
psychotropic medications, 66, 68, 171, 176–77, 180, 189, 344, 367n6

qi, 312
quality of life, 17

racism, 42, 50, 322
radical individualism, 90
Readers Guide to Periodical Literature, 65
Reagan, Ronald, 346
reciprocity, 230, 255, 285, 374n11
reconstruction, 13, 22, 71, 123, 158, 163, 333
reengineering, 325
Reinharz, Shulamit, 338
relaxation response, learning, 60
religion, 18, 119, 143, 165, 195, 216, 242, 297, 303, 317–18, 338, 345, 349, 368n1
religious conversion, 14, 173, 193, 203
see also spirituality
resistance stage, drug experience, 181, 182–88
responsibility, sense of, 269
Richter, Alice, 41
Riesman, David, 332
Rivers, Joan, 79
The Road Less Traveled (Peck), 30
role-take, 106, 111, 370n15
romantic love, 192, 329, 371n16
Rosenberg, Morris, 106

Rosenhan, D. L., 150
Rothman, David, 309
Rothman, Sheila, 210
Rubin, Lillian, 290
Rudy, David, 244

safety, social connection, 102–3
Samoa, 244
sampling, 349–54
demographics, 242, 324, 368n1
gender distribution, 350
generalization, 353–54
sample size, 353–54
saturated self, 333
Saving Normal (Frances), 29, 358n31–32
schizophrenia, 21, 36, 150–51, 312, 376n9
Schorr, Lisbeth, 343
Scientology, 317
SeaWorld, 55
second shift, 269
secrecy, depression, 107, 119–20
security, 91, 326
seizures, 153, 258–60
selective serotonin reuptake inhibitors (SSRIs), 22, 34
self, 2, 50, 71–73, 91, 170, 172, 203, 221, 314, 316, 329–30, 342
absorption, 210, 319, 328, 330
actualization, 320
awareness, 25
blame, 97
definition, 74, 118, 134, 136, 140, 160, 172, 182, 185, 188
description or identity, 55
-disclosure, 292
-esteem, 278, 323
-fulfillment, 151, 317
-hatred, 119–22
identification, 44, 144
isolation, 103
loathing, 105
mutable, 336
mutilation, 211
postmodern, 332–36
-realization, 317, 332
-reliant, 221
-revelation, 289

self (*Cont.*)
 sense of, 250
 -sufficient, 255
 transformation, 71
self-help
 backlash, 319
 books, 11, 56, 78, 317
 groups, 41, 43, 118–19, 205, 236, 243–
  44, 268, 318–19, 349, 370n13, 372n22
semen loss, 312
sensitivity, 67, 247, 291
serotonin, 22, 32, 34, 81, 366n2
service economy, 115
sexism, 42, 50, 322
sexual abuse, 286–87
sexual identity, 280
shame, 175, 186
shock treatments, 45, 133, 153, 155, 274
Shur, Edwin, 319
sickness vocabulary, 317
sick role, 210, 369n6
side bets, 188
Simmel, Georg, 233–34, 380n4
sin vocabulary, 317
situational involvement, Goffman's notion
  of, 296, 375n21
Skonovd, L., 189
sleep, 58
 difficulties, 53–55, 58–59, 61, 104, 142,
  147, 176, 208, 253
 medications, 63, 168–69, 200
 remedies, 17
sociability, 293
social bond, 91, 331, 378n44
social connection, safety, 102–3
social construction, 25, 132, 144, 214,
  359n49, 365n9
 illness identities, 131–34
 marriage, 144
 reality, 132, 214, 359n49
social integration, 90–91, 303
social isolation, 324, 363n5
socialization process, 62, 74, 91, 173, 179,
  197, 203–4, 207, 297
social movements, voices for
  change, 39–48
social order, 295–96, 304, 328

social withdrawal, 89–91, 101, 103–6, 121
The Sociological Imagination (Mills),
  64, 301
sociology, 2, 11, 49–50, 344
 changing values, 338, 344–46
 communitarian movement, 345
 depression, 70, 72, 303
 formal, 380n4
 human behavior, 64
 human beings, 89–91
 labeling theory, 370n13
 mental illness, 18, 63
 nature/nurture debate, 97
 scientific objectivity and
  detachment, 361n5
 scientific vision of, 4
 social connection, 89–92, 354
 value of social structures, 356n5
Sorokin, Pitirim, 344
spiritual advisor, 287
spirituality, 179, 224, 242–44, 248–49,
  287, 337–41
Spock, Benjamin, 269–70
spouse abuse, 318
SSRIs. *See* selective serotonin reuptake
  inhibitors (SSRIs)
stage, 73–74, 107, 134, 136, 164–65, 365n6
stage theories, 369n8
Steinem, Gloria, 356n8
stigma
 depression, 11, 26, 39
 emotional disorder, 182
 mental illness, 42, 107, 119–21, 144,
  152, 295, 313
storytelling, 5, 37, 39, 359n45, 359n48
strangers, 106, 256, 304
Strauss, Anselm, 72, 134–35, 180
Strauss, Murray, 369n11
Styron, William, 67, 89
subcultures, 120, 180, 188
suicide, 86, 114
 attempts, 69, 117, 127, 130, 179,
  265–66, 270
 North America, 311, 322
 Paul Lozano, 226
 study of, 90, 303–4
 Vincent Foster, 107

surrender, 64, 119, 156, 241, 318
symbolic interaction theory, 70–71,
    180, 243, 250, 307, 335, 341,
    367n6, 373n28
symbolic universe, 198
symbols, 79, 165, 249
sympathy, 75–76, 211, 254, 282, 297
    biography, 255
    boundaries, 253
    emotional economies, 255–56
    expressions of, 233
    margins, 256, 298
sympathy credits, 210
Szasz, Thomas, 32, 358n27–28, 358n36,
    360n2, 364n2, 370n13

Tannen, Deborah, 351
teenage pregnancy, 322
temp agencies, 325
temper dysregulation disorder, 29
tenure theory, 57
therapeutic culture, 118, 318–19, 329
therapeutic experts, 14, 66, 68, 136, 157,
    226, 313, 315
therapeutic state, 316
therapists, 18–19, 56, 60, 66, 114, 130, 317
    anger toward, 226
    finding right, 226–36
    see also psychiatrists; psychiatry
therapy, 9, 17–19, 25, 56, 119, 204, 215,
    222, 226, 241, 272, 289, 318
    drug, 157, 176–77, 191
    family, 142
Thomas, W. I., 90
Titicutt Follies (documentary),
    152, 358n29
Toennies, Ferdinand, 322
Toffler, Alvin, 333, 379n65
tough love conversation, 291
Toynbee, Arnold, 344
Transcendental Meditation, 317
Trazadone, 192, 194, 202, 216
trial commitment, drug experience,
    181, 188–90
tricyclic antidepressants, 34
trouble, micro politics of, 140, 365n9
true love, 371n16

Trump, Donald, 346
tuberculosis, 32, 210
Turner, Ralph, 316
turning points, identity, 10, 72, 74, 118,
    123, 128, 134–36, 144, 214
twelve-step programs, 243–44, 330

unemployment, 65–66, 212, 322–23
US FDA (United States Food and Drug
    Administration), 35

Valium, 16, 27, 171, 176
Van Gogh, Vincent, 245
Vaughan, Diane, 144
victimization, 160–61, 327
Vietnam War, 344, 346
viral encephalitis, 257–58
vocabulary of motives, 188

Wakefield, Jerome, 31
Wall Street (movie), 346
Warhol, Andy, 352
Weber, Max, 114, 197, 319, 322
Western medicine, 307–8, 340
When Harry Met Sally (movie), 293
Whitaker, Robert, 36–37, 47, 359n45
white collar workers, 326, 349
Wide World of Sports (TV series), 304
Williamson, Marianne, 316
Wilson, William Julius, 324
Wiseman, Frederick, 152, 358n29
withdrawal
    behavior, 218, 310, 327
    Klonopin, 16–17, 169
    medication, 21
    social, 89–91, 101, 103–6, 121
Within Our Reach: Breaking the Cycle of
    Disadvantage (Schorr), 343
womb to tomb, 325
women's movement,
    consciousness-raising, 42–43
work disconnection, 323–27
Wurtzel, Elizabeth, 67
Wuthnow, Robert, 377n32–33
Xanax, 16, 176, 178
Zborowski, Mark, 307
Zoloft, 22, 201

CPSIA information can be obtained
at www.ICGtesting.com
Printed in the USA
BVHW062157250919
559422BV00004B/13/P